Health Informatics

This series is directed to healthcare professionals leading the transformation of healthcare by using information and knowledge. For over 20 years, Health Informatics has offered a broad range of titles: some address specific professions such as nursing, medicine, and health administration; others cover special areas of practice such as trauma and radiology; still other books in the series focus on interdisciplinary issues, such as the computer based patient record, electronic health records, and networked healthcare systems. Editors and authors, eminent experts in their fields, offer their accounts of innovations in health informatics. Increasingly, these accounts go beyond hardware and software to address the role of information in influencing the transformation of healthcare delivery systems around the world. The series also increasingly focuses on the users of the information and systems: the organizational, behavioral, and societal changes that accompany the diffusion of information technology in health services environments.

Developments in healthcare delivery are constant; in recent years, bioinformatics has emerged as a new field in health informatics to support emerging and ongoing developments in molecular biology. At the same time, further evolution of the field of health informatics is reflected in the introduction of concepts at the macro or health systems delivery level with major national initiatives related to electronic health records (EHR), data standards, and public health informatics.

These changes will continue to shape health services in the twenty-first century. By making full and creative use of the technology to tame data and to transform information, Health Informatics will foster the development and use of new knowledge in healthcare.

More information about this series at http://www.springer.com/series/1114

Alan Davies • Julia Mueller

Developing Medical Apps and mHealth Interventions

A Guide for Researchers, Physicians and Informaticians

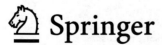 Springer

Alan Davies
University of Manchester
Manchester, UK

Julia Mueller
University of Cambridge
Cambridge, UK

ISSN 1431-1917   ISSN 2197-3741   (electronic)
Health Informatics
ISBN 978-3-030-47498-0   ISBN 978-3-030-47499-7   (eBook)
https://doi.org/10.1007/978-3-030-47499-7

This Springer imprint is published by the registered company Springer Nature Switzerland AG.
The registered company address is: Gewerbestrasse 11, 6330 Cham, Switzerland

This book is dedicated to the memories of:
Valerie Jane Davies 1955–2000
Bruce Nigel Davies 1953–2013

Preface

Using smartphone applications as a means of collecting research data and trialing and implementing medical/health interventions is becoming increasingly popular, due in part to the ubiquitous nature of mobile technology. A large swathe of the world's population has access to a smartphone, which is essentially a powerful hand-held computational device bristling with sensors. mHealth apps open up avenues for personalised interventions with the possibility of rich, high quality data acquisition. Data can be combined with modern scalable big data approaches, such as pattern mining and machine learning, which can be used to discover new insights into aspects of people's mental and physical health.

With all this potential, many domains are now moving into mobile technology and app development. Designing a medical or health intervention and deploying this on a mobile device in the form of an application is a task that requires expertise in many different disciplines. Between them, the authors of this book have worked in the fields of academic research, data science, software engineering, clinical practice and health psychology. We have worked on large and small interventions and have learnt many lessons along the way.

It is our hope that we can translate some of this experience into useful insights to help readers who are considering implementing a medical/health intervention to navigate the complexities of this area. This book is aimed at bridging the gap between researchers, developers and clinicians to highlight best practice and the steps involved in designing, building and evaluating mHealth interventions. We offer insights into the different aspects of such projects with additional case studies to help foster better understanding, communication and working practices between experts to work collaboratively and effectively on delivering mobile health interventions.

Manchester, UK   Alan Davies
March 2020

Acknowledgements

We would like to thank Alex Turner, Michael Lee and Jonathan Carlton for the helpful and constructive feedback provided. We also extend our gratitude to all the people and organisations that have allowed us to kindly reproduce images and other materials used throughout this book. Alan would like to thank Monika and Victoria Golaś for their continued patience and use of the flat's front room for the duration of the project. Julia would like to thank Nick for his invaluable patience and support. Julia would also like to thank her family Margrit, Ingo, Halina and Flora, without whom she wouldn't be where she is today. Finally, we would like to thank Dr Caroline Jay and Professor Simon Harper for their continued support of our careers.

Contents

About the Authors

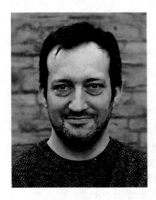

Dr. Alan Davies is a lecturer in Health Data Sciences at the University of Manchester in the Division of Informatics, Imaging and Data Sciences. Alan has a background in Computer Science (PhD) and Nursing Science (BSc) and has previously worked as a software engineer and app developer in industry.

Alan also worked in interventional cardiology, assisting with routine and emergency cardiac procedures where he authored several medical textbooks on electrocardiogram (ECG) interpretation. More recently he has worked for the University of Manchester as a Research Software Engineer (RSE) and Data Scientist prior to becoming a lecturer.

He delivers modules on the MSc in Health Informatics joint award delivered by UCL and the University of Manchester, where he is a module lead on the 'Usable Health Systems Design' module and the 'Modern Information Engineering' module. He also teaches on the MSc in Health Data Science on various modules, including 'Understanding Data and Decision Making' and 'Health Information Systems and Technologies'.

Alan's research is focused on mHealth interventions and how patients interpret medical data. Alan was a Data Science fellow at AstraZeneca, as well as a member of the Universities Research Ethics committee (UREC). Alan completed his PhD in the Interaction Analysis and Modelling lab at the University of Manchester using eye-tracking methods to examine how clinicians interpret ECGs.

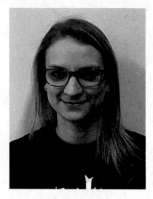

Dr. Julia Mueller is a Research Associate in the Medical Research Council Epidemiology Unit at the University of Cambridge. She works within the programme on Prevention of Diabetes and Related Metabolic Disorders in High Risk Groups.

Prior to this role, she worked as a Lecturer in Healthcare Sciences in the Division of Population Health, Health Services Research and Primary Care at the University of Manchester, leading a course unit on Digital Public Health on the Master of Public Health programme. Much of her research relates to digital health, with a particular focus on health-related behaviour change interventions such as mobile apps for chronic disease management. She is also a strong proponent of patient and public engagement and has organised and participated in various events and initiatives to help patients become involved in research and to disseminate research findings to members of the public.

Julia completed a BSc in Psychology at the Georg-August-University in Goettingen, Germany, and an MSc in Health Psychology at the University of St Andrews. Her studies piqued her interest in the links between psychological and physical well-being, and in the potential of Web-based interventions for improving health. In 2018, Julia completed a PhD research project at the University of Manchester about the role of Web-based information in help-seeking of those worried about lung cancer.

Acronyms

BM	body mass index
CBT	cognitive behavioural therapy
COPD	chronic obstructive pulmonary disease
DHI	digital health intervention
DHT	digital health technology
ECG	Electrocardiogram
EEG	electroencephalogram
FDD	Feature-driven development
GUI	graphical user interface
HCI	Human computer interaction
HCP	healthcare professional
IDE	Integrated development environment
MRC	Medical Research Council
NHS	National Health Service
OS	Operating System
PWA	progressive web apps
RCT	Randomised controlled trial
TDD	Test-driven development
UCD	User Centered Design
UI	User interface
UX	User experience
WHO	world health organisation
XP	eXtreme programming

Chapter 1
Introduction to mHealth

1.1 What Are Health Apps?

Health apps, or *mHealth interventions* are *mobile applications* that aim to promote and maintain health. Mobile applications, also referred to as *mobile apps* or simply *apps* are software applications that are designed to run on mobile (i.e. handheld) devices such as smartphones, tablets and wearable devices like smartwatches. Mobile apps run directly on the device, whereas web and desktop applications run within a web browser or a desktop machine, respectively.

Health apps aim to promote and maintain health by supporting behaviour change and/or decision making. This spans a wide variety of different interventions with different aims. In this book, we define health apps as interventions aiming to change behaviour, support patients, and improve patient outcomes, delivered via smartphones or other mobile devices [21]. They are typically used by patients, carers, or healthcare professionals.

Examples of typical health apps or mHealth interventions

- Apps to promote healthy lifestyles, like physical exercise or healthy diets
- Apps to assist decision-making, e.g. an app to help healthcare professionals decide whether to prescribe antibiotics
- Apps to help people with long-term health problems to self-manage their condition
- Apps to facilitate interaction and communication between patients (peer support), between patients and healthcare professionals (telehealth), or between healthcare professionals
- Apps to track patient outcomes over time to allow continuous assessment

---

© Springer Nature Switzerland AG 2020
A. Davies, J. Mueller, *Developing Medical Apps and mHealth Interventions*, Health Informatics, https://doi.org/10.1007/978-3-030-47499-7_1

Possible aims of health apps
- enabling users to be better informed about their health
- allowing users to share experiences with others in similar positions (e.g. other patients with the same condition)
- changing perceptions and cognitions around health
- assessing and monitoring specified health states or health behaviours
- improving communication between patients and healthcare professionals (HCPs)
- supporting users to change their behaviour to promote healthier lifestyles

1.2   mHealth, eHealth and Related Terms

Before delving further into mHealth and health apps, clarification of commonly used terminology in this field is helpful. There are several terms that are frequently used in the general field of digital health, often with considerable overlap and lack of clear definitions. Firstly, *eHealth* is often used synonymously with *digital health*. The World Health Organisation (WHO) defines eHealth as "the cost-effective and secure use of information and communications technologies in support of health and health-related fields, including health care services, health surveillance, health literature, and health education, knowledge and research" [42]. *Mobile Health* or *mHealth* is a sub-field within eHealth. It is concerned with "the use of mobile phones and other wireless technologies to support the achievement of health objectives" [44]. Thus, mHealth encompasses the use of mobile apps for medical care as well as prevention, health promotion and disease management. Related to the field of mHealth is *uHealth*, which is concerned with the use of ubiquitous technology in health care and health promotion. Ubiquitous technology refers to mobile devices or objects embedded with processors that enable them to connect via the Internet (e.g. smartphones, tablets, smartwatches, activity trackers, other wearable devices, or biometric devices). Increasingly, microprocessors and sensors are embedded in everyday objects (e.g. in hospital beds to allow real-time tracking of the availability of beds). Such technology is also referred to as *Internet of Things* or *pervasive technology*. As such, mHealth is a sub-field within uHealth. *Telemedicine* or *telehealth* (literally "healing at a distance") refers to the use of information and communication technologies to facilitate access to medical care and information [43]. It includes, for example, the use of text messaging, emails, telephone or video calls for consultations and other communications with healthcare professionals. Thus, there can be some overlap between mHealth/uHealth and telemedicine, for example in form of mobile apps that facilitate communication between healthcare professionals.

eHealth is also often used interchangeably with *health informatics*, though the two terms refer to different concepts. Health informatics specifically refers to the management and use of patient information, and as such is concerned with IT-based innovations in healthcare services [14]. It encompasses the generation, management, analysis, interpretation and communication of health data. *Data science* can be understood as a sub-domain of health informatics which focuses specifically on data analysis. It makes use of powerful programming systems, hardware and algorithms to obtain insights from structured and unstructured data [4]. Such advances are important given the large quantities of complex data generated through increasing digitisation. Data analysts are now often faced with health datasets of high volume and diversity which cannot be analysed using traditional database software tools, meaning that new algorithms, techniques and approaches are required [4].

Figure 1.1 provides an overview of definitions of important topics and concepts in the field of digital health.

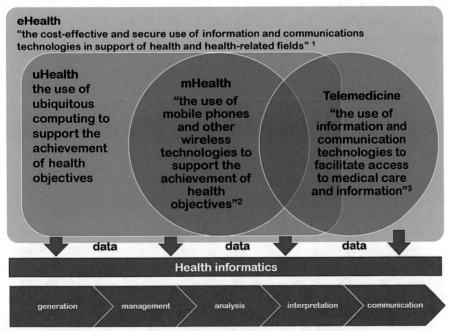

[1] *World Health Organization. eHealth, http://www.emro.who.int/health-topics/ehealth/ (accessed 1 November 2019).*
[2] *World Health Organization. mHealth: New horizons for health through mobile technologies. Geneva, Switzerland, http://www.who.int/goe/publications/goe_mhealth_web.pdf (2011).*
[3] *World Health Organization. TELEMEDICINE: Opportunities and developments in Member States, https://www.who.int/goe/publications/goe_telemedicine_2010.pdf (2010).*

Fig. 1.1 Overview of key concepts in the field of digital health

1.3   Why Do We Need Health Apps?

With improvements in treatments and overall quality of life, people are living longer. The World Health Organization (WHO) estimates that by 2050, 2 billion people (more than a fifth of the world's population) will be over 60 years of age. This means that noncommunicable diseases related to ageing such as cancer, respiratory conditions, diabetes and cardiovascular diseases are increasing.

Moreover, other determinants of chronic health problems such as obesity are increasing. In the UK, for example, the number of diabetes diagnoses increased from 1.4 million in 1996 to 4.5 million in 2015, and a further increase to 5 million is expected by 2025 [5]. Worldwide, diabetes is expected to affect 1 in 10 people by 2040 [5]. Globally, noncommunicable diseases account for over 70% of all deaths, and 80% of all premature deaths [45]. In addition to being the most prevalent global health problem, noncommunicable diseases are also the most costly. Costs extend beyond immediate treatment costs, for example in terms of reduced employment and productivity resulting in loss of income to individual households, and loss of national economic output. Effective and low-cost interventions are needed to address this growing burden.

Given these changes in the health profiles of the general population, paired with wider economic crises resulting in decreasing public spending on health and falling government commitment to health, financial pressures on health services are increasing [38].

According to the WHO, the majority (80%) of cardiovascular diseases, stroke and diabetes as well as 40% of cancers could be prevented through lifestyle changes in the population [42].

Developments in technology have often been cited as a potential solution to the healthcare crisis. Technology can help streamline processes, increase efficiency, and empower patients to manage their own health better. For example, infusion pumps have automated processes of giving injections which previously had to be undertaken manually by nurses. This frees up nurses' time and ensures more patients can be treated [37]. In the UK, the Topol Review, which was published in 2019, specifically explored how digital health technologies can be harnessed to tackle problems faced by the National Health Service (NHS) related to increasing demand coupled with financial constraints [23]. The review concludes that digital technologies will help improve services offered by healthcare professionals (rather than replace them) and will free up time which healthcare professionals can spend with patients.

Technology, and in particular mobile technology, is becoming increasingly prevalent across the world, further highlighting its potential to play a key role in tackling the global healthcare crisis. Globally, there are more than 3 billion smartphone users [31]. Among advanced economies, 76% of adults report owning a smartphone, with some countries such as South Korea reporting smartphone penetration as high as 95% [36]. Emerging economies are rapidly catching up, with a median 45% reporting smartphone ownership. Moreover, around 90% of the population in advanced economies and 60% in emerging economies are connected to the Internet [36].

Due to the widespread penetration of smartphone ownership and Internet connectivity, health apps present a cost-effective, scalable means of disseminating health interventions to large numbers of people. The Topol Review specifically highlights health apps as a key development that will help tackle pressures faced by the NHS. It estimates that smartphone apps will affect more than 80% of the NHS healthcare workforce.

Health apps could potentially empower people to self-manage their health rather than relying on over-stretched healthcare services. A systematic review on health apps designed to improve self-management of key symptoms of chronic conditions found apps for diabetes, chronic lung diseases, and cardiovascular diseases [41]. Several were associated with significant improvements in clinical outcomes, such as blood glucose levels in people with diabetes, improved physical functioning in people with cardiovascular diseases, or lung function parameters in people with chronic lung diseases [41].

Aside from allowing patients to self-manage their health conditions, health apps can also assist healthcare professionals with important tasks such as decision-making, health record management, and communication [40]. Again, this can free up resources and enhance efficiency to help under-resourced healthcare systems deal with increasing demands and pressures. For example, a study at Toronto General Hospital explored the implementation of smartphones for communication among medical teams, with different communication channels depending on the level of urgency [26, 46]. In subsequent surveys, the teams reported improvements in communications and reductions in disruptions to workflows. Although response time to emergencies did not change significantly following the implementation of the smartphone-based communication system, team members did report spending less time attempting to contact physicians, suggesting that time was potentially freed up for other processes [26, 46].

In another example, researchers in Boston developed an app which allows clinicians to capture and securely store clinical images in electronic health records [18]. Clinicians who used the app reportedly found it easy to use and helpful for clinical practice. Visual data can be extremely helpful for clinical diagnoses and monitoring of disease progression. For example, clinicians often ask patients to take regular photos of suspicious moles to document any changes indicating melanoma. The app was developed to streamline previous processes for recording visual data which involved clinicians taking photos on personal phones, emailing the photos to their email accounts, and then opening this email on a hospital workstation in order to copy and paste images from the email into the electronic health record.

App functions such as decision support and enhanced communication can also be harnessed to tackle other challenges facing healthcare systems worldwide including the global influenza pandemic, antimicrobial resistance, and vaccine hesitancy. For example, the "Antimicrobial Companion app" provides practitioners with access to clinical guidelines as well as facilitating decision-making [9].

It should be noted that, despite these promising findings, tangible impacts of health apps on wider healthcare utilisation and the efficiency of healthcare systems have not been systematically assessed. Therefore it is unclear whether the potential of apps to reduce pressures on healthcare services are realised in practice. In the UK, for example, a King's Fund review cautioned that, despite the potential of technology to deliver considerable savings for the National Health Service, they are often not implemented at the scale needed to realise their full potential [3]. Thus, further research is necessary to assess the extent and scale of the impact of mHealth on health services and health outcomes.

1.4   Types of Health Apps

The following sections introduce different types of health apps including apps for health promotion and prevention, disease management and remote access to treatment.

1.4.1   Health Apps for Health Promotion and Prevention

Many health apps target determinants of health to promote health and prevent health problems. There are currently thousands of apps available on app stores which claim to help users lead healthier lifestyles, for example by supporting users to stop smoking, adopt healthier diets, exercise, or drink less alcohol. This is of particular relevance given the increasing prevalence of non-communicable diseases which are largely attributable to lifestyle factors.

> **Case study: "Craving to Quit" – an mHealth intervention to support smoking cessation**
> "Craving to Quit" was developed by researchers from Yale University [8]. It drew on mindfulness training – based on ancient Buddhist practices – to reduce smoking rates among smokers motivated to quit, and to reduce the association between craving and smoking. The app used minfulness-based meditation practices to help users manage cravings and body sensations related to them, and to foster acceptance and retrain the mind. Additionally, the app made use of *experience sampling* to measure smoking, craving, and other factors up to six times per day.
> **Evaluation:** The app was evaluated by comparing it to a control app which had the same look and feel as Craving to Quit, but included only experience sampling [8]. The primary outcome was one-week point-prevalence absti-

(continued)

nence from smoking at 6 months. The authors found no significant differences between participants who received Craving to Quit, and those who used the control app, regardless of whether abstinence was self-reported or verified by CO-monitoring. The groups also did not differ in smoking rates. There was some preliminary evidence to suggest that the mindfulness app led to a reduced association between cravings and smoking.

1.4.2 Health Apps for Disease Management

Health apps are used frequently to help patients (and healthcare professionals) manage diseases, particularly long-term conditions such as diabetes, chronic respiratory conditions, cancer, and mental health problems. Health apps can help patients keep track of their symptoms, medication and other disease-related variables. They can also be used to provide patients with educational information about their condition. Features can be added to support patients with self-management. For example, automatic reminders can help patients adhere to treatments. Health apps can also support patients with the psychological difficulties associated with chronic diseases by drawing on psychological therapeutic methods like cognitive behavioural therapy and mindfulness meditation. For example, patients with chronic obstructive pulmonary disease often experience anxiety due to breathing difficulties, which can significantly impair quality of life. Health apps can help alleviate symptoms and reduce anxiety by helping users practice breathing techniques [2] as well as mindfulness-based meditations [25]. Such self-management interventions are particularly important in light of the increasing burden of non-communicable diseases paired with rising financial pressures on healthcare systems.

Importantly, not all health apps are patient-facing; apps may also support decision-making by healthcare professionals. For example, Tuon et al. [39] examined antimicrobial prescriptions at a university hospital before and after implementation of an app providing antimicrobial use guidance. The authors found significant reductions in prescriptions for several antibiotics, as well as a reduction in costs related to antibiotics.

Case study: An mHealth intervention for atrial fibrillation
Guo et al. [11] developed and tested an app for management of atrial fibrillation, with different versions for patients and healthcare professionals respectively. The app involved the following features:

(continued)

Personal health record: The app was able to record clinical features in a personal health record, including atrial fibrillation features, details about the patients' medical history, results from laboratory tests, and current treatments (e.g. drugs and other pharmacologic treatments).

Clinical decision support: The app automatically recommended different treatment methods based on entries to the personal health record. For example, the app calculated patients' stroke risk and recommended anticoagulants if indicated.

Patient's educational programme: The educational programme included self-support items which aimed to improve patients' knowledge of atrial fibrillation and to help patients manage their condition at home.

Patient involvement with self-care: Patients were encouraged to monitor and record their heart rate, blood pressure, and feedback on their treatment.

Structured follow-up: At regular intervals, the app assessed drug therapy, thrombotic events, bleeding events, quality of life, and treatment satisfaction with automatic reminder notifications.

Data security: Access to the app was protected by a user-sensitive password. The public health records were stored on a cloud platform.

Evaluation: A cluster-randomised controlled trial was conducted to test effects of the app. Participants who used the app showed significant improvements in knowledge of atrial fibrillation, quality of life, and drug adherence, compared to those in the control arm of the study [11].

1.4.3   Health Apps for Remote Access to Treatment

Health apps can facilitate remote access to treatment, by (a) providing users with effective treatments within the app itself (e.g. audio meditations) or (b) by facilitating communication with healthcare professionals (or other individuals who are able to provide support). This is important for those living in remote or underserved areas (e.g. in rural areas), those with mobility issues, as well as those with competing responsibilities (e.g. work, care-giving). For those who are well versed in the use of technology, health apps can offer easy access and round-the-clock availability at low cost. For example, the National Institute for Health and Care Excellence in the UK now recommends digital cognitive behavioural therapy for children and young people suffering from mild depression.

Case study: An mHealth telehealth intervention for posttraumatic stress disorder

Kuhn et al. [17] developed an app to support military veterans with post-traumatic stress disorder (PTSD) by facilitating psychoeducation and self-management. The app was developed using participatory design principles by conducting focus groups with people with PTSD and using their suggestions to develop content and features. Features requested by users included the ability to be used discreetly when PTSD symptoms arise (e.g. in a supermarket queue), and the ability to track PTSD symptoms.

The app included the following sections:

Psychoeducation: This section provided educational information about PTSD, its symptoms, progression, and available treatments.

Self assessment: In this section, users were able to record their symptoms using a validated self-report measure. Users were able to schedule assessments at regular intervals and set reminder notifications. After inputting information, the app provided users with an overview of their symptoms in form of a graph, as well as feedback on the severity and progression of their symptoms.

Coping mechanisms: This section provided users with various tools for self-management of symptoms, such as breathing exercises and progressive muscle relaxation.

Finding support: This section provided users with links and telephone numbers to help them find professional help. Users were also able to add contact details from their own support network (e.g. family, friends).

At the time of publication, the app had been widely used (over 130,000 downloads in 78 different countries) [17]. It was tested with 45 veterans with PTSD. Participants used the app for several days and then rated user satisfaction and perceived helpfulness using standardised questionnaires. They also discussed their perceptions of the app in focus groups.

1.5   Common Features of Health Apps

Health apps are typically complex interventions that include various different features and components that allow them to promote health, illness management, decision making and behaviour change.

Many health apps include *information and education* as a key component (Fig. 1.2). Patient education is becoming increasingly important as healthcare systems place stronger emphasis on self-care in order to manage rising demands.

Decision support aids are also commonly used in many apps. This often entails data input by the user, which the app then uses to return a recommendation for

Fig. 1.2 Example of an app
providing information about
lung functions to educate
patients with respiratory
conditions. App created by
the authors

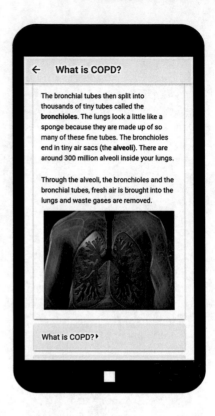

further action. For example, Figure 1.3 shows an app which healthcare professionals can use to make decisions about antimicrobial prescribing for urinary tract infections.

Health apps often include ***behaviour change support***. This can take many different forms. For example, in the app shown in Fig. 1.4, users receive a reminder when they are due to take or repurchase their medication. This "nudges" users to engage in the desired behaviour, i.e. adhering to a treatment regimen.

Health apps are also increasingly used as a platform for ***self-assessment and monitoring***. Both researchers and clinicians frequently rely on patients recalling past events accurately, often over a long time frame. However recall is typically imperfect or biased. For example, research suggests people are often unable to accurately report the amount of sleep they obtain [19] or the symptoms they have experienced over longer time frames [30]. Moreover, healthcare professionals often make decisions about treatment regimens based on patients' symptom profile when they present during consultations, but this "snapshot" may not provide an accurate picture of the general symptom profile.

Health apps are a useful tool to support self-assessment and monitoring because they allow *ecological momentary assessment* (EMA) (or *experience sampling*) as well as monitoring via sensors. EMA involves repeated sampling of participants' behaviours and experiences in real time, in their natural environments [33]. This

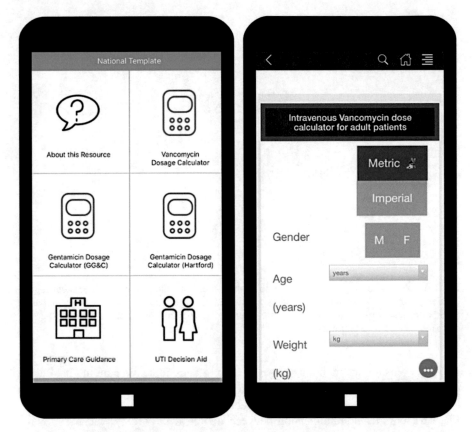

Fig. 1.3 Example of an app providing decision support to healthcare professionals on antimicrobial prescribing for urinary tract infections. (© Tactuum, https://play.google.com/store/apps/details?id=com.tactuum.quris.nes.antimicrobial&hl=en or https://qrs.ly/ykb0cmf. Screenshot reproduced with permission)

helps to build a more detailed understanding of patients' health. For example, the app shown in Fig. 1.5 sent users daily reminders to log their level of breathlessness over a timeframe of several weeks. This enabled users to view how their symptoms varied over time. This information could also be useful for healthcare professionals to support decision making on optimal treatment.

Another useful feature often incorporated into health apps is **communication and interaction**. Through text messaging and (video) call functions, health apps can enable rapid communication. The app shown in Fig. 1.6, for example, uses a secure messaging system to allow healthcare professionals to communicate medical information quickly and efficiently to other healthcare professionals. Messages and images are transferred using end-to-end encryption to ensure confidential information can be communicated securely. The app also uses two-factor authentication to enhance security. Figure 1.7 shows another example of an app which facilitates in-app consultations.

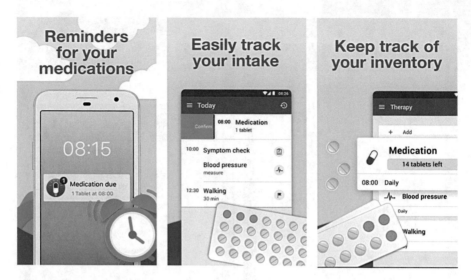

Fig. 1.4 Example of an app which aims to support users in adhering to their treatment regime by alerting them via automatic reminders when medication is due to be taken or repurchased. (© Smartpatient, https://play.google.com/store/apps/details?id=eu.smartpatient.mytherapy Screenshots reproduced with permission)

The two examples mentioned above relate to communication among healthcare professionals, and between healthcare professionals and patients. Health apps can also enable communication between patients as a form of peer support. The app in Fig. 1.8 facilitates communication between people with chronic pain by allowing users to interact and exchange advice. Peer support apps are particularly useful for patients who would otherwise struggle to identify peers (e.g. for rare conditions), or for those who are unable to access face-to-face support (e.g. if they have mobility issues or live in remote areas), or for sensitive conditions that people may feel uncomfortable discussing in person (e.g. if there is a perceived social stigma).

Finally, another note-worthy feature of many health apps is the incorporation of ***theory-based psychological interventions***. Many apps translate psychological interventions that were originally developed for face-to-face interactions into digital formats. For example, various apps incorporate established psychotherapy methods like *cognitive behavioural therapy* (CBT) or *mindfulness*. Figure 1.9 shows an app designed to reduce anxiety and stress which includes mindfulness-based components (e.g. recorded meditation exercises) and CBT-based components to challenge and reframe negative or anxious thoughts.

Fig. 1.5 Example of an app which used experience sampling/ecological momentary assessment to help patients monitor their breathlessness over time. App developed by the authors

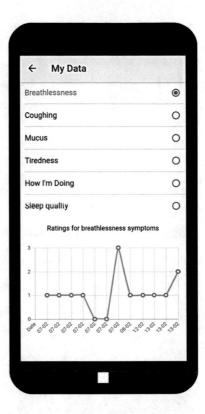

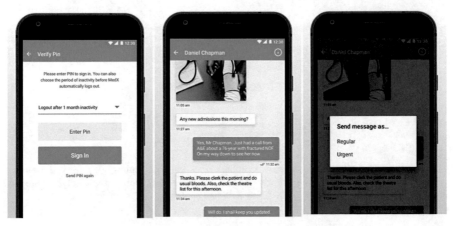

Fig. 1.6 Example of an app which uses secure messaging to facilitate communication between healthcare professionals. (© MedXAU, https://play.google.com/store/apps/details?id=com.medx. android&hl=en Screenshots reproduced with permission)

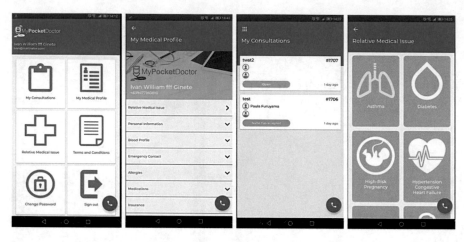

Fig. 1.7 Example of an app which can be used to access in-app consultations with licensed clinicians. (© MyPocketDoctor https://play.google.com/store/apps/details?id=com.mypocketdoctor. android Screenshots reproduced with permission)

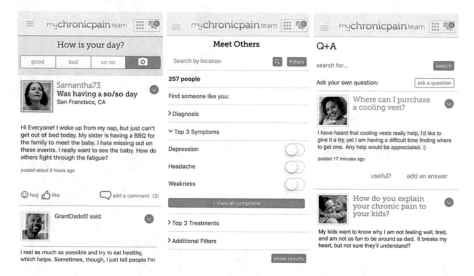

Fig. 1.8 Example of an app which facilitates peer support among people with chronic pain. (© Chronic Pain Support, https://play.google.com/store/apps/details?id=com.myhealthteams. mychronicpainteam. Screenshots reproduced with permission)

1.6   Advantages and Benefits of Delivering Interventions via Health Apps

Delivering interventions via mobile phones – as opposed to face-to-face settings or use of other media – can be advantageous for several reasons.

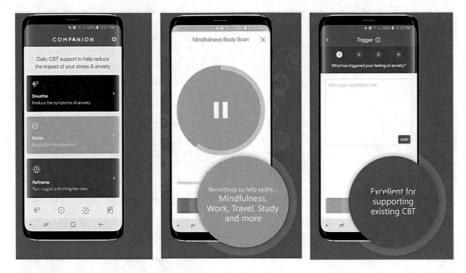

Fig. 1.9 Example of an app which uses psychological therapy methods like cognitive behavioural therapy and mindfulness. (© Stress & Anxiety Companion, https://play.google.com/store/apps/details?id=com.companionapps.anxietycompanion. Screenshots reproduced with permission)

Affordability: Interventions delivered via digital platforms are often cheaper than face-to-face interventions, and, apart from initial development costs, their maintenance and running costs tend to be low. A systematic review of economic evaluations of mHealth interventions found that 74% of the included studies found evidence for the cost-effectiveness of mHealth interventions, although recommended economic outcome items were frequently not reported [16].

Scalability: There is enormous potential for mHealth interventions to be scaled up to large audiences [21], whereas face-to-face interventions typically require more substantial logistical efforts and resources to be delivered to larger audiences, such as staff training and venue costs.

Flexibility: Health apps are accessible round-the-clock and from various locations (though an Internet connection may be required). This makes it easier for users to fit their use of the intervention to their unique schedule, as opposed to face-to-face interventions, which are administered at a specific time and place. This is particularly important for those with competing priorities such as work or caring responsibilities.

Tailoring and personalisation: Health apps can be adapted to specific characteristics and requirements of users, while traditional interventions are often static. For example, information presented via a leaflet is usually generic, while information presented via an app or a website can easily be tailored to user characteristics and preferences. Health apps can be tailored in terms of content (Fig. 1.10) and in terms of functionality (Fig. 1.11).

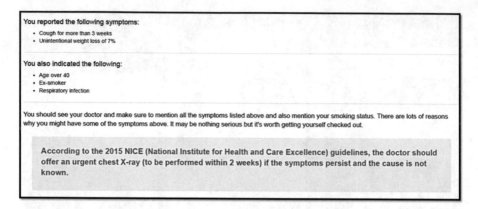

You reported the following symptoms:

- Cough for more than 3 weeks
- Unintentional weight loss of 7%

You also indicated the following:

- Age over 40
- Ex-smoker
- Respiratory infection

You should see your doctor and make sure to mention all the symptoms listed above and also mention your smoking status. There are lots of reasons why you might have some of the symptoms above. It may be nothing serious but it's worth getting yourself checked out.

According to the 2015 NICE (National Institute for Health and Care Excellence) guidelines, the doctor should offer an urgent chest X-ray (to be performed within 2 weeks) if the symptoms persist and the cause is not known.

Fig. 1.10 Example of web-based intervention that tailored content to users based on their reported symptoms and risk factors based on clinical guidelines. Website developed by the authors

Fig. 1.11 Example of an app which allows users to tailor features like reminders to their own preferences. App developed by the authors

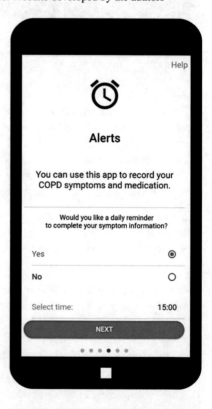

Interactivity: Apps offer advantages over static materials like leaflets and booklets by enabling interactivity. This can be in form of interactions with other users (e.g. other patients or healthcare professionals), or simply in form of interactions between the user and the interface. Simple interactions – like a change in the graphical user interface when a user taps a certain area of the screen – can help keep the user engaged and attentive.

Anonymity: Health apps can offer increased anonymity, which may be important for those with sensitive health concerns. For example, someone with moderate anxiety or depression may feel comfortable downloading an app, whereas they might not feel comfortable seeking face-to-face professional support due to the attached stigma. A systematic review on the factors affecting engagement with digital health interventions found that perceived anonymity plays an important role, e.g. for interventions relating to sexually transmitted diseases and mental health [24].

Widespread availability: With over 2.5 billion smartphone owners across the world and increasingly prevalent Internet penetration, health apps are nearly universally accessible, particularly in advanced economies, where approximately 76% of the population own smartphones [36]. Smartphones are almost ubiquitous among younger populations aged 18–34 years in advanced economies, with an average of (95%) owning a smartphone. Although smartphone ownership is lower among older populations (55% among those aged 50 years and above in advanced economies), the age gap between the generations has been decreasing noticeably since 2015 [36]. It is important to note, however, that smartphone ownership varies considerably by country, with only around 45% smartphone ownership in emerging economies. Unequal distributions of smartphone ownership and Internet access are further discussed in Sect. 1.7.

1.7   Disadvantages and Challenges of Delivering Interventions via Health Apps

Despite numerous advantages and benefits, there are also a number of important challenges and limitations that need to be taken into account when considering the delivery of a health intervention via mobile technology.

Lack of regulation: A main issue with health apps is that content is not officially regulated, which means that the accuracy and safety is not guaranteed. Virtually anyone who is technically able to develop an app can upload this to app stores, with no requirements for medical quality control. For example, Taki et al. [34] systematically assessed infant feeding websites and apps. Out of 46 apps, 78% were rated poor quality, and none were rated excellent. The reviewed apps showed issues with navigability, design, readability, accessibility (e.g. for those with visual impairments), and content. A lack of regulation and evidence base can lead to ineffective interventions, and, at worst, inaccurate medical information which can lead to serious negative consequences. For example, consider the pregnancy and diet app in Fig. 1.12, which encourages women to eat salmon and mackerel during pregnancy. The app fails to mention that these should be consumed in moderation

Fig. 1.12 Example of an app
providing medically
inaccurate and potentially
harmful information. The app
encourages pregnant women
to eat oily fish like mackerel
and salmon, without
mentioning that these can
contain harmful pollutants
like dioxins and
polychlorinated biphenyls.
Image created for the purpose
of this book, based on
existing apps.

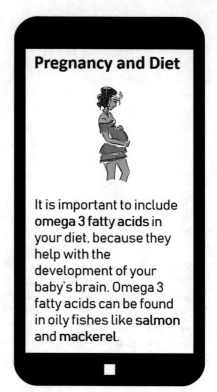

because they may contain harmful dioxins and polychlorinated biphenyls. Another example of apps providing inaccurate advice are apps that claim to promote safer consumption of alcohol by providing estimates of blood alcohol concentration to enable users to determine whether they are safe to drive. Such apps do not in fact have any capacity to estimate blood alcohol concentration. There are initiatives which aim to mitigate such issues by providing users with access to quality-controlled health apps, such as the NHS Apps Library of the UK National Health Service [22]. All apps in the library are required to meet standards sourced by NHS Digital, including evidence of clinical safety, security and technical stability.

Lack of face-to-face contact: Although remote consultations and support can be convenient and may sometimes be the only option open to patients, the importance of personal contact should not be underestimated. Face-to-face contact may be important when physical examinations are required, or to build trustful relationships between clinicians and patients with clear respective responsibilities [32]. Without this contact, patient engagement and compliance with treatments may decrease [32]. However, the extant literature shows ample evidence that healthcare delivered via telemedicine (i.e. video or messaging formats) has no detrimental effects on health outcomes, professional practice or satisfaction [6, 35]. For example, Tates [35] compared web-based versus face-to-face consultations for gynecological health problems and found no differences in information exchange, interpersonal relationship building, or shared decision making.

Digital divide: Not all population groups have equal access to digital technology, and almost half of the world's population are currently still cut off from the Internet [20]. Even where access is available, users may encounter further barriers, for example due to the high levels of (health) literacy often required for health app usage. Similar divides are apparent at a global level; in developed countries, 81% of the population have Internet access, whereas only 41.3% of people in developing countries use the Internet [15]. Apart from lack of access to Internet connectivity or mobile devices, there are further *accessibility* issues for specific user groups. For example, most apps do not include text-to-speech/speech-to-text features and are therefore not accessible to users who are unable to read or type, e.g. users who are blind, have manual dexterity issues, or are illiterate. Moreover, both chronic and acute health conditions are often accompanied by disability-like impairments that might affect mobility, cognition, or perception and thereby impact on people's ability to interact with mobile devices and interfaces [13].

Generally, those who are older, less educated, and of lower socio-economic status are less likely to have access to or use smartphones [36]. At the same time, these groups are often particularly vulnerable to health problems. As such, there are concerns over whether digital health interventions risk further isolating and disadvantaging those with the worst health outcomes, thereby widening health inequalities.

Rapid change of technology vs. slow pace of evidence-based development and evaluation: Aside from the lack of regulation, the availability of evidence-based apps is further hampered by lengthy processes involved in the evaluation of apps and publication of the findings. For independent evaluations by academic institutions, this will often involve several months or even years, from first applying for funding to undertaking the evaluation and finally publishing results in academic journals. Given the rapid pace at which technology changes, the evaluated technology will often be outdated by the time evaluations are completed and published.

Data security concerns: Health apps often involve input of personal, sensitive data by users. This can include for example names and contact details, demographic characteristics (age, gender...), health data (e.g. weight and blood pressure measurements, symptom tracking data...), and information about the users' location (e.g. GPS coordinates). In some cases these data are stored simply on the device itself, but in many cases, data are transferred from the device to remote databases (e.g. for research or data processing). As such, there is a considerable risk of data breaches, either through errors/oversights, or malicious attacks. For example, on reviewing security hazards related to digital communication between patients and clinical teams, Griffiths et al. [10] found that there is a risk of inadvertently disclosing sensitive information, for example when users accidentally send messages to the wrong recipient (oversight/error) or hacking and interception of communication (malicious attacks). Despite existing laws on data protection such as the European Union's General Data Protection Regulation (GDPR) and established guidelines for good practice, the majority of the most popular mobile health apps do not follow regulations and guidelines, entailing serious data privacy risks [27]. Data security is discussed further in Chap. 5.

Resistance to implementation: Many users as well as healthcare professionals may exhibit some resistance to implementing and using health apps. For example, there may be concerns among healthcare professionals that health apps do not meet guidelines for good medical practice, or that incorporation of mHealth may be disruptive to workflows and therefore time-consuming [7, 28, 32]. Users may resist uptake of health apps, for example if they are sceptical of their effectiveness in improving health outcomes, if they do not trust their accuracy and credibility, if they perceive health risks to using apps, or if they feel worried or fearful about taking an active role in their own health management [12].

Technical failures: As with all technology there is a risk of technical failures that could lead to errors or disrupt and thereby compromise patient safety or app functionality. For example, Griffiths et al. [10] evaluated digital communication strategies between young people with long-term health conditions and their clinical care teams. They identified important technical problems that could lead to barriers to communication, including lack of Internet access in certain situations, battery failures, freezing of apps, and limited storage on devices resulting in failure to record content. In Reade et al. [29] pilot study testing an app for tracking chronic pain, physical activity and weather data, participants' batteries depleted quickly because accelerometer data capture used a large amount of power. This led to potential data losses as well as user disengagement.

High dropout: Although the ease with which apps can be accessed – often free of charge and requiring no formal commitment – means that they are likely to be accessed by large numbers of users, this also means that user retention is often low. Users often decide within the first 3–7 days whether they will continue using an app, and most apps lose over three quarters of their users only 3 days after download [1]. After 3 months, only 5% of users remain. Although there are millions of apps on app stores, only a few thousand are able to sustain continuous engagement [1].

1.8   Summary of Key Points

This chapter introduced the field of mHealth and provided an overview of different types of mHealth interventions, including apps for health promotion and prevention of disease, apps for disease management, and apps which facilitate remote access to treatment. The importance of mHealth has surged over recent years and is likely to rise further, given increasing pressures on healthcare systems worldwide due to limited financial resources and demographic shifts in the population. mHealth involves many benefits that are likely to help support healthcare professionals and free up time to spend with patients, but they also involve limitations and challenges that require careful consideration to mitigate risk and harm.

- mHealth is concerned with the use of mobile phones and other wireless technologies to achieve health objectives
- Health apps (or "mHealth interventions") are mobile applications that aim to promote and maintain health by supporting behaviour change and/or decision making.
- Health apps are of particular importance in light of rising pressures on healthcare systems worldwide, with most healthcare systems struggling to meet the demands of an increasingly ageing population coupled with a surge in long-term health conditions such as diabetes.
- Health apps can span a wide array of aims, such as health promotion and prevention, supporting (self-)management of chronic conditions, tracking of health outcomes over time, supporting decision making, enabling remote access to treatment, and facilitating peer support.
- Apps can provide a means of disseminating interventions that is relatively affordable and scalable. They offer considerable advantages over more static materials through their flexibility and interactivity.
- Valid concerns remain regarding the lack of regulation, data security, technical failures, and barriers to access experienced by those who are unable or struggle to purchase or operate mobile devices and Internet connectivity (who also tend to be those most vulnerable to poor health outcomes). Further challenges include high dropout rates among users and potential resistance to innovation among stakeholders and/or users.

1.9 Quiz

1. An app which allows users to send text messages to their healthcare professionals would be considered. . .

   (a) an mHealth intervention
   (b) a telehealth intervention
   (c) a uHealth intervention
   (d) all of the above

2. Which of the following items is **not** an example of ecological momentary assessment (EMA)?

   (a) An app uses smartphones' in-built accelerometer to track physical activity levels of users as they go about their everyday lives.
   (b) An app asks users to rate their breathlessness levels after they have undertaken a physical exercise at a clinic as part of a study.
   (c) An app requires people with asthma to input their symptoms daily over a period of several months.

Answers to the quiz can be found in "Solutions to Quizzes".

1.10   Exercises

In this chapter, we discussed the concept of the "digital divide". Those who experience barriers to accessing technology and the Internet are often also those who are most vulnerable to poor health outcomes. What conclusion would you draw from this; should healthcare services refrain from implementing mHealth interventions? What measures could they take to mitigate the effects of the digital divide? Reflect.

Recommended Reading

1. Castle-Clarke S. What will new technology mean for the NHS and its patients? Four big technological trends. Technical report, The King's Fund and the Nuffield Trust; 2018.
2. National Health Service. The Topol Review: Preparing the healthcare workforce to deliver the digital future. Technical report; 2019.
3. Taylor K, Silver L. Smartphone ownership is growing rapidly around the world, but not always equally. Technical report, Pew Internet Research Centre; 2019.
4. Whitehead L, Seaton P. The effectiveness of self-management mobile phone and tablet apps in long-term condition management: a systematic review. J Med Internet Res. 2016;18(5):e97.

References

1. Andrewchen CA. New data shows losing 80% of mobile users is normal, and why the best apps do better.
2. Beattie MP, Zheng H, Nugent C, McCullagh P. COPD lifestyle support through self-management (CALS). In: 2014 IEEE International Conference on Bioinformatics and Biomedicine (BIBM). IEEE; 2014. p. 1–7. http://ieeexplore.ieee.org/document/6999281/
3. Castle-Clarke S. What will new technology mean for the NHS and its patients? Four big technological trends. Technical report, The King's Fund and the Nuffield Trust; 2018.
4. Consoli S, Reforgiato DR, Petkovic M. Data science for healthcare: methodologies and applications. Cham: Springer Nature Switzerland AG; 2019. https://doi.org/10.1007/978-3-030-05249-2
5. Diabetes UK. Diabetes Facts and Stats: 2015. Technical report; 2015. https://diabetes-resources-production.s3-eu-west-1.amazonaws.com/diabetes-storage/migration/pdf/DiabetesUK_Facts_Stats_Oct16.pdf
6. Flodgren G, Rachas A, Farmer AJ, Inzitari M, Shepperd S. Interactive telemedicine: effects on professional practice and health care outcomes. Cochrane Database Syst Rev. 2015;(9). Art. No.: CD002098. https://doi.org/10.1002/14651858.CD002098.pub2
7. Gagnon M-P, Ngangue P, Payne-Gagnon J, Desmartis M. m-Health adoption by healthcare professionals: a systematic review. J Am Med Inform Assoc. 2016;23(1):212–20. https://doi.org/10.1093/jamia/ocv052
8. Garrison KA, Pal P, O'Malley SS, Pittman BP, Gueorguieva R, Rojiani R, Scheinost D, Dallery J, Brewer JA. Craving to quit: a randomized controlled trial of smartphone app-based mindfulness training for smoking cessation. Nicotine Tob Res. 2018;22(3):324–331. https://doi.org/10.1093/ntr/nty126
9. Google Play. Antimicrobial companion; 24 Feb 2020. https://play.google.com/store/apps/details?id=com.tactuum.quris.nes.antimicrobial&hl=en

10. Griffiths F, Bryce C, Cave J, Dritsaki M, Fraser J, Hamilton K, Huxley C, Ignatowicz A, Kim SW, Kimani PK, Madan J, Slowther A-M, Sujan M, Sturt J. Timely digital patient-clinician communication in specialist clinical services for young people: a mixed-methods study (The LYNC study). J Med Internet Res. 2017;19(4):e102. https://doi.org/10.2196/jmir.7154

11. Guo Y, Chen Y, Lane DA, Liu L, Wang Y, Lip GYH. Mobile health technology for atrial fibrillation management integrating decision support, education, and patient involvement: mAF app trial. Am J Med. 2017;130(12):1388–96.e6. https://doi.org/10.1016/J.AMJMED.2017.07.003

12. Gurtner S. Modelling consumer resistance to mobile health applications. In: ECIS 2014 Proceedings; 2014. https://aisel.aisnet.org/ecis2014/proceedings/track09/7

13. Harper S, Mueller J, Davies A, Nicolau H, Eraslan S, Yesilada Y. The case for 'Health-induced impairments and disabilities'. In: W4A '20, 20–21 April 2020, Taipei; 2020.

14. Healthcare Information and Management Systems (HIMSS). Health informatics defined.

15. International Telecommunication Union. ICT Facts and Figures; 2017. https://www.itu.int/en/ITU-D/Statistics/Pages/facts/default.aspx

16. Iribarren SJ, Cato K, Falzon L, Stone PW. What is the economic evidence for mHealth? A systematic review of economic evaluations of mHealth solutions. PloS One 2017;12(2):e0170581.

17. Kuhn E, Greene C, Hoffman J, Nguyen T, Wald L, Schmidt J, Ramsey KM, Ruzek J. Preliminary evaluation of PTSD coach, a smartphone app for post-traumatic stress symptoms. Mil Med. 2014;179(1):12–8. https://doi.org/10.7205/MILMED-D-13-00271

18. Landman A, Emani S, Carlile N, Rosenthal DI, Semakov S, Pallin DJ, Poon EG, Poon EG. A mobile app for securely capturing and transferring clinical images to the electronic health record: description and preliminary usability study. JMIR mHealth uHealth 2015;3(1):e1. https://doi.org/10.2196/mhealth.3481

19. Lauderdale DS, Knutson KL, Yan LL, Liu K, Rathouz PJ. Sleep duration: how well do self-reports reflect objective measures? The CARDIA sleep study. Epidemiology (Cambridge). 2008;19(6):838–45. https://doi.org/10.1097/EDE.0B013E318187A7B0

20. Makri A. Bridging the digital divide in health care. Lancet Digital Health. 2019;1(5):e204–5. https://doi.org/10.1016/S2589-7500(19)30111-6

21. Murray E, Hekler EB, Andersson G, Collins LM, Doherty A, Hollis C, Rivera DE, West R, Wyatt JC. Evaluating digital health interventions. Am J Prev Med. 2016;51(5):843–51. https://doi.org/10.1016/j.amepre.2016.06.008

22. National Health Service. NHS Apps Library. https://www.nhs.uk/apps-library/

23. National Health Service. The topol review: preparing the healthcare workforce to deliver the digital future. Technical report; 2019. https://topol.hee.nhs.uk/wp-content/uploads/HEE-Topol-Review-2019.pdf

24. O'Connor S, Hanlon P, O'Donnell CA, Garcia S, Glanville J, Mair FS. Understanding factors affecting patient and public engagement and recruitment to digital health interventions: a systematic review of qualitative studies. BMC Med Inform Decis Mak. 2016;16(1):120. https://doi.org/10.1186/s12911-016-0359-3

25. Owens OL, Beer JM, Reyes LI, Gallerani DG, Myhren-Bennett AR, McDonnell KK. Mindfulness-based symptom and stress management apps for adults with chronic lung disease: systematic search in app stores. JMIR mHealth uHealth. 2018;6(5):e124. https://doi.org/10.2196/mhealth.9831

26. Ozdalga E, Ozdalga A, Ahuja N. The smartphone in medicine: a review of current and potential use among physicians and students. J Med Internet Res. 2012;14(5):e128. https://doi.org/10.2196/jmir.1994

27. Papageorgiou A, Strigkos M, Politou E, Alepis E, Solanas A, Patsakis C. Security and privacy analysis of mobile health applications: the alarming state of practice. IEEE Access. 2018;6:9390–403. https://doi.org/10.1109/ACCESS.2018.2799522

28. Puntis J. Health apps don't meet GMC advice on good practice. BMJ (Clin. Res. ed.) 2019;365:l1880. https://doi.org/10.1136/bmj.l1880

29. Reade S, Spencer K, Sergeant JC, Sperrin M, Schultz DM, Ainsworth J, ⋯ Dixon WG. Cloudy with a chance of pain: engagement and subsequent attrition of daily data entry in a

smartphone pilot study tracking weather, disease severity, and physical activity in patients with rheumatoid arthritis. JMIR mHealth uHealth. 2017;5(3):e37. https://doi.org/10.2196/mhealth. 6496

30. Schmier JK, Halpern MT. Patient recall and recall bias of health state and health status. Expert Rev. Pharmacoecon. Outcomes Res. 2004;4(2):159–63. https://doi.org/10.1586/14737167.4.2. 159

31. Statista. Smartphone users worldwide 2016–2021; 2019. https://www.statista.com/statistics/ 330695/number-of-smartphone-users-worldwide/

32. Stevens WJM, van der Sande R, Beijer LJ, Gerritsen MG, Assendelft WJ. eHealth apps replacing or complementing health care contacts: scoping review on adverse effects. J Med Internet Res. 2019;21(3):e10736. https://doi.org/10.2196/10736

33. Stone CJ, Skinner AL. New technology and novel methods for capturing health-related data in longitudinal and cohort studies. Technical report, MRC Integrative Epidemiology Unit; 2017. https://www.closer.ac.uk/wp-content/uploads/New-technology-and-novel-methods-for-capturing-health-related-data.pdf

34. Taki S, Campbell KJ, Russell CG, Elliott R, Laws R, Denney-Wilson E. Infant feeding websites and apps: a systematic assessment of quality and content. Interact J Med Res. 2015;4(3):e18. https://doi.org/10.2196/ijmr.4323

35. Tates K, Antheunis ML, Kanters S, Nieboer TE, Gerritse MB. The effect of screen-to-screen versus face-to-face consultation on doctor-patient communication: an experimental study with simulated patients. J Med Internet Res. 2017;19(12):e421. https://doi.org/10.2196/jmir.8033

36. Taylor K, Silver L. Smartphone ownership is growing rapidly around the world, but not always equally. Technical report, Pew Internet Research Centre; 2019. https://www.pewresearch. org/global/2019/02/05/smartphone-ownership-is-growing-rapidly-around-the-world-but-not-always-equally/

37. Thimbleby H. Technology and the future of healthcare. J Public Health Res. 2013;2(3):e28. https://doi.org/10.4081/jphr.2013.e28

38. Thomson S, Figueras J, Evetovit T, Jowett M, Mladovsky P, Maresso A, Cylus J, Karanikolos M, Kluge H. Economic crisis, health systems and health in Europe: impact and implications for policy. Technical report, WHO; 2014.

39. Tuon FF, Gasparetto J, Wollmann LC, de Moraes TP. Mobile health application to assist doctors in antibiotic prescription – an approach for antibiotic stewardship. Braz J Infect Dis. 2017;21(6):660–4. https://doi.org/10.1016/J.BJID.2017.08.002

40. Ventola CL. Mobile devices and apps for health care professionals: uses and benefits. P & T Peer-Rev J Formulary Manag. 2014;39(5):356–64. http://www.ncbi.nlm.nih.gov/pubmed/ 24883008 http://www.pubmedcentral.nih.gov/articlerender.fcgi?artid=PMC4029126

41. Whitehead L, Seaton P. The effectiveness of self-management mobile phone and tablet apps in long-term condition management: a systematic review. J Med Internet Res. 2016;18(5):e97. https://doi.org/10.2196/jmir.4883

42. World Health Organization. (n.d.). Chronic diseases and health promotion. Retrieved October 2, 2019, from https://www.who.int/chp/chronic_disease_report/part1/en/index11.html

43. World Health Organization. TELEMEDICINE: opportunities and developments in Member States. Technical report; 2010. https://www.who.int/goe/publications/goe_telemedicine_2010. pdf

44. World Health Organization. mHealth: New horizons for health through mobile technologies. Technical report; 2011. https://www.who.int/goe/publications/goe_mhealth_web.pdf

45. World Health Organization. Noncommunicable diseases; 2018. https://www.who.int/news-room/fact-sheets/detail/noncommunicable-diseases

46. Wu RC, Morra D, Quan S, Lai S, Zanjani S, Abrams H, Rossos PG. The use of smartphones for clinical communication on internal medicine wards. J Hosp Med. 2010;5(9):553–9. http://www.ncbi.nlm.nih.gov/pubmed/20690190 http://www.journalofhospitalmedicine.com/ jhospmed/article/127436/smartphones-clinical-communication

Chapter 2
Project Development Methodologies, Management and Data Modelling

2.1 Introduction

A project usually consists of a set of temporary activities that conclude with a specific goal. Projects tend to have finite resources and duration. They may involve putting together a team to meet the project's intended goals. Project constraints often hinge around cost, time-frame and available resources. Project management skills and techniques are essential to ensure the cost effective, time effective release of a project, especially as poor project management has been shown to have greater impact on medical/health research projects than methodology [27]. It is important when starting a new project to clearly define:

- *Scope*: What will the project cover/not cover?
- *Time frame*: How long will the project run for? Are there any hard deadlines?
- *Budget*: How much money is available to the project?
- *Resources*: This can include equipment, personnel, space, expertise and technology requirements

Some of the points above may be fixed, while others could be compromised to a greater or lesser extent. For example a project with a fixed end date might compromise on budget and spend more money in order to achieve the goals by the set date, whereas another project may run over time to save on a fixed budget and so on. It is a good idea when starting a project to consider which of these components are constrained, which could be optimised and which are negotiable to some extent.

© Springer Nature Switzerland AG 2020

A. Davies, J. Mueller, *Developing Medical Apps and mHealth Interventions*, Health Informatics, https://doi.org/10.1007/978-3-030-47499-7_2

Common reasons why projects fail

- Insufficient staff skill set
- People leaving before project completion
- Poor scoping or mission creep
- Poor allocation of funding, or underfunding
- Failure to define end points or to know when something was done
- Poor documentation making it hard for others to pick up work when people leave
- Poorly defined tasks
- Poor scheduling

Most people are probably familiar with the adage that work expands to fill the allotted time (Parkinson's law). Another similar phenomenon often experienced by students, hence the name 'Student syndrome' refers to the planned procrastination that students often partake in when an imminent assignment deadline is looming. This leads them to address the task at the last possible moment. Such observations relate to the psychological aspects of work that impact on humans. To mitigate against such things and to ensure that there are no unwanted surprises along the way, various project management techniques have been created and applied to projects along the way.

A lot of good project management revolves around identifying and mitigating risks that may prevent the project from realizing its objectives. This is very relevant for software projects given that around 19% of them are never completed and a further 46% have experienced a range of issues, such as running over time and/or budget or not matching original specifications [3].

2.2   The Software Crisis

In the 1960s it became apparent that there were significant issues with developing software systems (even small ones). This lead to software projects running over time and budget, being hard to maintain and of poor quality. They also often failed to meet the requirements they were built to address. In the wake of this crisis, different design methodologies were proposed and implemented. Many earlier systems were designed using the *waterfall* methodology (Fig. 2.1), so called because of the cascade of stages that are carried out in sequence resembling a waterfall. The first formal mention of the waterfall model has been attributed to Winston Royce who was involved in the creation of software for space mission planning. He does not call the model waterfall explicitly and uses it to point out the various flaws and risks in the use of such an approach [20]. Earlier methodologies like waterfall

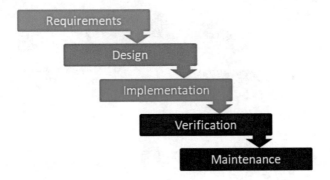

Fig. 2.1 Waterfall methodology

placed a strong emphasis on getting things right first time [30]. This meant that the cost of making changes to these systems increased dramatically along the project timeline [2].

This type of approach tends to involve 'big upfront requirements gathering' and a contract or terms of reference document to indicate what the deliverables for such a project would be. Developers then embark on the design and implementation of the system, with testing usually carried out towards the end of the project. Methods like this have certain disadvantages in that they are reliant on the customer knowing what they want and being able to accurately and completely describe these requirements. It might not always be possible for a customer to know how a new system might impact on their practices prior to implantation. As previously mentioned, changes made later on in the project life-cycle are subject to higher increases in cost. Such methods can however be appropriate if a project is very well scoped and any potential changes down the line are small and manageable, and therefore not too costly. A more recent alternative to these approaches is the Agile methodology.

2.3 Agile

Back in 2001, seventeen supporters of various lightweight methodologies came together and termed the commonalities among their approaches 'Agile' [30]. The Agile software engineering methodology has become an increasingly popular method for designing modern software applications (and project management in general). Agile features an incremental iterative approach (Fig. 2.2).

The main stages involve gathering requirements, planning regarding the prioritisation of requirements and how to deliver them. This is followed by development and testing. Testing is carried out early in Agile so that errors/bugs are identified and resolved rapidly. By "failing fast", early changes can be made to the product to improve it and ensure it adds value. After this the product will be deployed or reflected on with further specifications and adjustments before launching the next

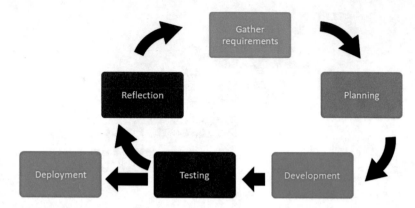

Fig. 2.2 Agile methodology

iteration. Deployment consists of small working versions of the product, known as a minimal viable product (MVP) that features the most essential or core functionality that is built upon in an incremental way. Agile has become a bit of a buzz word, with many organisations claiming to be Agile. The reality is that although people are aware of the terms and processes of Agile, to make it work they really need to change the way they think and act. This involves a paradigm shift for most people who may be used to thinking in a more linear way. In fact most western education follows a linear flow with assessment at the end of a course for example. Thinking in an iterative way and providing incremental versions of a system is not something that comes naturally. A system developed with Agile would provide an 'end-to-end' slice of functionality of the entire system, rather than producing it layer at a time as would have been the case with traditional methodologies. We want to ensure that we are placing real value at the heart of our processes. Quantifying what we mean by value can be difficult as it can mean different things in different settings. For many companies this can be profit. In healthcare settings this can apply to things such as improving patient health outcomes, quality of life and safety, reducing waste, improving efficiency, optimizing processes to reduce waiting times and improving performance and so on.

It is important for the team to have an understanding of what they mean by value so that they can ensure the work they produce adds value. When teaching the Agile methodology to students, we often find that they are aware of the terms and processes. However when we attempt to get them to apply Agile, they often have trouble adapting the Agile way of thinking and acting. This is because it is more than a methodological set of processes and requires adoption of an Agile mindset. Software engineers/developers often want to produce something that might be the quickest or easiest option on their list. This might not however add any value for the stakeholders/customers. For example producing a login page for an app is of little value to a customer if there is no app functionality to log into to use. Having a minimally functional app that implements the main basic functionality is of much greater value. Some seasoned developers also have to adapt their practices when applying Agile which values adaptability to the inevitable changes that occur with projects. Developers take pride in their work and want to produce the best and most efficient code instead of always focusing on the minimal functionality needed to add immediate value. This is not a new phenomenon regarding programmers' approach to their code and was highlighted as far back as the 1970s.

> *There is no doubt that the grail of efficiency leads to abuse. Programmers waste enormous amounts of time thinking about, or worrying about, the speed of noncritical parts of their programs, and these attempts at efficiency actually have a strong negative impact when debugging and maintenance are considered. We should forget about small efficiencies, say about 97% of the time: premature optimization is the root of all evil.* - Donald Knuth [17]

As mentioned, Agile is also a mindset. The progenitors of Agile produced a manifesto to document the values associated with Agile. The manifesto consists of the following values:

Agile manifesto [4]

- **Individuals and interactions** over processes and tools
- **Working software** over comprehensive documentation
- **Customer collaboration** over contract negotiation
- **Responding to change** over following the plan

The Agile manifesto promotes self organising team work and flattens the structure so that individuals working on the project are valued and trusted allowing developers to contribute to choices. This also extends to viewing the customer as a member of the team with equal status. The focus on working software is key to delivering real value and avoiding waste. Some developers may want to create the perfect feature but often a 'good enough' working feature adds more value to the overall system and means that working code can be shipped faster. The main benefit comes in the adaptability to change and seeing it as inevitability, rather than something to resist.

This way of working is helpful when building apps/systems where there is a lot of change and the project may change direction or focus rapidly as it continues. The rapid MVP development allows the customer to give regular feedback to shape the direction of the project. This especially lends itself to co-design approaches. In addition to the manifesto, Agile also has a set of guiding principles:

The 12 Agile principles [5]

1. Our highest priority is to satisfy the customer through early and continuous delivery of valuable software
2. Welcome changing requirements, even late in development. Agile processes harness change for the customer's competitive advantage
3. Deliver working software frequently, from a couple of weeks to a couple of months, with a preference to the shorter timescale
4. Business people and developers must work together daily throughout the project
5. Build projects around motivated individuals. Give them the environment and support they need, and trust them to get the job done
6. The most efficient and effective method of conveying information to and within a development team is face-to-face conversation
7. Working software is the primary measure of progress
8. Agile processes promote sustainable development. The sponsors, developers, and users should be able to maintain a constant pace indefinitely
9. Continuous attention to technical excellence and good design enhances agility
10. Simplicity – the art of maximizing the amount of work not done is essential
11. The best architectures, requirements, and designs emerge from self-organizing teams
12. At regular intervals, the team reflects on how to become more effective, then tunes and adjusts its behavior accordingly

Agile moves away from estimates and usually involves less documentation. It is more difficult to manage with distributed teams. For Agile to work, the management of an organisation has to buy into the idea and allow the self organising team approach that Agile requires. This can be difficult for teams using more traditional approaches to fully embrace. Healthcare is often seen by many as something different that stands apart from other domains. This could be in part because of its critical to health and life and so more caution is often rightly applied before adopting new practices and ways of working. Agile has however been used successfully in the healthcare environment, albeit usually for smaller scale software development tasks. An example of this is the work of Dafydd et al. who reflect on their creation of a digital training portfolio using Agile methods, which they were able to deliver at a lower cost point [8].

2.3.1 Agile Methodologies and Frameworks

Agile is an umbrella term for multiple different practices ranging from more lightweight single teams to heaver weight approaches that may utilise multiple teams. An overview of the single team lighter weight principles and practices and processes are presented here.

2.3.2 Scrum

Scrum is one of the most popular Agile frameworks currently in use. Scrum was founded on empirical process control theory [25] and is associated with various activities and artifacts that are involved in its application [26]. These include activities like *sprint planning*, *sprint review* and *retrospective*, as well as the daily Scrum meeting. Artifacts include the *product* and *sprint* backlogs. Work takes place in iterative cycles called *Sprints*, which are typically 1, 2, or 4 weeks in duration and add functionality and value in each step.

There are several key roles in a Scrum team. These consist of:

- **Scrum development team**: A small team, usually between 3–9 members. A self-organising team that shares accountability equally among its members
- **Scrum Master** (SM): Makes sure that the Scrum process is followed on behalf of the Scrum team. The scrum master role is **not** synonymous with the manger of the development team, and should be viewed more like a facilitator and coach who serves the teams needs
- **Product Owner** (PO): Represents the customer or other stakeholders and controls what is know as the Product Backlog. In some places this is more of a strategic role as a user/stakeholder advocate, in others, more of a task driven role involving the organisation of tasks and their priority.

The Product Backlog is a list with ordered items containing all of the project's requirements. This includes all the features, enhancements and any bugs that need fixing [25]. This is priority ordered by the PO, who also makes sure that it is clear and visible to the team. This can be displayed on a board (Fig. 2.3). These features/enhancements are often represented using *user stories* (see Sect. 2.5.1) to represent system requirements that are broken down in various levels of granularity. These items can then be transferred to a Sprint Backlog and can be broken down into smaller user stories or tasks and moved between relevant columns to show the current stage of the task(s). For example a task could be moved into a 'pending' column (e.g. sprint backlog representing all the units of work prioritised for the current sprint). This can then be transferred to the 'in-progress' column and finally upon completion into the 'done' column. There is also sometimes a 'done done' column used to indicate that that feature is finally finished and approved/signed off, rather than just complete. Boards like this offer a transparent snap-shot overview of

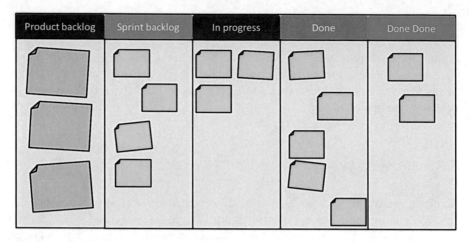

Fig. 2.3 Example Sprint Backlog showing typical columns that user stories or tasks (represented with the yellow notes) are moved between

the entire project. The prioritization of tasks is controlled by the Product Owner, who can update the backlog at any point at their discretion [25] in order to reprioritize the client's needs or anticipate their future needs.

The Scrum Master organises a daily stand up meeting of around 15 min called a daily Scrum to plan for the next 24 h [26]. The time limit must be adhered to and the team should remain standing. This keeps the team focused and prevents them becoming too comfortable and extending the meeting to talk about other issues. The aim is to synchronise activity and to inspect progress towards the goal of the current sprint. This is different to a status meeting where people often report back to a manger or team leader. The daily scrum is focused on the development team and their combined accountability and decision making to adapt the plan accordingly. This is fundamental to the self-organising team aspect of Scrum. The daily scrum should be seen as a collaborative planning session [22]. Figure 2.4 gives an overview of the framework. The Product Backlog is used in the sprint planning phase to generate the Sprint Backlog, detailing the tasks involved in the current sprint. The Scrum team work on the sprint (having a daily Scrum meeting) until the sprint is complete. They then embark on a *sprint review* where the stakeholders are invited to inspect the results of the latest sprint with the team. This is then shipped to the stakeholder and followed by a *sprint retrospective*.

The sprint retrospective is carried out after the sprint review to evaluate and plan future improvements. This includes reflecting on what the team wishes to continue to do, anything the team should stop doing and anything new the team should start to do (start, stop and continue doing). At the end of each iteration there must be a completed and usable increment that the customer can inspect and use. This moves the whole project a step closer to its overall goal.

SCRUM FRAMEWORK

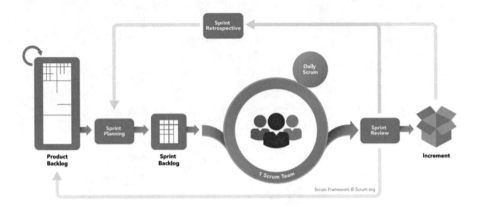

Fig. 2.4 Scrum framework, from [26] https://www.scrum.org/resources/scrum-framework-poster.
(Copyright Scrum. All rights reserved)

Example 1: Using the Scrum framework to prototype a Health and Wellbeing Platform

Keijzer-Broers et al. [16] employed a scrum approach (paired with an Action Research Approach) to develop a Web-based platform to provide health and wellbeing support to elderly users, to help them identify relevant smart living services.

In the first stage of this project (Problem Formulation), the authors conducted 70 stakeholders interviews and two focus groups. The aim of this stage was to engage potential stakeholders and clearly formulate the problem they wished to address.

The scrum approach was used in the second stage (Building, Intervention and Evaluation). This involved four scrum teams working in parallel to address the following aims:

- Specify the critical design issues of the platform
- Set up a project plan
- Create a first template of the platform architecture
- Design mock-ups to provide a basis for the design of the platform

To further inform the work of these different teams, the authors also conducted three workshops with the stakeholders identified in the first stage:

(continued)

- Workshop 1: In this first workshop, main features of the platform (established with stakeholders during stage 1: problem formulation) were evaluated together with stakeholders in order to verify the different requirements
- Workshop 2: In a second workshop, the technical architecture of the platform was further discussed and specified
- Workshop 3: In a third workshop, stakeholders discussed critical design issues, focusing on issues around trust and data privacy

Subsequently, insights derived from the workshops were used to develop initial mock ups of the platform. Potential end-users were included from the start to ensure issues could be identified and addressed early, and to ensure design features were validated iteratively throughout the process. Additionally, usability tests with potential end users were conducted.

Example 2: Using the Scrum framework to develop a self-help pregnancy Android app

Harris et al. [15] used the scrum approach to develop an Android app to help women achieve a healthy weight during pregnancy.

Roles

The team consisted of 5 people who assumed multiple roles. The authors define the following roles:

- Product Owner: This individual acted as a liaison between the customers, the project sponsors, and the development team, and was tasked with communicating the requirements of the project
- Scrum Master: This individual was tasked with communicating the development goals to the team and with liaising between the product owners and the team. The scrum master also organised each sprint by assigning items from the product backlogs into the sprint backlogs, and assessed the team's progress at the end of each week.
- Application development team: This group was tasked with coding and testing the application.
- User interface design team: This group was in charge of designing the look and feel of each individual screen of the application.

Product backlog

The team created a product backlog detailing the required components and functionalities of the application together with the customer. This included:

- UI component: all screens and UI elements

(continued)

- Notifications/reminders component: reminders for the user to input data into the app such as weight and activity
- Weight monitoring component: a feature allowing the user to input and monitor their weight over time
- Dietary information component: a feature allowing the users to input and monitor their food intake, as well as receiving feedback regarding the quality of their diet
- Activity monitoring component: a component allowing users to input and monitor their activity levels
- Google Health component: a component which interfaces with Google Health to enable the user to log weight, diet and activity information
- Feedback component: a component which provides feedback to the user based on the information they inputted
- Information library: a component containing information about food (e.g. portion sizes) and help screens
- User manual: a component providing guidance on using the application

Meetings and progress tracking
The following mechanisms were implemented to facilitate planning and progress tracking:

- Weekly meetings
- Frequent communication between individual team members via telephone to track progress
- Sprint planning meetings at the start of each sprint
- Weekly meetings with the customers to assess the product backlog

Work plan and sprints
The project spanned 21 weeks, split into three sets of seven-week terms:

1. The first term involved background research and literature reviews on weight gain during pregnancy as well as requirements gathering from the customers
2. The second term focused on software development and also involved conducting focus groups to facilitate the development of front-end components. It was split into three two-week sprints: Sprint 1 focused on the user interface and the notifications/reminder component; Sprint 2 and 3 focused on the weight tracking, nutrition tracking, and the activity tracking components
3. The final term involved completing the coding of the application and polishing the user interface. This term was also split into three sprints: Sprint 1 focused on the feedback component, the Google Health component, and the information library; Sprint 2 focused on the feedback component and

(continued)

the information library, and Sprint 3 focused on bug fixes, polishing the user interface, and developing the user manual

The team adapted the scrum approach to suit the aims and timelines of their project. Deviations from scrum included:

- No scrum burn down chart to assess the completed work per day was created, due to limited time available to the scrum master (who was also part of the development team) and because the product backlog did not change much throughout the project
- Weekly meetings were held instead of daily standup meetings (for the same reasons outlined above)
- No sprint retrospective meetings were held due to time constraints

For further details see Harris et al.'s comprehensive description in [15].

2.3.3 Kanban

Kanban is another of the most widely used of the Agile methodologies. Kanban is a Japanese word describing a visual board. It was adapted for use in Agile from Toyota. A kanban board is typically a large physical board that displays the current state of work visually. This is often split into columns where cards containing the 'work units' are moved between the columns to indicate their current state, for example moving a task from *pending* to *in progress* or *done*. These boards offer a transparent snapshot of the entire current state of a project in terms of the tasks or work units that can be seen by the entire team. This can be a wall mounted board with cards or post it style notes that are physically moved between columns. Kanban boards can also be represented digitally with various software.

Whereas Scrum teams work in sprints pulling tasks from the product backlog into a sprint backlog, Kanban teams implement a continuous process rather than breaking tasks down into sprints. The tasks are instead limited by a Work In Progress (WIP) limit. Each column on a Kanban board has a WIP limit that is dependent on the capacity and resources of the team. Completing a task and transferring it to another column on the board initiates another task being pulled from the backlog to replace the completed one. This ensures a continuous stream of work. As Kanban does not utilise iterations, it is best used for short-cycle deliverables.

There are some similarities and equivalents to Scrum in Kanban. These include the use of a board called a Kanban board rather than a scrum board (although these are sometimes also referred to as Kanban boards). The equivalent of a Scrum master is referred to as an 'Agile coach' in Kanban and the daily Scrum meeting is called a 'stand up'. The sprint review is referred to as a 'demo'.

Some people confuse a product backlog with a Kanban board. The backlog is essentially a pool of potential pending tasks that are usually ordered according to priority from essential features to "nice to haves". The Kanban board in contrast shows all the tasks that will be initiated imminently. Thus the backlog can be used to represent a subsection of a Kanban board.

Example: Using a Kanban approach in the development of a mobile app to promote a vegetarian diet
Festersen [11] combined waterfall methodologies with agile methodologies and also used a Kanban chart to manage the coding stage of the development of a mobile app to promote adoption of a vegetarian diet. The Kanban chart was created using Kanbanpad (a free online tool) and detailed the functional requirements of the app and tasks needed to accomplish these.

The project was managed by combining the Kanban chart with a Gantt chart. The Gantt chart provided an overview of the overall project and the higher-level tasks (e.g. "complete literature review" or "usability testing") as well as their timelines. The Kanban chart on the other hand detailed smaller, more specific tasks (e.g. "Find studies on mobile nutrition tracking" or "Find participants for usability test").

2.3.4 Extreme Programming (XP)

Extreme Programming focuses on producing high quality software. It is based on a number of values (communication, simplicity, feedback, courage and respect). Managers, customers and the developers are all part of an XP team, which usually has somewhere between 2 and 12 developers [29]. As with Scrum, XP also focuses on self organising teams and daily communication. Pair programming (see Sect. 2.4.4) is one of the core practices in XP [3]. The testing of software code is seen as another core component of XP with one of the rules being that all code written should have unit tests. XP applies practices that include the use open plan working environments to improve team communication and the co-location of a cross-functional team. The customer must be regularly available to the team and actively engaged, and ideally become part of the team.

Applying Extreme Progrmaming to the development and implementation of a biosecurity health care application

Fruhling et al. [12] conducted a study to evaluate whether agile methods such as extreme programming (XP) could help improve the development and implementation of telehealth services, specifically a biosecurity telehealth project. The project involved a secure, dedicated web-based telecommunication network system that connected clinical health laboratories in Nebraska. XP was chosen for this project because:

- It is flexible
- It allows rapid prototyping
- It involves low overhead costs
- It is suited for small/medium-sized projects

Two teams worked on this project:

- Information technology/development team: consisted of two part-time developers (two further developers joined later as the demands of the project grew), an on-call senior research technologist professional, and a project manager
- User team: consisted of the Director of the University of Nebraska Center for Biosecurity, the Assistant Director of the Nebraska Public Health Lab and two health professionals

At an initial meeting at the start of the project, the user team provided details of their requirements, i.e. how they would use the network system and how they would expect it to function to facilitate communication between the different laboratories.

Following this initial meeting, the development team researched which technologies could be used for the development of the system, and developed a system prototype based on the requirements. The prototype was developed in the form of unit test plans before coding commenced. Two developers worked together on all coding (pair programming).

The first functioning prototype was running within a few weeks, and overall 10 prototypes were developed over a 21-month period.

Evaluation of the method:

Overall, the authors conclude that XP was successfully implemented in this telehealth project. Five out of the main nine principles of the approach were implemented fully. The principle of pair programming was modified (a lead developer was assigned who reported on progress) and the principle of having an on-site customer throughout development was not feasible because the customers had competing responsibilities (i.e. working in a health laboratory).

(continued)

The authors note that the rapid prototyping principle was critical in achieving customer buy-in for the project. Although the customers showed some reservations regarding the new technology, this was quickly diffused when the developers were able to produce a running prototype within a few weeks. This also facilitated gaining user feedback, and helped avoid major issues before too much time had been invested in development.

The authors also conclude that the iterative development allowed the customers/users to become better acquainted with the technology and related terminology, thus facilitating engagement and feedback mechanisms.

Additionally, the authors note that the iterative development process had positive impacts on group synergy and cooperation.

Finally, the authors observed that the iterative approach was conducive for the incorporation of newly developing technologies due to its high level of flexibility [12].

2.3.5 Feature Driven Development (FDD)

Unlike some of the other Agile approaches mentioned, Feature driven development (FDD) is more of a top-down approach that was designed to work with larger development teams on larger projects. FDD consists of 5 principle steps:

1. Develop a model (model the domain)
2. Build a list of features
3. Plan by feature
4. Design by feature
5. Build by feature

The approach was designed to work with Object Orientated Programming (OOP) paradigms. And starts with initial modelling which describes the overall model of the system (often using class diagrams). This then determines the list of features needed to realise the system. Once a feature list is generated, each feature can be planned and then designed and built. Modelling in FDD is iterative with more detail added over subsequent iterations. The level of detail in the modelling stage needs to be sufficient to derive good estimates. This allows for requirements to evolve during the course of the project. There is also the concept of a *Class* owner in FDD. This refers to individuals being responsible for class ownership. These individuals are assigned ownership of a class and are responsible for ensuring its performance and consistency. The definition of a feature is very specific in FDD and refers to some function of value to the customer. This takes the form of:

< action > < result > < object >.

An example could be *Calculate average Emergency Department waiting time of a user.*

As with other approaches, FDD is an iterative process that aims to deliver working software frequently.

Example: Using FDD to develop a virtual reality intervention for veterans with mild traumatic brain injury

Levy et al. [18] used an FDD approach in their development of an intervention for veterans with mild traumatic brain injury. The intervention consisted of a virtual reality grocery store which, when used under the guidance of a therapist, can be used to assess and treat cognitive and emotional impairments associated with mild traumatic brain injury or post-traumatic stress disorder. Within the virtual reality store, users can pick up and buy items (using a virtual wallet) and even hold conversations with virtual sales assistants.

The authors proceeded in 4 steps:

1. **Step 1:** A model of the software to be developed was created collaboratively between clinical and technical teams in a series of meetings. The model included the context and look and feel of the software, as well as a list of potential features.
2. **Step 2:** The list of features to be developed was selected from the list of potential features through discussions between the clinical and technical teams. Features were prioritised based on their potential utility (input from the clinical team) and the feasibility of developing them given available time and resources (input from the technical team).
3. **Step 3:** Each individual feature was then specified by **(i)** planning the milestones and timelines for their development, **(ii)** assigning each feature to a specific developer who was in charge of designing and planning the implementation of the feature and **(iii)** building, implementing and testing the feature in the software (undertaken by the assigned developer).
4. **Step 4:** The features were then reviewed in joint meetings between the clinical and technical teams, and the clinical team assessed whether the features met their requirements and expectations and, if applicable, how the features should be adapted.

Steps 3 (i)–(iii) were cycled through iteratively until the clinical team was satisfied with the set of features. Steps 1–4 were repeated until all feature sets had been developed and implemented to satisfaction.

2.3.6 Lean Software Development

Lean focuses on "just in time production". This is achieved by reducing development costs whilst simultaneously increasing the speed of development. Lean originates from Lean manufacturing principles used by the Toyota production system. The 7 primary principles of Lean include:

1. **Eliminating waste**: If something does not add any value to the end product for the customer it is removed. This can include things like additional features that were not asked for and partially completed work
2. **Decide as late as possible**: This refers to keeping options open and not to engage in extensive planning and not to commit without knowledge and understanding of requirements and their value
3. **Deliver as fast as possible**: Lean also focuses on delivery of a Minimum Viable Product (MVP) without over engineering solutions to get a minimal but working version of the software to the customer as soon as possible
4. **Amplifying learning**: Promote retention of learning through things like documentation and code reviews, commenting code and knowledge sharing sessions
5. **Team empowerment and respect**: Including the team in the decision making process. Motivating the team and trusting them to do the job
6. **Building in integrity/quality**: To ensure this is built in practices like Test-driven development and pair programming along with incremental development based on regular feedback are intrinsic to the Lean project
7. **Optimization of the whole**: Larger systems may interact with other teams and components. Optimization of these factors can improve the overall efficiency and improve interactivity between components

> **Example: an agile and lean process model for mobile app development**
> Vallon et al. [28] conducted case studies with several mobile-app-centric companies (one of which specialised in developing apps for people with diabetes) to develop an agile and lean process ("ALP-mobile") model for mobile app development. Industry experts from the companies were asked to review the model and assess strengths and limitations.
>
> Their agile and lean process, ALP-mobile, combined elements of Scrum, Kanban and eXtreme Programming. It involved the following elements:
>
> 1. **Preliminary meeting:** First, a meeting is held with the customer to discuss the specific mobile software project.
> 2. **Kick-off meeting:** In this meeting, the development approach is discussed and specified.
> 3. **Requirements engineering:** Next, the product owner formulates user stories based on the requirements of the customer (as discussed in the previous meetings). Note that, because this is an agile and lean approach, not all user stories have to be specified at the beginning of the project; additional user stories may be added as the project progresses.
> 4. **Planning meetings:** The product owner also schedules planning meetings for estimation of the user stories (see Sect. 2.5.3 for details on estimation).

(continued)

These meetings are iterative, as new user stories may be added throughout the project.

5. **Early prototyping:** ALP-mobile encourages early prototyping to facilitate obtaining early feedback from customers
6. **Close communication with the customer:** This is encouraged in ALP-mobile and facilitates the lean approach.
7. **Ongoing weekly retrospective meetings:** These are helpful in order to review progress
8. **Daily standup meetings:** These meetings help coordinate efforts within the team (max. 15 min).
9. **Lean-style kanban board:** This allows transparency and provides an overview of progress.

For the lean-style Kanban board, the authors recommend including the following columns:

- **Backlog:** i.e. the user stories
- **Selected:** a list of user stories selected by the product owner based on their priority and feasibility
- **Work in Progress:** a limited number of work items are pulled in this column; new ones are pulled in once resources free up, facilitating a continuous flow as stipulated by the lean approach
- **Pending:** all work items that have been implemented and tested; the items in this column represent the current version of the software
- **Done:** work items are pulled into this column once the software has been distributed

The authors conclude that, overall, industry experts' appraisal of their ALP-mobile model was very positive, particularly regarding the enhanced flexibility of the process. Their evaluation also highlighted that any model will always need to be adapted to the individual company's requirements and constraints. This individualised tailoring can be undertaken as part of retrospective meetings and can be expedited through an "agile coach" [28].

2.3.7   Crystal

The Crystal family of methodologies are a set of methodologies for object-orientated development that were developed by Alistair Cockburn [7] in 1991 for IBM. The method applied is dependent on the size of your team, the priority of the project and its criticality (the level of danger posed by the system if not performing as intended).

The 7 properties of Crystal [7]

1. Frequent delivery
2. Reflective improvement
3. Osmotic communication (co-location of team to share information)
4. Personal safety (no ridicule or reprimand for sharing ideas)
5. Focus (clear priorities)
6. Easy access to expert users (get frequent user feedback)
7. Technical environment (needs to be supported by appropriate technical environment, including continuous integration)

The Crystal family is colour coded depending on the team size. There are five colours which represent five different Crystal methodologies:

- Clear: up to 6 people
- Yellow: up to 20 people
- Orange: up to 40 people
- Red/Maroon: up to 80 people
- Maroon/Diamond/Sapphire: up to 200 people

The method applied is designed to scale with the size of the project. For example, a small project involving less than six people would use the Crystal Clear methodology, whereas a larger project with up to forty people would be better suited for the Crystal Orange methodology. According to the Crystal method, a small project which increases in size should begin utilising a new methodology (e.g. switch from Crystal Yellow to Crystal Orange) rather than trying to expand the existing methodology. When deciding on the appropriate methodology, however, not only the group size but also its criticality needs to be taken into account. For example, any project which could potentially involve risk to human life would be classed as *Sapphire*. The priority of the project would also need to be considered when selecting a methodology.

Another key characteristic of this approach is that it is *lightweight*, meaning that it does not involve large amounts of documentation, management and reporting.

As Fig. 2.5 shows, the factors affecting the choice of which method to follow depends on team size as well as Comfort (e.g. how many hours team members are comfortable to work), Discretionary Money (how much money is available for the project), Essential Money (how much money is required to complete the project), and Life of the project (e.g. how long the project needs to run).

For example, for any given project, the developers might initially consider how much money is available, how much is needed, how many staff members are available, how many hours they are able to work, and how long the project would take. If these factors do not add up satisfactorily, the developers may e.g. increase the team size, and then select the appropriate Crystal methodology. Alternatively, if

	Clear	Yellow	Orange	Red	Maroon
Life (L)	L6	L20	L40	L80	L200
Essential Money (E)	E6	E20	E40	E80	E200
Discretionary Money (D)	D6	D20	D40	D80	D200
Comfort (C)	C6	C20	C40	C80	C200
	1-6	7-20	21-40	41-80	81-200

Project criticality

People involved in project

Fig. 2.5 Overview of the dimensions of Crystal. Criticality is shown in rows for the teams sizes. Each column represents a different Crystal methodology. (Modified from: Alistair Cockburn. Crystal Clear: A Human-Powered Methodology for Small Teams. Addison-Wesley Professional, Boston, MA, USA, 2004 [7]. Used with permission)

the team size is fixed, the developers may consider adjusting other elements, such as how much time the project will need to be completed.

2.4 Agile Practices

Several of the Agile methods previously mentioned use the same or similar common practices. These include:

2.4.1 Minimum Viable Product (MVP)

This refers to developing and releasing just as much of the product as is needed to provide some real value to the customer. There is also sufficient product to trigger a feedback loop of continual improvement until the product is fully featured. The MVP is more than just the smallest amount of deliverable functionality, it is also an opportunity to see how real users/customers interact with the product to see how effective it is and that it meets the intended needs/value.

2.4.2   Testing in Agile

When applying Agile, people often say "test early and fail fast". This refers to adding testing to every phase of planning and development so that issues and bugs can be identified and fixed early on so they do not end up being discovered later at greater cost.

2.4.3   Test Driven Development (TDD)

Test driven development places writing tests at the heart of program design with tests being written before the code that requires the test is created. By writing code to pass the test, testing is driving the development process. This also ensures a comprehensive test suite is created by default. Test driven development is covered in more detail with examples in Chap. 4. This can also be carried out using *pair programming*, where one developer will write a test and the other will write code to pass the test.

2.4.4   Pair Programming

This practice involves a pair of programmers working together on a single machine to develop code. This usually involves one typing whilst the other observes. There are different combinations, such as 2 senior coders, a junior and a senior and 2 juniors. This can be combined with other practices such as test driven development where one can write a test and the other writes the code required in order to get the test to pass. The evidence on the effectiveness of this practice is not definitive. Many earlier studies, such as [21] suggest that there was a statistically significant difference between a control group and a experimental group applying pair programming. This was evaluated both in terms of scores generated for readability and functionality of the coded solutions. Findings suggest that collaborative programming was a more enjoyable experience which increased the confidence of those involved. It was also faster than individual coding (41% faster for groups) [21]. Further work in this area, in the form of a meta-analysis showed that there was a lot of variation between the different studies that were included with signs of publication bias [14]. It appears that it can be time effective when the complexity of the task is lower, but it yields results of lower quality. When the complexity is high, the solutions are of a higher quality when pair programming is applied [14]. This improvement in quality is however offset by increased effort [14]. For success in pair programming, active task engagement is required from both parties, and there should be no relationship issues between the pair [1]. From a personal perspective, this can work very well if applied appropriately (not every task requires two people). This approach can work well for problem solving and designing algorithms. It does require buy-in from both members of the pair who should be open to constructive criticism and learning from one another. As such it may not be suitable for all personality types.

2.4.5   Continuous Integration (CI)

CI is used to automate the process of testing and building the code of development teams using a version control system (see Sect. 2.6.4.1 for more details). This focuses on automatically integrating changes made to a codebase by multiple developers. The code is first tested before it is integrated. This uses version control with additional checks and tests. This manages developers merging their code with the master code in the project repository. This can be done at various intervals (usually several times a day). This works when the developer commits their changes to the repository. This in turn is detected by the CI server, which then runs unit tests and integration tests on the committed code. When the code is built successfully the team is automatically informed, if not the team is alerted to the errors detected by running the failed tests so they can fix the code as soon as possible.

2.4.6   Code Review

This process involves review of software code by someone other than the one who wrote it. It is useful for maintaining the quality of the code shipped. A reviewer typically looks for aspects of the code that include those highlighted below by Google.

- **Design**: appropriateness for system and structure
- **Functionality**: works as intended?
- **Complexity**: how easy is it to understand (could it be simplified)?
- **Tests**: are automated tests present, correct and designed well?
- **Naming**: are variable names, functions/methods and classes etc. well named? Are they clear and representative?
- **Comments**: Is the code well commented with clear and useful comments?
- **Style**: does the code follow an established institutional convention or style guide?
- **Documentation**: has the relevant documentation been updated to reflect changes where appropriate?

Adapted from [13].

Code reviews can be used in any development methodology and can add value to the quality of the overall product. A code review can also be a good opportunity for the professional development of junior developers by providing a mentorship opportunity.

2.5 Requirements Gathering and Representation

All of the methodologies described above include some process for 'gathering' the system requirements from users/customers. There are different ways in which these requirements can be elicited and who they are obtained from. In some cases this could be the commissioner of the project and in others the end-users themselves. Requirements gathering is particularly important in the context of *user-centred design*, because it allows you to understand, specify and take into consideration the requirements of the users throughout the product cycle. This will enhance the success of the product and it will ensure the product adds value to the customers and end-users. User-centred design is discussed in further detail in Chap. 7, Sect. 7.3, and means of engaging users and understanding their needs and preferences are also described in Chap. 3, Sect. 3.8.

2.5.1 User Stories

One method for eliciting specification requirements is by example. One way to do this is through the use of *user stories*. A user story is a structured statement that shows how a certain type of user might interact with the system to carry out a specific goal or task. For example:

> As a **\<type of user\>** I want to **\<some feature/goal\>** so that \<value\>.

If we were making software for a school or university, for example, one of the users might be a teacher or lecturer. They might want to use the system to view their students' grades:

> As a **course teacher** I want to **see my students' grades** so that **I can see who is top of the class**.

There may also be different users of the system that interact with it to perform very different tasks based on their perspectives e.g.:

> As a **student** I want to **see my grade** so that **I know how well I am doing in this subject**.

> As a **course administrator** I want to **see student attendance per subject** so that **we can plan room allocation for timetabling**.

The work involved in generating the required features can be expressed in 'story points', with more complex stories being split into smaller stories. Large stories are called *epics*. An example could be:

> As a **Clinical Commissioning Group manager** I want **an interactive digital medication prescribing dashboard** so that **I can plan resource allocation for different primary care surgeries in the region**.

This is an example of an epic user story that represents a significant amount of work that is represented at a fairly high level. This dashboard project could be broken down into multiple user stories spread over a number of iterations. Each of the user stories may also be broken down into a subset of specific tasks required to complete the story. User stories are much less formal than an official contract and are a friendlier way of communicating requirements. They do not represent a formal contract or specification. They are in essence also a reminder to converse with the end user or stakeholder. User stories are useful because they implicitly include the nature/type of user the feature is aimed at, the overall purpose of the task the user is trying to accomplish (what the feature will be) and what value this particular feature has. This last point is very useful for prioritising and for making the user or customer really think about the value of the feature instead of just asking for things they might quite like but that don't add any real value.

2.5.2   Personas

Another way of generating user stories is to first create personas for the type of users that you intend to use your system. This is a similar idea to creating a vignette (Fig. 2.6).

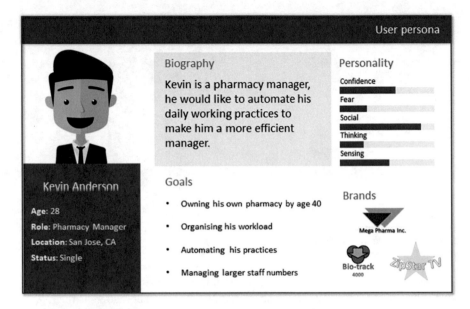

Fig. 2.6 Example user persona

User personas can be used to create archetypal users of the system. A number of user stories for each of these personas can then be generated to represent a 'typical' user's interaction with the system. Personas often contain some background information about the character, such as demographics, a quote that sums up the character and some personality traits. This may also include likes, dislikes and favourite brands.

2.5.3   Estimating

In order to know how much output is possible in each sprint to plan future releases and for the purposes of continuous improvement, it is necessary to measure a team's *velocity* (rate of change over time) to get a consistent measure output per sprint. Rather than use time for this, which people are poor at estimating, we instead use *story points*. One of the issues with using time is that it takes different people different amounts of time do things as they may have different levels of experience. In fact even the same developer may complete the same task or similar task faster in the future due to learning from the previous task.

In the early 1980s it was found that traditional estimation resulted in something called "the cone of uncertainly" [6]. This describes the phenomenon where the degree of uncertainty in estimation reduces over time as there are less unknowns emerging as the project progresses.

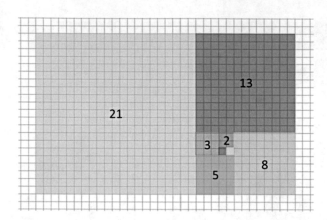

Fig. 2.7 First 8 numbers of the Fibonacci sequence displayed as squares to illustrate relative difference between the numbers

A standard estimation method is to use numbers from the Fibonacci sequence. This is because the actual numbers don't matter as such, what matters is the *relative difference* between the numbers. For example, we want to ensure the user story requiring the least effort is estimated at a relatively smaller size compared to the user story requiring the most effort. Numbers from the Fibonacci sequence are therefore used because they have a relative difference:

$$F_n = F_{n-1} + F_{n-2}(F_0 = 0, F_1 = 1)$$

$$0, 1, 1, 2, 3, 5, 8, 13, 21, 34, 55, \ldots F_n$$

This relative difference is probably best illustrated visually as seen in Fig. 2.7.

This is used in what is called *planning poker*. This estimation game is often used in Scrum and Extreme Programming to estimate the size of stories in points. A user story is chosen and presented by the Product Owner and discussed with the team. Each team member estimates the size of the task using a number on the Fibonacci scale, and writes this number down on a card. The purpose of using cards is to prevent developers from influencing each others' estimates. Each team member then turns over their estimation card simultaneously. Outliers (those with very high/low estimates) explain the reason behind their choice. The process is repeated iteratively until consensus is reached.

2.5.3.1 Story Points

Story points can be used as an abstracted measure for a team's output. As such, they serve as a measurement unit that can be used for estimating the size of a user story. The value of the points is often derived by using a reference user story, usually the story identified as taking the least effort. Subsequent points are assigned to stories based on this reference story.

Factors commonly used to estimate the size of user stories [19]:

- Complexity
- Business value
- Risks
- Amount of work
- Dependencies

It can be helpful to conceptualise the assignment of story points using clothes sizing as an analogy [19]. You can do this by assigning numbers of the Fibonacci sequence to the different categories of clothes sizing, e.g.

- XXS → 1
- XS → 2
- S → 3
- M → 5
- L → 8
- XL → 13
- XXL → 21

You can now conceptualise your user stories according to their size, and then assign the corresponding Fibonacci sequence number as the number of story points. For example, a medium-sized user story (i.e. a story requiring medium effort to complete) would be assigned 5 user story points, whereas the largest, most complex user story should be assigned 21 points. Other values can also be assigned in place of the Fibonacci sequence depending on the type of projects and relative size of jobs.

A team's *velocity* is the amount of work a team can produce in a sprint over time. For example, if a team can complete 25 points per sprint, and there are user stories totalling 100 story points in the backlog, we can estimate that the team will require 4 sprints to complete the project. Note that velocity should be applied to a team, not on an individual basis.

Consider the 3 stories shown in Table 2.1. We only count completed stories for the purposes of measuring velocity for a given sprint.

Table 2.1 Story points assigned to stories with completion status for a sprint

Story	Story points	Status
1	5	Done
2	2	Done
3	3	Incomplete

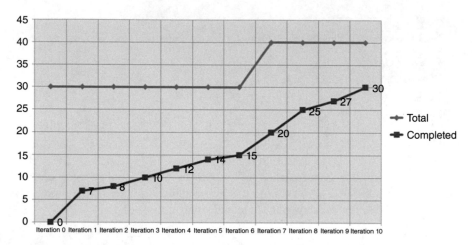

Fig. 2.8 Example burn-up chart. The blue line represents the total points in the project. The red line shows the current work done

2.5.4 Burn-Up Charts

This type of chart can be used to show and track work completed on a project (or smaller unit such as an iteration). The unit of work is displayed on the vertical axis. This could be story points, hours worked etc. On the horizontal axis the time is displayed. This could be dates, days or sprints. Figure 2.8 shows an example of a burn-up chart. The red line shows the number of completed story points at each iteration. The blue line shows the total number of story points for this project (30). We can see how the red line should come up to meet the blue line at the end of the project. This gives an immediate visual representation of the current progress in relation to the end point. We can see that in iteration 7 the blue line suddenly goes up from 30 to 40. This represents extra work being added to the project increasing the amount of effort.

2.5.5 Burn-Down Charts

In contrast to a burn-up chart where we see progress steadily climbing toward completion, a burn-down chart works in the opposite direction. A burn-down chart shows the ideal completion of tasks over a time period mapped against the actual progress towards meeting this ideal. Figure 2.9 shows an example of this. The vertical axis represents the total effort in terms of time, story points, tasks etc. The horizontal axis represents time in terms of days, sprints or dates. The blue line represents the target or ideal task completion over time. The red line shows the actual completion. This is useful to see if the actual progress is matching the

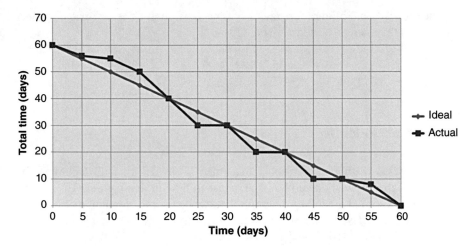

Fig. 2.9 Example burn-down chart showing ideal and actual task completion

expected progress. If the red line falls below the blue line, it indicates that progress is faster than expected. If the red line is above the blue line then the progress is slower than expected and we can see how far off we are from where we should be. Extra lines can also be added, such as forecast time, which might be different to ideal or target time.

Both burn-up and burn-down charts can be used together in a single project. Burn-down charts are perhaps more appropriate for providing an overview of a single sprint, whereas burn-up charts can show the entire project over each sprint. Both types of chart are very useful for communicating the status of the project or current iteration rapidly and again can be used to communicate with a variety of stakeholders.

2.5.6   PERT

The Program Evaluation and Review Technique (PERT) can be used to help to provide project estimates. It works by generating a weighted average of 3 values comprised of:

1. *pessimistic* case (P), where all aspects are the worst case; essentially where everything goes wrong.
2. *optimistic* case (O), where everything goes according to plan.
3. *most likely* outcome (M), where there are no extremely good or bad factors influencing work and it runs as expected.

The values can be hours or days or some other unit. The estimated project completion time is represented with the formula:

$$\frac{O + 4M + P}{6}$$

2.6   Data Modelling

Another useful method of project management is to design and document the structure of the application and how the data will flow in that system. This can be achieved with formal modelling diagrams that can be used to communicate between stakeholders and developers. Some of the most commonly used diagrams include Data Flow Diagrams (DFD) and Unified Modeling Language (UML).

2.6.1   Data Flow Diagrams (DFDs)

Data flow diagrams can be divided into *logical* and *physical* DFDs. They are used to visually present processes that handle data and are used as a communication tool, for example between developers and stakeholders. There are 4 basic notation symbols used to represent:

- **Process**: changes the data in some way producing an output
- **Data store**: stores data (i.e. a database table, repository, filing cabinet)
- **Data flow**: the route data travels in the system can be in one or both directions
- **External entities**: something external to the system (i.e. another system, a person, organisation)

DFDs are represented at different levels of granularity. This begins with level 0, which provides a simple high level view of the entire system. The convention is to label the levels upward starting from 0, also known as a *context diagram*. Further levels decompose the system into sub levels showing progressively more detail. In reality most DFDs do not go beyond level 2. Level 1 breaks down the main process into sub-processes, level 2 breaks these down further. An example can be seen in Fig. 2.10 which shows a simple digital symptom entry system on a symptom logging app. The main box in the center represents the main *process*. The name of the process is added to the box. In this case "Symptom Entry System". The box to the left, labelled "User" is an *entity* that interacts with the process. The black arrows represent *data flows* showing the direction of travel, in this case from the user entity to the process and from the process to the data store. Data flow arrows can be uni or bidirectional to show data travelling in a single direction or both directions. The data flow arrows are also labelled to display details of the type of data flowing. Finally the box on the right represents a *data store*. In this case it is labelled as a "Database".

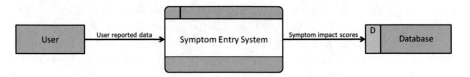

Fig. 2.10 A level 0 (context) data flow diagram for a simple digital symptom entry system

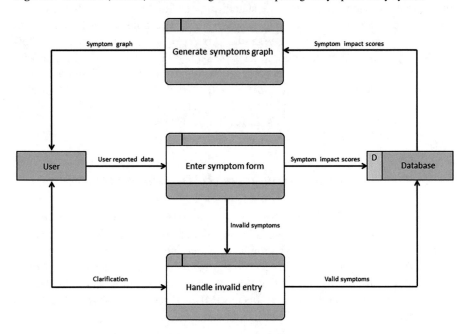

Fig. 2.11 A level 1 data flow diagram for a simple digital symptom entry system

This could also have been a non digital data store, such as a filling cabinet or other storage medium. This provides an overview of a system that takes some data from a user in the form of some user reported data. This in turn is processed by the symptom entry system and the generated symptom impact scores are stored in a database.

The second example from the same system shows the level 1 diagram of the same system (Fig. 2.11). In this case we can see the sub-processes, such as handling an invalid entry and generating a symptom graph that is displayed to the user. A level 2 diagram could break these processes down further, for example showing sub-processes involved in generating the user data graph. A more complex system would have multiple entities and data stores.

Such diagrams are useful for communicating with developers, who can see the main processes in a given system and the flow of data. They can also communicate proposed system designs with stakeholders. There are a couple of different DFD notations in existence. The one used here is called *Gane and Sarson* named after the creators. The second is called *Yourdon and Coad* and features circles used to represent processes and no segmented areas in the data store notation.

There are some basic rules for using DFDs. These include the rule that entities and data stores cannot have data flows between each other and other entities or data stores without a process being between them. Incorrect use can lead to outcomes such as *black holes*, where there is input with no output, or *grey holes*, where the input is not sufficient to generate the stated output. Finally there are also *miracles*, where there is output with no input to generate it. The other point to note about DFDs is that they only show the essential processes of a system and unlike flow charts, they do not detail any conditional expressions (i.e. if then, else). Dealing with choice takes place inside the process itself and is not detailed on the diagram. Further diagrams and details would need to be used to document any logical selection processes and specific detail of processes. They are however very useful for visual communication of the main processes of an entire system.

2.6.2   Unified Modeling Language (UML) Diagrams

UML provides a set of diagrams that can be used to model systems and interactions with those systems. This is especially useful before commencing development because, as mentioned previously, the cost of making changes increases dramatically as the project progresses. UML was created by the Object Management Group (OMG) [23] and provides a standard way of modelling systems that is not tied to any specific methodology. There are (as of UML 2.0) 13 different types of diagram available:

Types of UML diagram, adapted from [24]
Structure diagrams:

- Class
- Component
- Composite
- Structure
- Package
- Deployment

Behaviour diagrams:

- Use case
- Activity
- State machine

(continued)

Interaction diagrams (a sub-set of behaviour diagrams):

- Sequence
- Communication
- Timing
- Interaction overview

Examining each diagram in turn is beyond the scope of this book. We will instead look more closely at two of the more widely used diagrams from the structured and behavioural categories.

2.6.2.1 Use Case Diagrams (UCDs)

The UCD is a form of behavioural diagram and is often used for requirements gathering and communicating these requirements to developers and stakeholders. Figure 2.12 depicts an example of a system where a user can interact with a system by logging their medication use, viewing their test results and viewing messages. A lab can also send messages to the user and add details of their test results to the system. This could be an app that allows a patient with certain condition to interact with a laboratory.

Figure 2.13 details the various components of a UCD. This type of diagram displays the functional requirements of an intended system. We can use them to see how different entities with defined roles interact with the system through various use cases unique to that actor/role. Here a system is represented by a rectangle with the border defining the system boundary. Actors (users of the system) are represented with stick men and use cases with text bubbles (oval) describing the use case. Lines

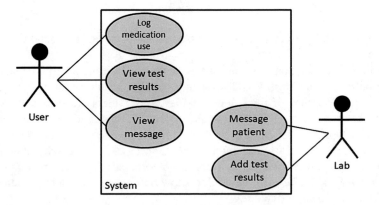

Fig. 2.12 Example UCD showing 2 'actors' interacting with a system

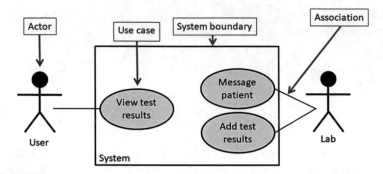

Fig. 2.13 Labelled UCD highlighting the diagrammatic components

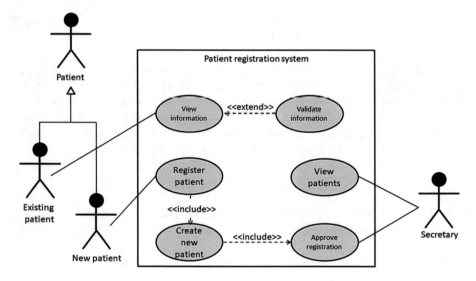

Fig. 2.14 Use case diagram for a simple patient registration system

between actors and use cases represent associations between actors and the system use cases.

Additional association notation can be used to indicate inherited behaviour, to add optional functionality and to include additional functionality. Figure 2.14 shows some examples of this. Here we see 2 sub-patients (a new and existing patient) that are inherited from the main patient. This is used for generalisation. This can be applied to use cases as well as actors themselves. For example we could have a general 'search' use case with some child cases like 'search patients' and 'search staff' that derive behaviour from the general case. Dashed arrows with the words *extend* and *include* can be used to show optional functionality (extend) and additional functionality (include).

There are some guidelines for drawing UCDs. Names used in use cases should be verbs as they model some form of action. The main actors are usually placed on the left of the diagram. Actors are used to represent a system external to the main system being represented. Actors do not interact directly with each other. Actors should be used to model the roles they have when interacting with the system rather than their more general business role.

2.6.2.2 Class Diagrams

Class diagrams model classes that exist in the Object Orientated Programming (OOP) paradigm. They are used to show the different classes in a system and how they relate to one another. Unlike UCDs they are structural diagrams that model the system itself rather than the interaction with the system.

A class is like a blue print that determines how an object created with that class will behave and what types of data they contain. Classes are used for creating *instances* of objects in programming languages that support object oriented methods. Languages like C++/Java and Python, to name a few, support OOP.

These class diagrams can then be directly implemented in a programming language that supports OOP. Many of the other diagrams available in UML are built on the initial class diagram. Figure 2.15 shows an example of a class diagram representing a single class. The name of the class is placed in the top of the diagram using Pascal case (capitalized words joined together). The next section details the variables (called attributes) and their associated data types. For example the variable called 'breathing' is an integer (whole number) data type. This could store a score for a user's rating of their symptoms for breathing, coughing and pain. The date recorded is a date type, and there is a free text comment option stored as a string (text type). The final section details the associated functions of the class called methods. Here we can see functionality for logging the symptoms, adding the text comment and closing the symptom logging class.

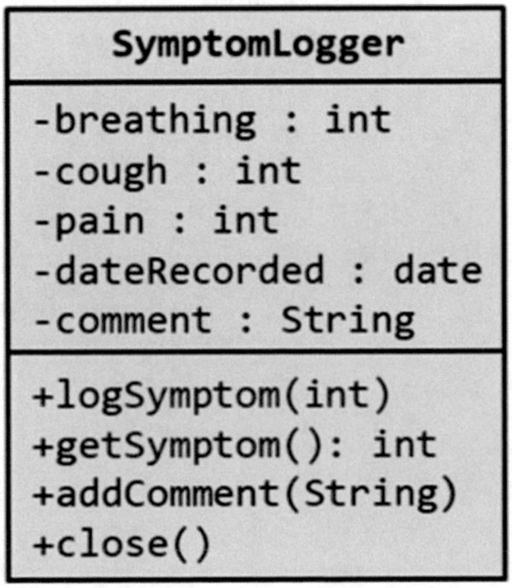

Fig. 2.15 Basic class diagram representing a single class for logging symptoms

Different programming languages support different case types:

- snake_case
- camelCase
- PascalCase
- kebab-case

The minus sign (−) indicates that an attribute or method is *private*, the plus symbol (+) indicates an item is *public*. A hash sign (#) is used to denote protected visibility. We can also see any data types passed into and out of the methods, such as *getSymptoms()* which returns an integer, or *addComment()* that expects a String type parameter for function input. Listing 2.1 shows how one might go about translating the class diagram into a working class in a language that supports OOP, in this case Java. The diagram shows the expected input and output for the class methods as well as the data it contains (attributes) and if these are publicly or privately available. The diagram does not however detail how one would specifically implement the methods in terms of their inner workings and logic.

```java
import java.time.LocalDateTime;

// sysmptom logging class
public class SymptomLogger{
    private int breathing;
    private int cough;
    private int pain;
    private LocalDateTime dateRecorded = LocalDateTime.now();
    private String comment;

    // log symptom method
    public void logSymptom(int SymptomScore, int symptomType){
        if(!(SymptomScore >= 0 && SymptomScore <= 3)){
            System.out.println("Score must be between 0 and 3");
            return;
        }
        if(!(symptomType >= 1 && symptomType <= 3)){
            System.out.println("Sypmtom type must be between 1 and 3");
            return;
        }
        switch(symptomType){
            case 1: this.breathing = SymptomScore; break;
            case 2: this.cough = SymptomScore; break;
            case 3: this.pain = SymptomScore; break;
            default: break;
        }
    }

    // additional methods ...
}
```

Listing 2.1 Example of starting to implementing the class diagram in Java

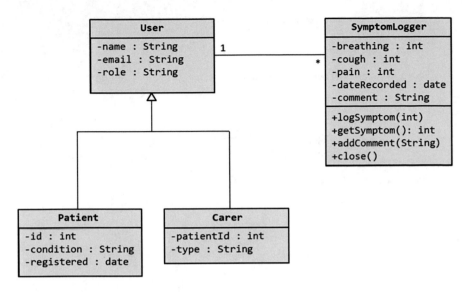

Fig. 2.16 Several classes interacting

Classes can be connected to one another with relationships (associations). Associations are often bi-directional unless otherwise indicated (i.e. uni-directional where an arrow head is used to show direction). Multiplicity can be indicated by adding details to the association line. Figure 2.16 shows a 1 to many relationship. Numbers are used and separated with 2 periods. For example, a zero to one would be 0..1 and a one or more would be 1..* and so on. Figure 2.16 also shows how generalization is indicated with two sub-classes (Patient and Carer) that are derived from the main class (User).

2.6.3 Data Journey Modelling

Researchers at the University of Manchester in the UK have developed another lightweight approach to data modelling that combines both the technical and social factors related to a system [10]. This approach also captures the costs involved in transferring or sharing data between different organisations. The model is constructed in 7 steps (Figs. 2.17, 2.18 and 2.19):

1. Generate containers for the data (rectangles used to show paper based or other physical storage medium like a desk or pigeon hole. Databases represented with the standard cylindrical notation).
2. Connect these containers with numbered lines to indicate the legs of the journey the data will take. Arrow heads are used to denote direction of travel.
3. Add the data entities being moved along each journey leg, for example "blood sample" or *test results*.

Step 1: Identify data entities of interest

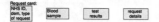

Step 2: Create the data containers where data is stored.

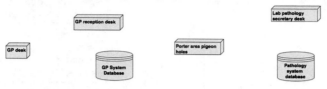

Step 3: Connect containers to form journey legs and number them.

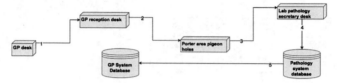

Step 4: Add the data entities being moved by each journey leg.

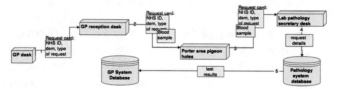

Step 5: Identify the actors interacting with the containers.

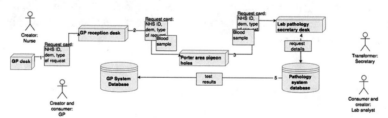

Step 6: Connect each actor with the container it interacts to use the data.

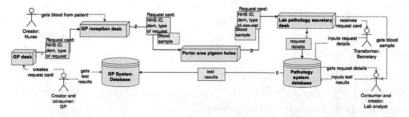

Fig. 2.17 Data journey modelling stages. (Reproduced with permission from [9], and adapted by permission from Springer Nature Customer Service Centre GmbH: Springer Nature. *Data Journey Modelling: Predicting Risk for IT Developments* by Iliada Eleftheriou, Suzanne M. Embury, Andrew Brass. © IFIP International Federation for Information Processing, 2016)

Phase A: Model existing landscape

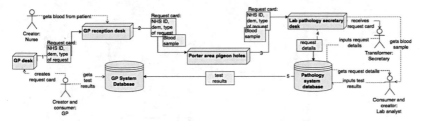

Phase B: Add to the model the new journey

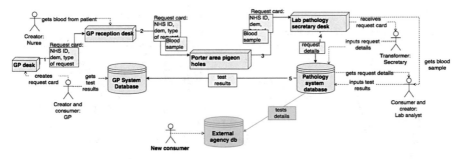

Phase C: Overlay on the model the boundaries

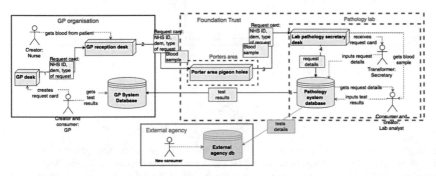

Fig. 2.18 Data journey modelling stages. (Reproduced with permission from [9], and adapted by permission from Springer Nature Customer Service Centre GmbH: Springer Nature. *Data Journey Modelling: Predicting Risk for IT Developments* by Iliada Eleftheriou, Suzanne M. Embury, Andrew Brass. © IFIP International Federation for Information Processing, 2016)

4. Add *actors* to identify how interaction occurs with the data containers. This uses the same notation as Use Case Diagrams (role labelled stick men).
5. Connect actors to containers they interact with. A labelled dashed line is used to indicate the actions they undertake with the data container, for example "gets

Phase D: Identify journey legs crossing the boundaries.

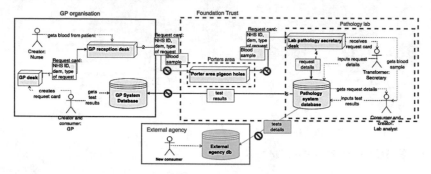

Phase E: Report findings using heatmap

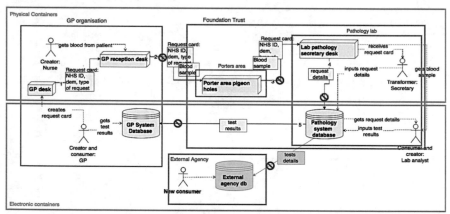

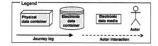

Fig. 2.19 Data journey modelling stages. (Reproduced with permission from [9], and adapted by permission from Springer Nature Customer Service Centre GmbH: Springer Nature. *Data Journey Modelling: Predicting Risk for IT Developments* by Iliada Eleftheriou, Suzanne M. Embury, Andrew Brass. © IFIP International Federation for Information Processing, 2016)

blood from patient" which is then placed on the "GP reception desk". Again the arrow head denotes the direction of activity.

6. Form boundaries. This is done by drawing boxes to represent the boundaries and labelling the clusters (i.e. their organisation or department).
7. Identify any legs of the data journey that cross those boundaries.

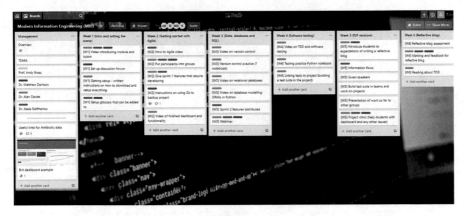

Fig. 2.20 Example Trello board for managing an MSc course on Modern Information Engineering. https://trello.com/. (Screenshot reproduced with permission. This publication is not affiliated or associated in any way with, or endorsed by, Trello, Inc)

2.6.4 Project Management Tools

Tools like *Trello* can be used to organise and manage tasks, as seen in Fig. 2.20 which shows a screenshot from a 'Trello' board depicting the tasks associated with a masters level university course module teaching software engineering and databases. Here the cards representing work units can be moved by dragging in between the columns to update the projects task status.

Some additional tools for managing projects and teams can be seen in Table 2.2. A combination of such tools are often useful depending on the methodology applied. Some projects may favor artifacts like Gantt charts for project planning whereas others will favor Kanban style project boards. Instant messaging platforms like *Slack* or *Teams* can also be useful for sharing files and communicating with team members rapidly. Version control is another essential tool for software projects with more than one developer, or where a solo developer wants to backup or share their code (possibly with a customer or for reproducability).

2.6.4.1 Version Control

Version control is a software tool that helps to manage the storage of code (and other files) and monitor any changes made to the code when working on modern software projects that share a code base between multiple developers.

One of the most popular version control tools is *GitHub* or *Git* for short. We will give examples of version control using GitHub for context. GitHub is a distributed version control system. Projects are typically organized in *repositories* and contain all the code and other resources of a project (data files, images, etc.). Once you have

Table 2.2 Some additional tools for managing projects and teams

Tool name	Description	Link
Slack	Cloud based instant messaging with channels. Connects to other apps and allows file sharing	https://slack.com/intl/en-gb/
Trello	For web-based Kanban-style project boards	https://trello.com/
GitHub	Version control tools and hosting	https://github.com/
Asana	Management platform, includes lists, task board, progress tracking and calendar	https://asana.com/
TeamGantt	Online Gantt chart software	https://www.teamgantt.com/
GanttProject	Gantt chart software	https://www.ganttproject.biz/
SmartSheet	For collaborative work management. Assigns and monitors task progress, manages calendars and allows sharing of documents	https://www.smartsheet.com/
OpenProject	For project planning and scheduling and support for Kanban and Scrum	https://www.openproject.org/

made a repository (repo for short), you can *commit* your files to it and thus backup your project.

```
1  git add *
2  git commit —m "my first commit"
3  git push
```

Git commands are prefixed with the word *git*. In this example we add all the files in our target directory with the asterisk (*). These can also be named individually. We then commit those changes. The optional *-m* allows us to add a message to the commit to state what its purpose was. This is typically something short and meaningful, such as 'implemented load feature' or 'fixed file sync bug'. Another advantage of version control is the ability to roll back changes to previous versions. This has the advantage of undoing any errors and restoring a project to a previous stable state. Repositories can be shared publicly or privately with selected collaborators and can be used as a means to distribute you code. For some research projects an academic paper may provide a link to a public repository to download data and analysis scripts as part of transparent and reproducible 'open science'. The concept of *branching* is used to point to a specific commit of a repository that can be copied to a local machine to work on. Repositories have a default branch in GitHub called the *master* branch. Each commit is a node on the branch. An example of this would be to create a development branch separate from the stable release branch where new features could be developed and tested. Once completed these branches can then be recombined.

```
1  git branch myBranch
2  git checkout myBranch
```

The first command makes a new branch called *myBranch*. We then tell git to switch to this branch using the *checkout* command. To switch back to master we could type *git checkout master*. We can also create a new branch and switch to it in one go with the shortcut *git checkout -b myBranch*. If a developer wanted to collaborate with another developer, then the second developer could create a branch of the project to develop a specific feature. When they have finished they can combine (merge) these branches together.

```
1  git merge myBranch
```

My merging the branches, the entire project work is combined so there are no commits unique to either branch. Another way of merging that gives a cleaner linear look to the commits is *rebase*. This makes the commits look like they were made sequentially.

```
1  git rebase master
2  git rebase myBranch
```

Another important concept in Git is *HEAD*. This is essentially a pointer to the most recent commit in a branch and represents the commit that is currently checked out. The HEAD can be detached and made to point at a specific commit rather than a branch. This is shown in the example below where instead of using *checkout* to switch between branches we use it to point to a specific commit. This is done by specifying the commit hashes (the long string of letters and numbers).

```
1  git checkout 1e0f187d250c430c0a3c31b8c7305769b70167a9
```

Fortunately you only need to specify a minimum of these letters and numbers up to the point where it can be uniquely identified rather than typing in the entire string (i.e. 1e0f187d). An alternative to this is to use relative referencing where you can traverse the tree of commits by moving up either one commit at time or in specified batches. The first line in the snippet below uses the caret operator ($\wedge$) to move up one commit at a time. The second line show how a number (in this case 3) can be used to specify how many commits to move up using the tilde operator (~).

```
1  git checkout myBranch^
2  git checkout myBranch~3
```

A common workflow for collaborative work using Git would involve creating a *feature branch* in order to develop a new feature. A developer would create a new branch each time they introduce a new feature. This way all updates and commits can take place on this branch as the developer works on implementing the feature. For example:

```
1  git checkout -b feature-x
2  git add *
3  git commit -m "My new feature"
4  git push -u origin feature-x
```

When several people are changing the same bit of code, conflicts can arise. To deal with this Git has a tool that allows you to compare the different versions of the same code side by side and choose which changes to accept or reject. To run this type:

```
1  git difftool
```

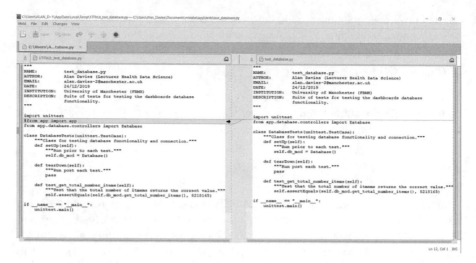

Fig. 2.21 Screenshot of the gitdiff tool for dealing with code conflicts in Git. https://git-scm.com/

This will launch the tool that allows you to visually compare the code changes. In the example seen in Fig. 2.21, you can see the green line shows a line of code that was subsequently removed. We can choose to accept or reject the change.

There may also be various files that you do not wish to include in the code base of the version control system. For example you would probably not want to commit your database or various other files that are not required. To do this you can create a file that must be called *.gitignore*. In this file you can add specific file names of files not to include that you do not want to send to your repository. You can also select entire types of files (e.g. all png images). In the example below we exclude all database and pyc files by using the asterisk followed by a period.

```
1  *.db
2  *.db-journal
3  *.pyc
```

Listing 2.2 Contents of .gitignore file

2.7 Summary of Key Points

We would recommend that for any project regardless of its size, there should be some level of project management applied. The level of project management you apply, and any methodology you may choose to use should be proportionate to the size of the project and the resources available for project management. Applying some of these methods will help to plan and deliver an intervention in an achievable and realistic way taking into account factors that can influence the successful and timely delivery of the intervention.

- The methods and techniques presented in this chapter could be used to manage most types of projects
- The agile methodology, which features an incremental, iterative approach and self-organising teamwork with flattened structures has become an increasingly popular method for designing modern software applications
- Requirements gathering can be undertaken using methods like user stories and personas; this is important because it facilitates a user-centred design, ensuring the product adds value to the customers and end-users
- Estimating the required effort for a project (rather than time, which people are bad at estimating) is useful for planning and resource allocation
- Data modelling can be used to design and document the structure of the application and how the data will flow in that system, and to facilitate communication between stakeholders and developers
- Version control tools can help manage the storage of code and files, and help monitor any changes made to the code when working on software projects involving multiple developers

2.8 Quiz

1. Which one of the following is **not** a common reason why projects fail?

    (a) Poor scoping or mission creep
    (b) Poorly defined tasks
    (c) Using an iterative design methodology
    (d) Failure to define end points or to know when something was done

2. A minimal viable product (MVP) is. . .

    (a) A smaller than usual end produce
    (b) A minimal end-to-end slice of functionality that adds some value
    (c) Over 50% of a developed feature

3. The Agile manifesto promotes self organising teams with a flatter structure where individuals are valued and trusted.

    (a) True
    (b) False

4. Which of the following are typical roles in a Scrum team?

    (a) Scrum master, Project Manager, Development team
    (b) Kanban master, Product Owner, Development team
    (c) Scrum master, Product Owner, Development team

5. A product backlog...

    (a) contains a list of all the project's current requirements
    (b) is a list of user stories or tasks currently being worked on for the current sprint
    (c) is a work limited item

6. Pair programming and code review are only used in Agile software design methods/frameworks.

    (a) True
    (b) False

7. A user story should contain the following components...

    (a) Background information about the user/client
    (b) Type of user, feature or goal and value/reason
    (c) Who wants it, when and how?

8. Data flow diagrams can be used to show the logical flow of a conditional expression (if/then/else).

    (a) True
    (b) False

9. Which of the following is **not** a correct Git statement:

    (a) git commit -m "Initial project commit"
    (b) git push
    (c) git pull then push with commit

Answers to the quiz can be found in "Solutions to Quizzes".

2.9 Exercises

1. Go to https://github.github.com/training-kit/downloads/github-git-cheat-sheet. pdf to get the Git cheat sheet. Follow the instructions to install Git. Then go to https://github.com/IAM-lab/britain-breathing-app and using the cheat sheet, check out a copy of Britain Breathing app code-base onto your local machine.
2. Create a class diagram to represent the following classes and their interaction:

```python
class Doctor:
    def __init__(self, name, role):
        self.name = name
        self.role = role
        self.patients_processed = 0

    def admit_patient(self, patient):
        print(self.name, "will admit patient", patient)
        self.process_patient()

    def diagnose_patient(self, patient):
        print(self.name, "will diagnose patient", patient)
        self.process_patient()

    def discharge_patient(self, patient):
        print(self.name, "will discharge patient", patient)
        self.process_patient()

    def process_patient(self):
        self.patients_processed += 1

    def number_of_times_patients_processed(self):
        return self.patients_processed

class Patient:
    def __init__(self, name, hospital_number,
    presenting_complaint):
        self.name = name
        self.hospital_number = hospital_number
        self.presenting_complaint = presenting_complaint
        self.PMH = []
        self.diagnosis = None

    def add_medical_history(self, medical_history_item):
        self.PMH.append(medical_history_item)

    def get_medical_history(self):
        return self.PMH

    def show_diagnosis(self):
        return self.diagnosis

    def update_diagnosis(self, diagnosis):
        self.diagnosis = diagnosis

    def whats_wrong(self):
        return self.presenting_complaint

class Surgeon(Doctor):
    def do_brain_surgery(self, patient):
        print(self.name, "will do a frontal lobotomy on
    patient", patient)
        self.process_patient()
```

3. Using the PERT calculation $\frac{O+4M+P}{6}$, think of a small project that you are involved in, and apply the PERT calculation. This could be a personal project (e.g. buying the weekly shopping) or a professional project. After you complete the small project, see how accurate your estimation was.
4. Create a "use case" diagram for a weight logging app. This lets a user record their weight and view trends regarding their weight over time. Consider what the different use cases may be for the users of such an app.

Recommended Reading

1. Williams L. What agile teams think of agile principles. Commun ACM. 2012;55(4):71–6.
2. Visual Paradigm. What is unified modeling language (UML)? https://www.visual-paradigm. com/guide/uml-unified-modeling-language/what-is-uml/. Accessed 13 Dec 2019.
3. Schwaber K, Sutherlan J. The scrum guide: the definitive guide to scrum: the rules of the game; 2017.

References

1. Agile Alliance. Pair programming: does it really work? 2020. https://www.agilealliance. org/glossary/pairing/#q=~(infinite~false~filters~(postType~(~'page~'post~'aa_book~'aa_ event_session~'aa_experience_report~'aa_glossary~'aa_research_paper~'aa_video)~tags~(~ 'pair*20programming))~searchTerm~'~sort~false~sortDirection~'asc~page~1)
2. Ambler S. Examining the Agile cost of change curve; 2018. http://www.agilemodeling.com/ essays/costOfChange.htm
3. Balijepally V, Mahapatra R, Nerur S, Price K. Are two heads better than one for software development? the productivity paradox of pair programming. MIS Q. 2009;33(1):91–118.
4. Beck K, Beedle M, van Bennekum A, Cunningham W, Fowler M, Grenning J, Highsmith J, Hunt A, Jeffries R, Marick B, Martin R, Mellor S, Schwaber K, Sutherlan J, Thomas D. Manifesto for agile software development; 2001. http://agilemanifesto.org/
5. Beck K, Beedle M, van Bennekum A, Cunningham W, Fowler M, Grenning J, Highsmith J, Hunt A, Jeffries R, Marick B, Martin R, Mellor S, Schwaber K, Sutherlan J, Thomas D. Principles behind the Agile Manifesto; 2001. http://agilemanifesto.org/principles.html
6. Boehm BW. Software engineering economics. Englewood Cliffs: Prentice-Hall Inc; 1981.
7. Cockburn A. Crystal clear: a human-powered methodology for small teams. Boston: Addison-Wesley Professional; 2004.
8. Dafydd D, Williamson R, Blunt P, Blunt DM. Development of training-related health care software by a team of clinical educators: their experience, from conception to piloting. Adv Med Educ Pract. 2016;7:635–40. https://doi.org/10.2147/amep.s108426
9. Eleftheriou I, Embury S, Brass A. Data Journey: a tool for identifying costs and risks; 2016. http://www.cs.man.ac.uk/~elefthi9/datajourney/.
10. Eleftheriou I, Embury SM, Brass A. Data journey modelling: predicting risk for IT developments. Cham: Springer International Publishing; 2016.
11. Festersen PL. VeggieMetrics: A nutrition tracking mobile application for facilitating the switch to a vegetarian diet [Internet]. Edinburgh Napier University; 2015. Available from: https://s3.amazonaws.com/academia.edu.documents/41054463/VeggieMetricsFinal. pdf?response-content-disposition=inline%3Bfilename%3DVeggieMetrics_A_nutrition_ tracking_mobil.pdf&X-Amz-Algorithm=AWS4-HMAC-SHA256&X-Amz-Credential= AKIAIWOWYYGZ2Y53UL3A%2F2020022

12. Fruhling A, Tyser K, de Vreede G-J. Experiences with extreme programming in telehealth: developing and implementing a biosecurity health care application. In: Proceedings of the 38th annual Hawaii international conference on system sciences, Big Island. IEEE; 2005. p. 151b–151b. http://ieeexplore.ieee.org/document/1385543/

13. Google. Eng-practices: Google's engineering practices documentation; 2020. https://google.github.io/eng-practices/review/

14. Hannay JOE, Dybå T, Arisholm E, Sjøberg DIK. The effectiveness of pair programming: a meta-analysis. Inf Softw Technol. 2009;51(7):1110–22. https://doi.org/10.1016/j.infsof.2009.02.001

15. Harris B, Duderewicz E, Miyauchi K, Ng M, Jenkins T. Mom-O-Meter: a self-help pregnancy Android app; Mar 2011. https://digitalcommons.wpi.edu/mqp-all/2333

16. Keijzer-Broers W, Florez-Atehortua L, de Reuver M. Prototyping a health and wellbeing platform: an action design research approach. In: 2016 49th Hawaii international conference on system sciences (HICSS). IEEE; Jan 2016. p. 3462–71. http://ieeexplore.ieee.org/document/7427616/

17. Knuth D. Structured programming with go to statements. Comput Surv. 1974;6(4):261–301. https://doi.org/10.1145/954127.954136

18. Levy CE, Miller DM, Akande CA, Lok B, Marsiske M, Halan S. V-Mart, a virtual reality grocery store. Am J Phys Med Rehabil. 2019;98(3):191–98. https://doi.org/10.1097/PHM.0000000000001041

19. Mahapatra N. Agile estimation for user stories. 2020. https://agiledigest.com/agile-digest-tutorial-2/agile-estimation-2/#STORYPOINT

20. Managing the development of large-scale systems. Proceedings of IEEE WESCON; 1970. p. 328–38. https://doi.org/10.1016/0378-4754(91)90107-E

21. Nosek JT. The case for collaborative programming. Commun ACM. 1998;41(3):105–8. https://doi.org/10.1145/272287.272333

22. Ockerman S. Scrum Myths: daily scrum is not a status meeting; 2019. https://www.scrum.org/resources/blog/scrum-myths-daily-scrum-not-status-meeting

23. OMG. About the unified modeling language specification version 2.5.1; 2017. https://www.omg.org/spec/UML/

24. OMG. What is UML; 2019. https://www.uml.org/what-is-uml.htm

25. Schwaber K, Sutherland J. The scrum guide: the definitive the rules of the game. Technical report; Nov 2017. http://www.scrumguides.org/docs/scrumguide/v1/Scrum-Guide-US.pdf

26. Scrum.org. Scrum.org; 2019. https://www.scrum.org/resources/what-is-scrum

27. Usherwood T. Introduction to project management in health research: a guide for new researchers. Buckingham: Open University Press; 1996.

28. Vallon R, Wenzel L, Brüggemann ME, Grechenig T. An agile and lean process model for mobile app development: case study into Austrian industry. J Softw. 2015;10(11):1245–64. https://doi.org/10.17706/jsw.10.11.1245-1264

29. Wells D. When should I use extreme programming; 1999. http://www.extremeprogramming.org/when.html

30. Williams L. What agile teams think of agile principles. Commun ACM. 2012;55(4):71–6. https://doi.org/10.1145/2133806.2133823

Chapter 3
Designing an mHealth Intervention

3.1 Introduction

Development of health apps should always be preceded by careful consideration
and planning. Although this involves additional investment of time and resources,
a rigorous approach to the development of ideas and content, taking literature,
user perspectives, relevant theory, and existing solutions into account will ensure
maximal benefits and efficiency as well as reduced risks.

The purpose of health apps is to "assess, improve, maintain, promote or
modify health, functioning or health conditions" [37]. They thus constitute "health
interventions" according to the International Classification of Health Interventions
developed by the World Health Organization. The digital technology underlying
mobile apps acts as a medium for conveying these interventions. This chapter
focuses on the development of interventions, whereas Chap. 4 examines the development process from a technical point of view. As such, the present chapter focuses
on the mechanisms which health apps use to bring about change.

This chapter will outline some of the crucial processes that should be involved
in the development of digital health interventions (DHIs). DHIs are interventions
that employ digital technology to promote and maintain health, through supporting
behavior change or decision making of the general public, patients, or healthcare
practitioners [22]. Mobile health apps are a specific form of DHI. It is important to
note that the processes described below do not represent a 'step-by-step' approach,
with a fixed start and end point or a prescribed order. Instead, the approach should be
cyclical, involving several iterations of each process. This ensures that problems can
be identified and addressed early on, that the intervention can be revised and refined
continuously, and that it remains grounded in the needs of its user group [38].

© Springer Nature Switzerland AG 2020
A. Davies, J. Mueller, *Developing Medical Apps and mHealth Interventions*, Health
Informatics, https://doi.org/10.1007/978-3-030-47499-7_3

3.2   Challenges to DHI Development

As outlined in Chap. 1, the field of mHealth entails a number of important challenges and limitations. Michie et al. [22] highlight the following key challenges involved in the development of DHIs:

- Incongruity between the rapid pace at which technology is developed, and the relatively slow pace of evidence-based development and evaluation
- Engagement is often low and attrition tends to be high, which may limit effects on behaviour change. Of particular concern is the fact that engagement may be lower among particular user groups (often those with the poorest health outcomes) and thus DHIs may contribute to health disparities
- Mechanisms of behaviour change and how DHIs bring about their effects are often unclear
- Testing the effectiveness of DHIs can be challenging because DHIs tend to be complex and, moreover, the data they generate are often heterogeneous and difficult to analyse. It is also difficult to control the testing environment (for example those assigned to the control group may download other apps)
- Lack of suitable methods for evaluating cost-effectiveness meaningfully
- Quality standards and regulatory processes are often unclear

Careful consideration should be given to each of these points prior to and during development of a DHI to ensure appropriate resources can be allocated to address and mitigate these challenges.

3.3   Developing Ideas and Specifying Aims

DHI development usually begins with the identification of a problem that the DHI is intended to address. Initial ideas will require significant consideration and refinement before they can be translated into a DHI. For example, healthcare professionals might notice that a large proportion of their patients are overweight or obese and have health problems associated with their weight (such as diabetes or cardiovascular diseases), resulting in significant burden and costs to the healthcare system. Based on these observations, they may decide to develop an intervention to tackle this problem. Specifically, they may decide to use an mHealth approach due to its cost-effectiveness and scalability. In order to develop this initial idea into an appropriate and effective intervention, however, several key aspects need to be considered and clearly defined (see box below). This is not to say that these aspects need to be set in stone; rather, they should be considered and explicitly addressed early on. This will ensure efficient use of time and resources.

The example above highlights another crucial aspect to developing initial ideas: those suffering from health problems, or those in close contact with those afflicted (such as health professionals) are usually well placed to identify relevant problems and possible solutions. Therefore their opinions and expertise should be sought early on. User and stakeholder engagement is discussed in more detail in Sect. 3.8.

The first key aspect to define is the issue the app aims to target, and relatedly, what outcomes it aims to produce. While most health apps tend to address several outcomes, it is helpful to identify a *primary outcome* to focus the development process. This may seem obvious, but interventions are often developed without clarifying these key questions first. For example, in the scenario described above, the developers of the intervention would need to decide whether the app intends to improve nutrition, decrease sedentary behaviour, or increase physical activity (or a combination of these). Depending on their choices, different mechanisms of behaviour will be at play which will be amenable to different strategies. Moreover, the intervention developers will need to decide which outcomes they want the app to bring about, and how they will know whether it has been successful. This could involve behaviours (e.g. amount of calories consumed or number of minutes of exercise per day), health outcomes (e.g. BMI, blood pressure), or healthcare outcomes (e.g. healthcare costs associated with obesity).

Aspects to consider when specifying aims of the app

- What specific behaviour(s) should it target?
- Who will be using the app?
- What outcomes does it aim to change?
- How do you aim to change the behaviour?

In addition to defining aims and targeted outcomes, intervention developers will need to clearly define their target population. This is crucial, as users' needs and perspectives should always be central to the development of any intervention. Different population groups will have different needs and preferences and face unique challenges. An intervention targeting obesity among adolescents, for example, is likely to involve very different features to an intervention targeting adults aged 65+.

A clear definition of the target population is particularly important in light of the "digital divide". The terms "digital divide" or "digital exclusion" denote the issue that not all population groups have equal access to digital technology. Access issues may relate to [34]:

- **Mental access**: lack of elementary digital experience (e.g. because of a lack of interest/anxiety)
- **Material access**: no possession of computers and network connections
- **Skills access**: lack of digital skills (e.g. lack of education)
- **Usage access**: lack of usage opportunities

For example, research indicates that age, education, income, social isolation, socio-economic status, ethnicity, and, in some countries, gender, are related to Internet access [9, 39] and smartphone usage [28]. Even among those who own smartphones and have access to the Internet, there is still a sociodemographic divide between those who use these technologies for health-related purposes, with an increased likelihood of eHealth and mHealth use among those who are younger and those who have higher incomes and education levels [15, 16]. Importantly, those who are less likely to have access to health-enhancing technologies and information also tend to be those with the poorest health outcomes. Therefore, if characteristics of the user population are not taken into account, we risk increasing health inequalities with the implementation of health apps. For example, consider the development of a nutrition app aiming to reduce risk of type 2 diabetes. The risk of having type 2 diabetes is higher among those from deprived socioeconomic backgrounds [5]. An app involving medical jargon and complex scientific terms is not likely to be attractive to the at-risk population. Instead, it is likely to be used by those with high education levels from socioeconomically advantaged backgrounds, thus further isolating those who need help the most, and widening existing inequalities.

For these reasons, it is very important to consider your target population carefully before designing your app. This will be covered in more detail in Sect. 3.8 on user engagement.

As mentioned above, initial ideas need not, and indeed should not, be set in stone. At this early stage, it is best not to develop any specific features or content of the app in order to stay flexible, so that insights obtained from reviewing previous approaches and user engagement can be incorporated flexibly.

3.4 Ethical Considerations

While DHIs aim to promote and improve health, there is also a potential for harm that requires careful consideration during development, particularly as many DHIs could be classed as medical devices. DHIs could entail detrimental effects if they [22]:

- **Provide inaccurate information**. For example, an app providing dietary advice to pregnant women could potentially cause harm to the mother or the baby if inappropriate advice is provided regarding safe and harmful foods.
- **Involve behaviours or interactions that are incompatible with or attenuate desired behaviours**. For example, there is concern among experts that apps designed to help those suffering from insomnia through sleep-tracking could actually induce anxiety and thereby exacerbate sleeping problems by heightening users' focus on their lack of sleep.
- **Displace more effective behaviour change interventions**. For example, pulmonary rehabilitation is recommended for people with certain lung conditions. This supervised programme entails training and education over several weeks. An app to promote physical activity in people with lung problems may be

perceived as less cumbersome and time-intensive and therefore deter patients from taking up the more effective existing intervention.

- **Compromise data protection standards/laws**. For example, an app may share data with third parties without gaining consent or by obfuscating consent processes. This is particularly concerning when data collected by the app is sensitive and potentially personally identifying, e.g. information about sexual partners in a HIV management app.

It is important to consider ethical aspects early during development of DHIs because this may entail adapting typical work flows and processes used in engineering. Modern software development often aims to be "agile", meaning that work is conducted iteratively, constantly cycling through development, testing, and adaptation phases (for details see Chap. 4). This often entails a "fail fast, fail often" approach whereby solutions are implemented and tested quickly rather than aiming for perfection prior to implementation, with the rationale that quick failings can lead to quick learning and improved solutions. Such agile approaches may at times be at odds with more rigid, risk-averse procedures and policies employed in the field of health care [22].

Importantly, early development stages of a DHI should involve identification of relevant regulatory frameworks. For example, in the UK the Medicines and Healthcare Products Regulatory Agency has issued guidance on when software applications are considered to be a medical device and how they are regulated [18]. Similarly, the Department of Health in Australia provides guidance on regulations that apply to software and apps that meet the definition of a medical device in the Therapeutic Goods Act [1]. In the US, the Federal Trade Commission has developed an interactive tool to help those developing mobile health apps identify the federal laws they need to adhere to [10]. At an international level, the International Medical Device Regulators Forum set up a working group dedicated to Software as Medical Device in 2013. The working group has published several technical documents relating to the regulation of software that is classed as a medical device [13].

Aside from regulations, clinical governance and legislations, there are other less clear-cut ethical considerations regarding data ownership [22]. Some apps store collected data locally on the user's device whereas others will store user data on external servers. In such cases, it is unclear who owns these data, and whether and in what form they may be shared. Some business models might see app usage provided for free in exchange for the users' data. As such, commercial and ethical interests can be at odds and require thorough review and thought during development stages.

It may be useful to consult tools for reviewing apps created by the Organisation for the Review of Care and Health Applications (ORCHA) [27] during the development of applications. By consulting such tools during development (rather than at the end when the application is considered complete), potential issues can be identified and addressed early on.This can help ensure, for example, that your app adheres to published data privacy and user experience standards [13].

3.5   Reviewing Existing Evidence and Approaches

Once initial ideas have been developed, a crucial first step involves reviewing the available evidence. A plethora of health apps already exist, some with an extensive evidence base. By reviewing the evidence base before developing your intervention, you ensure that you build on existing knowledge, and that your app addresses a "need-gap" which has not been filled by previous approaches (Fig. 3.1). This will help avoid devoting time and resources to ineffective strategies, or duplicating existing efforts. This can involve reviewing academic literature, but should also entail systematically examining app stores and app libraries such as the "NHS Apps Library", a repository developed by the National Health Service in the United Kingdom to help consumers and professionals find evidence-based digital health tools [26].

3.5.1   Reviewing the Literature

A review of the literature (e.g. academic research articles and reports) can help you understand the evidence base underpinning your chosen health issue or health behaviour. For example, a review of the literature on mobile apps aimed at

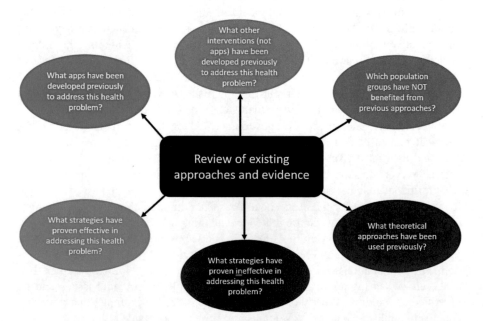

Fig. 3.1 The figure highlights how a review of existing approaches and evidence can help to address important questions prior to intervention development

increasing physical activity found that apps are more effective when they target physical activity in isolation, rather than in combination with nutritional advice [31]. The review also highlighted that impacts of physical activity apps are more evident in shorter time frames, suggesting that future apps need a stronger focus on strategies to sustain engagement over time. By reviewing this information, those interested in developing physical activity apps can gain useful insights into app features that have proven successful or not successful in the past, and features that have not been tried but might be promising. Therefore, any plan to develop a new app should begin with a literature review.

There are different methodologies and techniques for effectively identifying and reviewing literature, depending on the aims [12]. Initially, reviews will be broad in scope and will involve different combinations of search terms in order to obtain a general overview of the extant literature and to identify key concepts and gaps in existing research. For example, if you are interested in research on the effectiveness of smartphone apps for enhancing physical activity in children aged 5–10 years, you might initially search different databases with various search terms like ("smartphone" AND "physical activity" AND "children"). This would help you obtain a general overview of the literature. If you found a large number of studies involving child populations, you might then begin to narrow your search to your specific age group. Once you have ascertained that literature is available for your specific area of interest, it is then often helpful to turn to more systematic strategies for finding, reviewing and synthesising literature, to ensure you take all available evidence into account before making further decisions.

3.5.2   Systematic Reviewing

Following an initial scoping review, a "systematic review" can be useful to identify relevant evidence and limit bias. Systematic reviews constitute the most thorough, objective and comprehensive approach to reviewing the literature [3]. This entails a rigorous, systematic approach, with the aim of identifying *all* literature related to a specific question, including peer-reviewed journal articles and grey literature such as dissertations and conference abstracts. This involves using reproducible methods and objective criteria. Usually, researchers will identify a list of key words and design a specific search strategy which is used to query different databases. Subsequently *all* records returned via the search must be reviewed against a set of specific criteria by at least two independent researchers. Included records then need to undergo a quality appraisal, and finally reviewers must extract and synthesise relevant information into a coherent review.

If studies are sufficiently similar, their results can even be statistically combined or "pooled" to determine effects of interventions across different studies in a *meta-analysis*. Meta-analyses provide a more robust estimate of the effect of an intervention because, by pooling data from several studies, they involve much larger sample sizes than single studies alone. More details on conducting systematic reviews are provided in the Centre for Reviews and Dissemination's guidance for undertaking reviews in health care [3].

Another important resource for those conducting systematic reviews and meta-analyses is PRISMA (Preferred Reporting Items for Systematic Reviews and Meta-Analyses), see for example [23]. The PRISMA Statement consists of a checklist and a flow diagram. The checklist is used to identify whether all important items have been reported in a systematic review (e.g. the eligibility criteria used to identify studies that are to be included or excluded from the review). It should also be used during initial preparation stages of the review, as a guide of aspects that should be considered and recorded. The Flowchart (Fig. 3.2) shows the different stages of the study identification process, and highlights what numbers need to be recorded and reported in the final review. The PRISMA checklist and flowchart as well as the accompanying PRISMA Explanation and Elaboration document can be downloaded from the PRISMA website (http://prisma-statement.org/).

Flores-Mateo et al. [11], for example, systematically reviewed the literature on apps to promote weight loss and increase physical activity and found 12 relevant studies. Eight studies examined body mass index and were pooled together in a meta-analysis, resulting in an overall sample of 1047 participants. Across the different studies, they found that mobile phone apps are associated with statistically significant reductions in body mass index, although several individual studies showed no effect on their own. This highlights how meta-analysis can show different results than individual studies through their increased statistical power through larger sample sizes.

Apart from helping us to identify whether interventions are effective or not, systematic reviews are also very useful because they provide an overview of the extant literature, and of interventions that have been previously evaluated. This will prevent "reinventing the wheel" and will ensure we build on rather than duplicate past efforts.

3.5.3 Reviewing Apps

The systematic reviewing technique can be applied to other forms of evidence, apart from research articles. Similar methods can be employed to systematically browse through app stores and app libraries (e.g. the NHS Apps Library from the UK National Health Service). For example, Sucala et al. [32] used the *Power Search function* to search iTunes and Google Play for apps relating to anxiety, using a specific set of key words such as "anxiety" and "worry". They then assessed all returned apps against a set of inclusion criteria (e.g. apps involving psychological techniques, apps focused primarily on anxiety). Their search returned over 4,000 apps, and 52 were included in their final review. These 52 apps were analysed in terms of the features and psychotherapy techniques they included and the empirical evidence to support them.

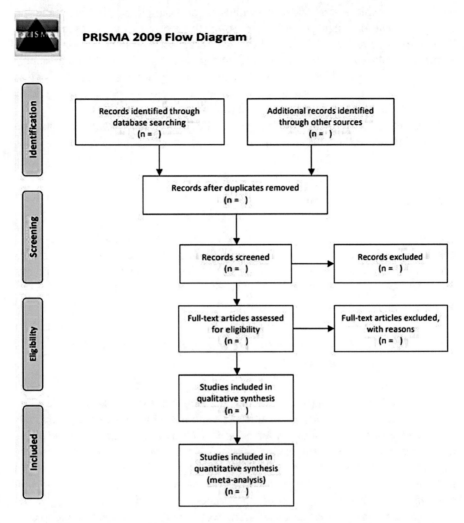

Fig. 3.2 The figure depicts the flow of information through the different phases of a systematic review [23]. http://prisma-statement.org/. (The image is distributed under the terms of the Creative Commons Attribution License)

3.5.4 Rapid Reviewing

While the review methods described above clearly provide a solid basis for the development of new mHealth interventions, it may not always be possible to undertake a full systematic review due to time or resource constraints. A systematic review of the literature typically takes at least six months. However, in recent years "rapid review" techniques have become more popular and accepted among the research community. Rapid reviews entail adapting standard systematic reviewing methods to enable faster evidence synthesis, for example by limiting inclusion criteria by date or language, employing only the most relevant keywords rather than an exhaustive list (determined based on initial scoping of the literature), and employing only one reviewer while a second reviewer verifies only a sub-sample of records etc. [33]. The use and publication of rapid reviews have increased exponentially in the last decade and good quality rapid reviews are now widely accepted for publication in peer reviewed journals [24].

Remember that following your review of the literature and available apps, you may need to revisit the aims and objectives of your proposed intervention.

3.6 Frameworks and Approaches

Frameworks and established approaches can help streamline intervention development, ensuring the process is efficient and comprehensive. Below we highlight potentially useful approaches which are used widely in the research community. These approaches are not mutually exclusive and can be combined.

3.6.1 The MRC Guidance for Developing and Evaluating Complex Interventions

The Medical Research Council (MRC) has developed a framework for the development and evaluation of complex health interventions. This framework is relatively broad and general, and therefore lends itself well as an overarching structure to frame the intervention development process. This framework was initially presented as a series of steps from development to final evaluation. However, as awareness of and interest in the methodology underlying the development of complex interventions increased, it became clear that the process is not characterised by a series of sequential steps. A revision of the framework published in 2008 now depicts a cyclical approach, to demonstrate that successful intervention development needs to involve several iterations to enable learning and "fine-tuning".

The MRC Framework involves four elements:

1. **Development**: This element should involve the identification of the evidence base and relevant theories, as well as any modelling required to refine the intervention and identify suitable outcome measures for evaluation (e.g. economic modelling to assess whether rolling out your app would be cost-effective).
2. **Feasibility and piloting**: In this element, interventions should be tested to assess their feasibility, to make sure everything "runs smoothly", and to obtain estimates for parameters needed to design the full evaluation. For example, if your app

aims to target a heard-to-reach group, you will need to test whether you are able to identify and engage this group, and what kind of recruitment rates you can expect (i.e. how many of the people that you approach actually download and use your app).

3. **Evaluation**: Any health intervention – including health apps – should undergo rigorous evaluation. This is necessary to test whether the intervention leads to expected improvements, and whether it is cost-effective. Any health app is tied to ongoing costs (for example costs for software engineering, updating, promotion), and if health systems and patients are to carry these costs, it is ethically unjustifiable to implement apps long-term without testing their effectiveness.

4. **Implementation**: This should only ensue following at least some initial testing to ensure the app is safe to use. This element will involve dissemination (e.g. marketing and promotion of the app) as well as long-term follow-up. This will help to demonstrate effects of the app "in the field", as opposed to the more controlled, experimental conditions likely to be used in the evaluation element.

It is expected that intervention developers will cycle through each element multiple times, with all elements interlinked, and no prescribed sequence. For example, you may begin by developing an initial draft of your app, and then pilot-test it. This may uncover issues, meaning you will need to return to the development phase before you can move on to evaluation. Likewise, evaluation and implementation can uncover further problems or opportunities, requiring more development and pilot-testing.

3.6.2 The Behaviour Change Wheel

The Behaviour change wheel (Fig. 3.3) is a framework which aims to facilitate the development of evidence-based behaviour change interventions through a structured approach [21]. It provides an overview of different factors that may play a role in behaviour change at individual level (e.g. capability, motivation and opportunities) and at policy level (e.g. fiscal measures, guidelines and regulations), and highlights intervention strategies that have proven effective in targeting these factors previously. As such, it provides a broad and comprehensive overview of behaviour change theory and available evidence. Readers who are interested in using this approach may want to read the book by Michie, Atkins and West [21] and view the accompanying website (www.behaviourchangewheel.com). The website shows an interactive image of the wheel, and clicking on any field within the image will show you a definition and an example, as well as highlighting which other fields are likely to be relevant. For example, clicking on any of the intervention functions will highlight policy measures that are likely to be relevant to support these.

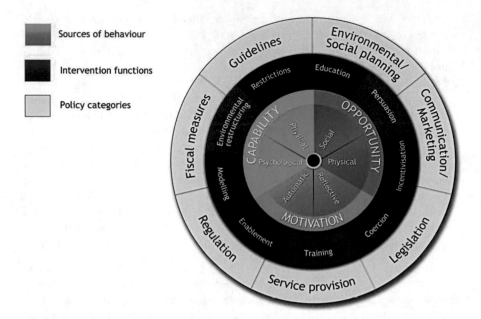

Fig. 3.3 The figure depicts the Behaviour Change Wheel, developed by Michie et al. [20]. (The image is distributed under the terms of the Creative Commons Attribution License) (http://creativecommons.org/licenses/by/2.0)

3.6.3   The Person-Based Approach

The person-based approach was developed by Yardley et al. [38] as a guide for those developing digital health interventions. It aims to ensure that intervention developers take the needs, priorities and preferences of their users into account and develop interventions jointly with users.

The person-based approach places a strong emphasis on conducting qualitative research to involve users from the outset, starting by asking users about perceived barriers and facilitators to behaviour change. It may also be beneficial to consult experts and other stakeholders. Throughout intervention development, members of the intervention target group should be engaged at all stages (i.e. generating initial ideas, operationalising ideas, testing prototypes/draft versions, design of the study to evaluate the intervention) by conducting interviews and/or focus groups.

Alongside user engagement, this approach also involves creating a set of guiding principles to make sure the intervention stays focused on its aims. These principles should be based on user engagement, theory, and previous research. The guiding principles will state what the aim is, who the target group is, and what characteristics of the target population are relevant (see box below for an example).

Table 3.1 provides an overview of the person-based approach.

Table 3.1 Overview of the person-based approach. (Adapted from [38])

Stage	Aim	Processes
Planning	Identification of challenges and problems the intervention must address/formulation of intervention aims	Review and synthesise qualitative evidence on user experience; conduct qualitative exploration of user views on planned intervention
Design	Creation of guiding principles	Formulation of guiding principles based on evidence identified in Planning stage
Development and evaluation of acceptability and feasibility	User evaluation of intervention components	Test intervention by observing users as they navigate the intervention using "Think Aloud" techniques to verbalise their thoughts. Carry out case studies of users using the intervention independently over longer periods of time
Implementation and trialing	Evaluate intervention in real-life contexts; undertake modifications to improve implementation	Conduct process analyses, using mixed (quantitative and qualitative) methods to understand how users use the intervention "in the wild" and focusing on acceptability, feasibility & effectiveness

An example of guiding principles for the development of an app for people with chronic obstructive pulmonary disease (COPD).

1. **Intervention objectives**: To allow people with COPD to track their symptoms over time, and to see how their symptoms vary with medication intake. To improve adherence to treatment regimes.
2. **Relevant aspects of users in the context**: People with COPD tend to be older (65+), of lower socioeconomic/education level, and less technically literate. Many do not own smartphones, or don't use them on a regular basis.
3. **Key behavioural issues, needs, or challenges that the intervention needs to address**: People with COPD often take medication incorrectly and do not adhere to physicians' recommendations. For example, patients often take medication only when symptoms worsen, even if instructed to use it regularly. The app needs to visualise how symptoms vary with medication intake in an intelligible way, to help patients understand how best to use their medication.

(continued)

4. **Intervention design features that can address the barriers and achieve the aim**: We tested some basic visualisations with users during user engagement events. Patients preferred line graphs and were able to interpret these if kept simple. Patients suggested depicting data points as circles, which would be filled in when medication was taken, and empty if medication was not taken. Nudge theory suggests users should be sent regular reminders (notifications) to complete and view their symptom information.

Importantly, the person-based approach should not be viewed as a series of "steps", but rather as a cycle of user engagement and intervention development, resulting in an iterative, user-centred process. For example, in a project aiming to develop an online intervention to encourage people with potential lung cancer symptoms to seek medical advice early, myself and colleagues cycled through a series of user engagement and development stages, with a clear set of guiding principles to ensure a focused, purposeful process [25], as shown in Fig. 3.4.

3.7   Behaviour Change Theories

Health apps are closely linked with human behaviour. They often involve attempts to change behaviour (for example, when using a health app to promote physical activity or healthy eating), and their effectiveness depends on whether they are correctly used. Human behaviour is complex and depends on a multitude of factors, such as cognitions, emotions, attitudes, individual characteristics, predispositions and experiences as well as environmental factors. Thus, predicting behaviour is extremely difficult. Therefore, health app development should be underpinned by a model or theory of behaviour and the factors that influence it. Psychological theories can help us identify the variables that we need to target in order to increase the likelihood of successful behaviour change. They are useful because they help us understand behaviour on a more abstract, conceptual level, which in turn allows us to make predictions and form hypotheses about behaviour.

It should be noted, however, that most theories of behaviour explain only small to moderate amounts of variation in that behaviour. Moreover, most theories have been developed in Western contexts and may therefore be less applicable in other cultural contexts. Finally, it should be noted that many behaviour change theories focus on the conscious, rational drivers of behaviour. Emotional, irrational or sub-conscious processes are often not accounted for. As such, no theory explains behaviour perfectly. In some cases, it may be more useful to figure out what works best in a specific situation and a particular target group, rather than trying to make

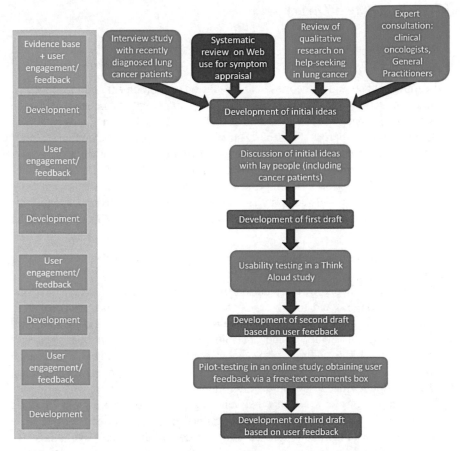

Fig. 3.4 The figure shows how we developed an online intervention for people with potential lung cancer symptoms, to encourage them to seek help early [25], using an iterative approach

an overarching theory fit into a specific context. Nevertheless, a consideration of the underlying mechanisms of the behaviour and the more abstract concepts that drive the behaviour is usually beneficial.

Health apps are often developed without an evidence-based, theoretical basis. Instead, they tend to be based on implicit commonsense models of behaviour, i.e. people assume they know what other people will do based on what they consider commonsense. However, commonsense assumptions often do not hold true in practice. Moreover, a systematic review of the literature found that Web-based behaviour change interventions have stronger effects when they are based on psychological theory [35].

3.7.1   Selecting a Theory

There are a multitude of different theoretical approaches which can be used to design health apps. The four main perspectives on (health) behaviour change are:

1. Learning and cognitive theories which focus on reinforcement and incentives
2. Stage models which identify different factors important for behaviour change based on the stage of "readiness to change" an individual is in, e.g. the "Health Action Process Approach", or the "Transtheoretical model of behaviour change"
3. Affect-based approaches which recognise that people do not always process information rationally and account for affect-driven behaviour, e.g. the "Protection Motivation Theory" which postulates that fear can motivate behaviour
4. Social cognition models that predict behaviour based on perceived consequences and perceived social acceptance of the behaviour, e.g. the "Theory of Planned Behaviour".

For more detail on individual theories, a useful overview is provided by Conner and Norman [4].

The choice of theory will depend on the behaviour you are trying to change, the target population, and the wider context. This is where your prior literature reviews, user engagement and/or qualitative research with users will come in useful. By synthesising this evidence and analysing it for conceptual themes, you will most likely be able to identify higher-level concepts that are likely to influence the behaviour you wish to target. You can then map these onto existing theories, to identify a theory that best captures the concepts you identified.

For example, in our research on developing an online intervention for those worried about lung cancer, we initially examined qualitative research on reasons why people with lung cancer delayed seeing a doctor about their symptoms. By synthesising findings across several studies, we found that beliefs appear to play a key role, such as "doctors will think I'm a time-waster if I make an appointment for a cough". In particular, people seemed concerned with what other people – such as doctors and family members or friends – would think if they sought medical advice for their symptoms. Based on this observation, we decided to go down the route of social cognition theories [25]. There may be other good rationales for choosing a theory; the important thing is to have a sound justification, rooted in evidence and user engagement.

3.7.2   Translating Theory into Practice

There is generally rather little practical guidance in the literature on how to go about developing behaviour change interventions, and how to translate theory into practice. There is a plethora of studies evaluating interventions, but not much published work to show how authors got to this point. "Intervention development" is often dismissed with a few lines, or simply described as "a creative process".

Interventions are often merely described as "based on XYZ theory", with little detail on how theoretical constructs were operationalised and implemented. Fortunately, there has been a recent trend from journal editors and reviewers to require more detail, but guidance is still scarce. For example, the Health Belief Model postulates that, in order to change behaviour, one needs to change people's perceptions of the benefits and barriers, perceptions of whether the health problem is an actual threat, and perceptions of one's own ability to perform the behaviour (self-efficacy). However, it is unclear how one would go about changing perceptions, and which techniques might work best in what context.

A useful approach is offered by Michie and colleagues. The researchers undertook a series of exercises to collate a comprehensive list of concrete, specific *behaviour changer techniques* (BCTs) that have been used in various interventions to change behaviour. This included systematically reviewing the literature and relevant textbooks and "brainstorming" among behaviour change experts [19]. Examples of BCTs include "role-play" and "rewards, incentives". This ultimately resulted in a hierarchically grouped taxonomy of 93 BCTs [4]. Michie et al. mapped these BCTs onto behavioural determinants (i.e. constructs that have been theorised to predict behaviour across a range of psychological theories, such as "beliefs about capabilities", "knowledge" or "social identity") by asking experts to rate the likelihood of different BCTs leading to changes in the different behavioural determinants. In a later study, Cane et al. [2] used grouping tasks with behaviour change experts and Discriminant Content Validity to map BCTs onto behavioural determinants. These mappings can be a useful tool for those developing behaviour change interventions, because they can provide us with a framework and rationale for selecting concrete BCTs to target specific theoretical constructs.

3.8 User and Stakeholder Engagement

So far, we have mainly discussed the incorporation of theories and formal frameworks into app development. Another crucial aspect that should always form a key part of digital intervention development is *user engagement*.

There are different user groups as well as wider stakeholders that need to be considered in health app design. Arguably the most important group tends to be the end-users, i.e. those who will ultimately use the app. Those commissioning app development will also play a central role in determining the general direction of the work. Additionally, wider stakeholders who may not be involved directly but who may be affected need to be considered. For example, when developing an app to facilitate cancer symptom detection by patients, you will need to consider:

- **End-users**, i.e. patients or lay members of the public. The app needs to be designed in a way to facilitate easy usage, using intuitive features and intelligible, lay language.
- **Commissioners**, e.g. the National Health Service. The app needs to fulfill commissioners' aims of helping people detect worrying symptoms and seeking help where appropriate, while avoiding unnecessary usage of healthcare services.

- **Wider stakeholders**, e.g. clinicians who will have direct contact with patients who seek medical services based on advice received in their app. The app needs to be aligned with clinicians' expertise. Other relevant stakeholder groups include professional bodies, e.g. the National Institute for Health and Care Excellence (NICE) in the UK. The app needs to be aligned with NICE clinical guidelines for suspected cancer.

End-users and stakeholders (referred to in the following as "users") should be involved in the process from the start, i.e. from initial stages of identifying problems to target and formulating the core aims of the app. This engagement is important for several reasons, including:

- **Identifying relevant problems to target:** Users are usually best placed to identify relevant problems, because they are able to draw on their own lived experience and the challenges they encounter in everyday life.
- **Developing solutions**: Following the same logic, users are often well placed to come up with innovative and feasible solutions, as they are aware of the constraints and opportunities that present themselves in practice. Users are often able to identify problems and issues that external persons would not be able to foresee.
- **Enhancing acceptability:** Apps are more likely to be acceptable to users if they have been co-designed. Without such input, apps risk including components that may be offensive, unsafe, confusing, or otherwise unhelpful.
- **Enhancing credibility:** Co-design with users can enhance credibility by signaling endorsement and approval from trusted sources. For example, it is easy to see why parents are more likely to use an app on child health if it has been developed together with health professionals.
- **Testing:** Features that might seem feasible or effective in theory may prove challenging, burdensome or downright annoying to users. Without testing your app with actual users, these kinds of issues can be difficult or impossible to foresee.

Case study: Engaging users to develop an app for monitoring and managing chronic obstructive pulmonary disease (COPD)

Myself and colleagues were involved in an mHealth project which aimed to improve self-management of chronic obstructive pulmonary disease (COPD) [7]. We involved users in the following ways:

Generating ideas: In the early stages of the project, we visited several events for patients with COPD, such as medical centres, Breathe Easy Support Group Meetings and other respiratory information events. We spoke to over 40 people with COPD as well as carers in various stakeholder meetings and focus groups. We also consulted 22 healthcare professionals in two stakeholder meetings. During these early meetings, we explored users' general interest

---

(continued)

in a potential COPD app, problems that people were facing in self-managing their disease, people's opinions on using sensors such as temperature and humidity sensors in their homes, and people's opinions on using "smart inhalers" which can connect to a smartphone app. Importantly, we did not enter these meetings with fixed, pre-defined notions, but instead used them as an open discussion space to gauge general interest and preliminary ideas. We used *vignettes* to facilitate discussions. The vignettes consisted of brief (ca. 250 words) descriptions of patient scenarios, including patients' age, diagnoses, symptoms, and particular issues they struggle with. For example:

> Peter is a 55 year old ex-smoker who has had COPD for 5 years. He works as a delivery driver. He owns a smartphone and an X-box, but doesn't use a computer regularly. Doctors have told Peter that his COPD is moderate. For Peter, this means that he has no problems walking on a flat surface, but struggles with stairs and is beginning to feel out of breath if there is even a little bit of a slope.

Paper prototyping: After gauging overall interest, we then invited people with COPD for focus group meetings to create paper prototypes for a COPD smartphone app. To facilitate engagement, we provided paper, pens, and paper cut-outs of smartphone screens onto which users could draw and write. One of the generated prototypes is shown in Fig. 3.5.

Prototype usability testing: Based on users' input and the paper prototypes, we created a scaled-down version of the planned app, which served as a prototype for usability testing. We undertook this intermediate step to avoid developing a full app only to find various usability issues. By working with a prototype, we were able to conduct initial usability testing while work on the main app continued. We tested our prototype in one-to-one sessions with people with COPD, to enable all users to contribute and avoid monopolisation of discussions by more vocal individuals. In one-to-one sessions, we asked users to navigate the app while vocalising their thought processes, prompting whenever we observed signs of users struggling ("Think Aloud" method). We identified several key problems during this process that we would not have otherwise foreseen, including:

- Users were required to enter a username and password to use the app, to protect the privacy of sensitive, personal data. Users struggled with this immensely because they were often not very experienced with smartphone usage, and many had visual and/or manual dexterity issues. For the main app, we therefore recommended a simpler 4-digit passcode system.
- Our prototype used sliders to enable users to enter their symptom details daily (Fig. 3.6). We considered this a standard app feature, and initial testing with other researchers in our lab highlighted no problems with this. During user testing, however, users struggled with sliders and became increasingly frustrated.

(continued)

- Our prototype also included toggle-switches such as the one shown in Fig. 3.6. We assumed this would be an intuitive feature, but users disliked the toggle switches (a) because they were difficult to use for those with visual and manual dexterity issues, and (b) because users struggled to interpret when they were switched on or off, as most were not very familiar with smartphone usage. We therefore decided to use simple, large, and clearly labeled buttons instead for this particular user group.

Further details regarding our methods and results can be found in [7].

3.8.1 Research and Patient and Public Involvement (PPI)

There are different ways to involve and engage users during your app development. First, it is important to highlight a few definitions and differences between approaches. When acquiring user input, we usually rely on *qualitative methods* because they allow in-depth, open-ended exploration (see Chap. 8). Rather than asking closed-ended questions about what we expect to see, qualitative research

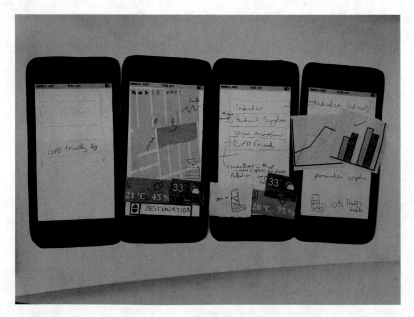

Fig. 3.5 The figure shows paper prototypes for a COPD self-management app created during user engagement

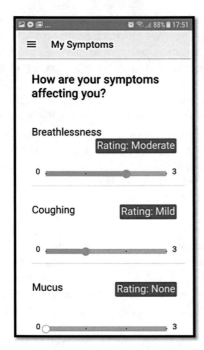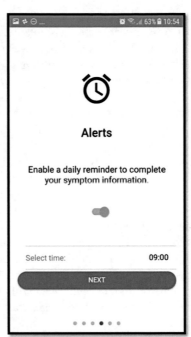

Fig. 3.6 The figure shows two screenshots from our prototype app. Left: The app featured sliders which users could use to indicate the severity of their symptoms. Users struggled greatly with sliders due to visual and manual dexterity issues. Right: Our prototype app made use of toggle switches to switch features such as notifications on and off; users had difficulty interpreting this feature, and struggled to use it due to visual and manual dexterity issues

emphasises open-ended questions to allow users to input their experiences, opinions and viewpoints. This enables us to explore unexpected and unintended aspects. For example, consider the following scenario: A researcher wants to find out what issues lead to inappropriate antibiotic prescribing among doctors. The researcher may have some initial ideas based on her experience. If she used a questionnaire with closed-ended questions to explore issues, she might simply ask things like "Do you struggle to keep up to date with prescribing guidelines?" (yes/no). However, this way she might miss other crucial aspects, such as pressures from pharmaceutical sales representatives, or problems calculating correct dosages on busy wards.

For these reasons, exploring user perspectives for app development should draw on qualitative methods. Mixed-methods approaches may also be beneficial. For example, you may begin with qualitative explorations to gain an insight into the relevant themes and topics, and then use a questionnaire (with closed-ended questions) to assess how prevalent these topics and themes are in a larger sample. Using the example above, the researcher might begin with interviews and focus groups, and then use a questionnaire with a larger sample of healthcare professionals to understand what proportion are affected by the different issues. Whether 1% or whether 80% of users report a problem may have a bearing on how you address it.

It is important to distinguish between *research* and *patient and public involvement* (PPI). Both are means to involve users in app design, but the approach is quite fundamentally different.

In research, we study characteristics and behaviours of the user. The user assumes the role of "research subject" or "research participant", while the researcher assumes the role of investigator. PPI, on the other hand, denotes research conducted *together with* members of the public (e.g. patients). Users take on an active role and contribute to study and app design. PPI work can usually be undertaken without gaining ethical approval (though different regulations may apply and the reader should familiarise themselves with relevant regulations in their area). This is because, in this case, users are not acting as research subjects, but rather as advisers contributing knowledge and expertise.

To conduct PPI for your app development, you could, for example, organise a meeting with user representatives, and you can discuss ideas and plans. You can approach the meeting with initial ideas and materials (see "paper-prototyping" below), but you should be able and willing to change plans based on user feedback. Meeting notes and any material generated during the meeting can then be used for app development.

In research, on the other hand, we would use methods to collect data about the participants (i.e. the users), and we would analyse and synthesise these data. Rather than meeting with users and discussing ideas, we would conduct interviews or focus groups, capture these in some way (e.g. through audio or video recording) and then analyse the data. This type of approach usually requires ethical approval.

There are advantages to both approaches. PPI work enables users to take an active role in the development of the app, whereas qualitative research allows a more detailed, in-depth exploration of user experiences and perspectives. Ideally, health app development will involve a combination of both, e.g. initial research to understand the health problem and its facilitators and barriers, and subsequent PPI work to actively engage and involve users.

3.8.2 Interviews and Focus Groups

There are different methods that can be used to explore user perceptions and experiences both in PPI work and research. *Interviews* are typically conducted in one-to-one sessions, with the aim of transferring information from one person (interviewee) to another (interviewer). Interviews are often structured using an *interview protocol* or *topic guide* consisting of a list of topics or questions to guide the interview. Questions should be open-ended to allow users to explain and elaborate on their views. For example, the question "Do you like this feature on the app?" is likely to elicit only a brief yes/no response, whereas the question "What do you think about this feature on the app?" is much more likely to invite elaboration and explanation.

Focus groups are also a useful tool to elicit users' views. In focus groups, a group of participants (or users) will discuss a particular issue, usually facilitated by a group moderator [29]. The moderator should ensure the discussion remains focused and does not veer off-topic, and they should strive to create a relaxed atmosphere which stimulates open and honest discussions. A note-taker may also be present to capture observations. The clear advantage of focus groups is that interactions and discussions within the group can highlight new insights. However, this depends on whether members of the group feel comfortable sharing. In group settings, there is a risk of some members being subdued by other, more vocal members. Therefore, careful consideration should weigh into the decision of whether to use an interview or a focus group approach. For example, pre-existing groups where members know and are comfortable with each other are more suitable for focus groups. Sensitive and personal issues are unlikely to be discussed in a focus group consisting of strangers. A combination of focus groups and interviews is sometimes advisable to provide all participants with a chance to contribute.

Both focus groups and interviews will generally benefit from a topic guide to prevent discussions from deviating from the topic. The degree to which interviews or focus groups are structured can vary considerably, from in-depth interviews with very little structure, to structured interviews which follow a fixed set and order of questions [14]. Semi-structured interviews are often used because they involve preset open-ended questions and therefore allow inquiries into specific topics, while still retaining the flexibility to explore unexpected topics. The degree of structure will depend on your aims. If you wish to brainstorm and generate ideas, a less structured approach is likely to be fruitful, whereas more structure may be beneficial to explore specific topics, such as participants' views on particular app features.

You should bear in mind that interviews, focus groups and engagement meetings may need to include not only app end-users, but also other stakeholders like healthcare personnel, carers and individuals from organisations that represent people who use services (e.g. charities).

The information you glean from interviews and focus groups is variable and will depend on your aims. Interviews and focus groups can be recorded and transcribed verbatim, and then analysed, e.g. for recurring and important themes [29]. Observation may also be useful, and observational notes can form an important supplement to transcriptions, as the following excerpt shows:

Participant: "Well, I was just going to ask you, can you not do this? No." **[tries to zoom into the text by pinching screen]** *"Because I find it difficult because I can't read small print."*

More details on interviews, focus groups and observation studies and how to conduct them are provided in Chap. 8. Further details on analysing data from these study types is provided in Chap. 9.

3.8.3   Paper Prototyping, Storyboarding and Digital Prototyping

Once you have developed some initial ideas and you have defined your aims and target outcomes, it is often beneficial to undertake some *paper prototyping* using *wireframes* (i.e. paper-based templates of smartphone screens). In its most basic form, this simply means drawing up drafts of the different screens to be displayed in your app. It is best to undertake paper prototyping together with users and/or stakeholders. Wireframes are useful because they visually represent app content, navigation, features and core functionalities [8]. They provide visual material that helps concretise and substantiate discussions with users (both end-users and commissioners). They also provide software engineers with specific reference material to guide development of graphical user interfaces. Figure 3.5 shows a set of wireframes created during user engagement activities to develop an app for people with COPD.

Wireframes can be tied together into a coherent narrative using *storyboarding*. Storyboarding is a useful *declarative* (i.e. non-programming) technique to facilitate app development as it helps bring prototypes together in a consistent, organised and meaningful way. It essentially involves writing a plan of how your app will function, which pages it will display to users in what order, and how users will transition through the content.

In storyboarding, individual screens of the app are referred to as *scenes* and the transitions from one screen to the next are called *segues*. The storyboard outlines the overall structure of the app, and ties together the scenes into a coherent "story". Figure 3.7 shows an example of a brief, simple storyboard. Note that storyboarding can be facilitated by the use of user stories and personas, which are described in more detail in Chap. 7. Developing storyboards using user stories helps to ensure that user requirements form the fundamental basis of app development.

3.8.4   Using Think Aloud to Refine Interventions

Once you have obtained user input (e.g. through interviews and focus groups) to develop your initial ideas including wireframes and storyboards, you will most likely develop a first iteration of your app. As discussed above, intervention development should ideally form an iterative process with continuous refinement based on user input. It can be extremely useful – and ultimately time-saving – to obtain user input on these initial drafts. This helps not only by enhancing usability and acceptability, but also by increasing the likelihood that the app will bring about intended outcomes.

The *Think Aloud* or *cognitive interviewing* technique is a key method used in usability studies and intervention development [38]. It involves users vocalising what they are thinking, feeling or doing as they navigate through the app, prompted

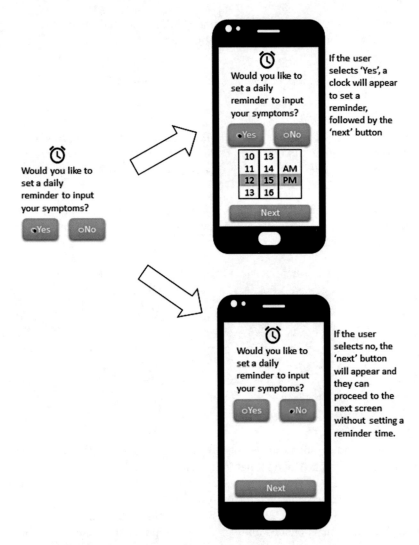

Fig. 3.7 Example of a brief, simple storyboard

by the observer if necessary [6]. This allows the observer to obtain insight into the processes underlying the users' decisions and actions.

Prompting the user to maintain a running commentary of their app usage is crucial to successful Think Aloud evaluations, as this kind of verbalisation of thoughts and actions does not typically come naturally to most people. Observers should pay particular attention when users appear confused, hesitant, or irritated. Importantly, prompts should be open-ended to allow the user to room to elaborate and to avoid "leading" the user in a preconceived direction. For example, consider the following two interactions taken from a Think Aloud study to evaluate an app which displays information to users about their symptoms in a graph:

Example 3.1 (closed-ended)
Observer: *"...Do you think this might be useful; this graph?"*
User: *"Yes, I do."*

Example 3.2 (open-ended)
Observer: *"So, if you could just describe what you think it [the graph] might show?"*
User: *"Just showed the ratings for breathlessness symptoms, it's giving me a graph of how my ratings would be over a day. Or maybe a few days. But yeah, it just shows how variable breathlessness can be."*

As the examples above highlight, open-ended prompts encourage the user to provide more detail than closed-ended questions, and they allow insight into the users' understanding of the app and its features.

Useful prompts for cognitive interviewing/Think Aloud

- How did you go about completing this screen?
- How did you arrive at that answer?
- What went on in your mind when you were clicking through this screen?
- Can you tell me what you were thinking when you were looking at this?
- I noticed you were looking here (and here). What were you thinking? / What lead you to do that?

The important advantage of testing the usability, acceptability and feasibility of an app using Think Aloud is that, due to the qualitative and flexible nature of the approach, *unexpected* and *unintended* outcomes and processes can be assessed. While a questionnaire with a fixed set of questions (such as the System Usability Scale, see Chap. 7) can be useful in assessing predefined outcomes, it will not allow the exploration of unanticipated findings. This is important because users will often behave in unexpected ways or use app features in ways the developers did not intend. Consider the following interaction taken from a usability study myself and colleagues conducted to test an app designed for people with COPD. While the user set up their profile on the app, we noticed that they switched off the reminder feature that would remind them to input their symptom data daily. The following interaction ensued [7]:

Interviewer 2: *"So, can I just ask, does that mean you prefer not to have a daily reminder?"*
Participant 1: *"No."*
Interviewer 2: *"Or would you like to have one?"*
Participant 1: *"Yes, the daily reminder would be good."*
Interviewer 2: *"Okay."*

Participant 1: *"So, the green means that it's set to remind?"*
(Source: Davies et al. (2020) [7]).

The reminder feature in this case involved a small toggle switch which turned green when it was switched on, and grey when it was switched off. While developing this app, we assumed this feature would be easy to use and intuitive. During our Think Aloud evaluation, however, it transpired that users were much less familiar with smartphones and technology in general than we had expected. In the example above, the user accidentally switched the reminder off although they would have liked a reminder, and they were not entirely sure how to interpret the grey/green colouring of the switch. As this example highlights, using exploratory, qualitative methods like Think Aloud is crucial to ensuring successful app development.

3.8.5 Identifying and Engaging Users

So far, we have talked about the importance of involving users in app design and testing. An important consideration in implementing this approach in practice is how to identify and engage with relevant user groups. As mentioned above, "relevant user groups" can entail both end-users as well as commissioners and wider stakeholders.

Example of users and stakeholders
When developing an app for parents of under 5 year old children to provide information about child health in order to reduce unnecessary emergency attendance, one would need to consider the following groups (not an exhaustive list):

- End-users, i.e. parents of under 5 year old children, with particular consideration for groups among whom unnecessary emergency attendance is high
- Commissioners, e.g. clinical commissioning groups in the United Kingdom
- Healthcare professionals in emergency care services
- Healthcare professionals in primary care services (who may see a rise in attendance as a result of parents being diverted from emergency care)
- Practice managers, healthcare professionals and others who would assist with app dissemination (e.g. Health Visitors, midwives, staff at Children's Centres)

For health apps in particular, this can be challenging as people with the relevant health problems may either be difficult to find (e.g. if the disease is rare) or they may be reticent to engage (e.g. if the health problem is sensitive or attached to stigma). Even if the app is for use by the general public rather than a specific patient group (e.g. a weight loss app), it is still important to engage with *lay* members of the public, as opposed to those who are particularly familiar with technology, research or health-related topics. While it may be useful to undertake some initial testing with colleagues or other professionals, a lay insight is often invaluable. If the app is targeted towards professionals (e.g. an app to help healthcare professionals make decisions on optimal treatment), views of those who are not familiar with the project and its aims should be sought.

Developing relationships with patient groups can be a lengthy process that requires time and resources, and this should be taken into consideration during project planning stages. Most groups or channels that could be used to access community members (such as those listed in the box below) are safeguarded by some form of "gatekeeping" to protect members. Gatekeepers could include, for example, leaders of support groups, practice managers of clinics, or administrators of online groups. Substantial time needs to be invested to build rapport and trust before individuals are likely to consent to helping out with app design and usability testing.

For example, while social media provides a means to reach potentially thousands of individuals with relative ease by posting in public support groups, group members often do not take kindly to posts seeking to recruit members. Such groups often experience a high level of unsolicited posts advertising products or services, and therefore such posts are often quickly removed by admin. Before posting in such groups, therefore, it is always useful to approach admin first and request approval.

Similarly, support groups are frequently solicited for research purposes and those wishing to engage members need to invest time and resources into building a relationship first. This will usually involve reaching out to group leaders initially, and, with the group's prior approval, attending meetings to introduce oneself and the proposed work, before groups will consider getting involved. Such processes will often take several months. Additionally, financial resources will be required, as individuals will need to be reimbursed for their time and efforts (see invo.org.uk for details). Moreover, simple gestures like providing free lunches can have a substantial impact on relationship-building, providing the basis for fruitful exchanges.

Importantly, when attempting to engage user groups, efforts should be made to reach out to those who's views are less frequently heard. For example, patients who are members of support groups tend to be generally well-informed about their health and well-integrated into the local community. However, those who are least informed and/or linked up with their community are often those who need the most support, and who would most benefit from health interventions.

Reaching out to these "seldom heard" individuals can be challenging. Substantial time and resources will need to be invested to seek out such individuals and build trust. A useful way to achieve this is via pop-up stalls in community settings (e.g. shopping centres) or via "lay health volunteers". For example, in a community intervention which aimed to raise awareness of cancer warning signs and symptoms in Greater Manchester, lay members of the public were initially recruited and trained in providing information on the signs and symptoms of cancer as well as in the delivery of public engagement games [36]. These "lay health volunteers" then engaged with local communities in settings they were familiar with, such as local pubs, thereby recruiting further volunteers. This was useful because the lay volunteers had valuable knowledge, skills, and cultural understanding (such as speaking minority languages) that helped them connect and engage with vulnerable groups.

Another important consideration is *diversity* and *representativeness*. Particularly when developing an app for patient use, it is important to ensure a diverse range of views and opinions are heard, including those from minority ethnic groups and low-income groups. For example, in preparation for a clinical trial on preterm birth, Rayment et al. contacted mothers through clinics as well as churches in Local Authorities that were among the most deprived in England and convened discussion groups to actively involve women in discussions about the trial design [30]. This ensured inclusion and involvement of women across the diverse community, which was particularly important due to the high incidence of preterm births among women from minority ethnic communities and those from socioeconomically deprived groups. It should be noted, however, that mothers not attending churches were not reached through this recruitment method, thus potentially limiting the representativeness of the recruited group.

Example strategies to reach out to patient groups and lay members of the public

- Contacting patient support groups
- Reaching out to organisations or institutions such as schools, companies or charities
- Reaching out to community groups or clubs e.g. churches, sports groups, choir groups, theatre/arts groups. . .
- Social media (including online support groups), newsletters and listservs
- Posters/flyers in relevant clinical or community settings (given prior approval) e.g. hospital ward, pharmacies, clinics, libraries
- Stalls or pop-up stands in community settings e.g. shopping centres, markets, fairs, pubs, social clubs, leisure centres, libraries, museums. . .
- "Snowballing" recruitment: Recruiting "community champions" or "lay health volunteers" i.e. members of the public who can then recruit further community members, see e.g. [17], or using links via (health) professionals
- Contacting professional membership bodies (if your app is targeted for professionals)

3.9   Sufficient Engagement

Engagement with mHealth interventions is often low and attrition can be considerable. Only about a third of users who download an app will open the app on the following day. After two weeks, only about a tenth of users will still engage with the app. This is also known as the "app churn rate". Even when users download and use an app, they may not utilise all of its functions as intended. User engagement is not a unitary construct; it involves many different dimensions and qualities. Table 3.2 shows different dimensions of user engagement with health apps.

Such considerations are important because they may impact on the effectiveness of the intervention. Prior to and during app development, it is therefore worth thinking about the types and levels of engagement that you expect will lead to behaviour change. For example, some apps may only require user engagement over a short, intense period of time, whereas others will only be effective if used regularly over longer time frames. Determining these parameters early on will help ensure sufficient resources are allocated to promoting the required engagement levels, and will also be invaluable when assessing the effectiveness of the intervention. It is therefore important to establish empirically what engagement is expected to achieve behaviour change in the context of a particular intervention and for different user groups [22].

3.10   Evaluation

It is important to note that evaluation needs to be considered early on during developmental stages of an mHealth intervention, so that the app can be designed in a way that is conducive to evaluation. For example, it may be helpful to present different theoretical components in separate modules within the app, so that they can be tested separately. In our previous research on developing and testing a website to encourage people with potential lung cancer symptoms to seek timely help, we implemented this "modular approach". Our intervention involved two factors which we hypothesised would increase intention to seek help: (i) a component based on the Theory of Planned Behaviour which was designed to influence people's beliefs

Table 3.2   A selection of different measures of user engagement with health apps

Measure of engagement	Examples
Frequency	How often do users open the app or use a certain feature?
Duration	How long do users engage with the app during a session, or how long do they use the app overall before ceasing to use it?
Intensity	How does the frequency of use relate to the duration?
Completeness	How many of the available features does the user use?
Regularity	Does usage occur in regular patterns or irregular bursts?

about the target behaviour (seeking timely medical advice), and (ii) personalised content tailored to the individual users' symptoms and risk factors to enhance perceived personal relevance [25].

We presented these two components separately on separate pages of the website:

1. To address beliefs, users were presented with quotes by healthcare professionals and (fictional) patients and their family members, as well as practical advice on seeking medical advice.
2. For personalisation, users were presented with a page providing personalised information about their symptoms and risk factors, and a page providing personalised advice on whether an urgent referral for a chest x-ray would be indicated for them based on UK clinical guidelines.

By presenting these factors separately, we were then able to test them in a factorial study design, meaning that study participants were randomly allocated to one of four study groups, with different combinations of the factors in each group (Fig. 3.8).

This study design allowed us to compare whether the two factors were effective on their own, whether they were more effective when combined, and also how these compared to having neither of the factors. This provides much more valuable insights than simply testing an intervention against a single control group, as it allows an exploration of which individual components are effective, and in what combination.

As this example highlights, it is useful to think about evaluation during early stages of development of an intervention, to ensure intervention components are incorporated in a way that renders them testable.

Evaluation of mHealth interventions is discussed in further detail in Chap. 8.

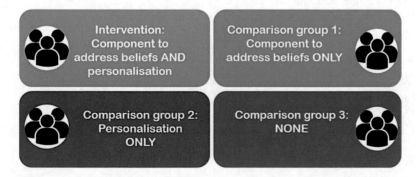

Fig. 3.8 Factorial study design used in our study to test the effects of different components of a website to encourage timely help-seeking for potential lung cancer symptoms

3.11   Summary of Key Points

This chapter provided an overview of the processes that should underlie the development of mHealth interventions to ensure the interventions are acceptable to users and likely to bring about desired improvements in health outcomes. Importantly, the intervention development process should not be viewed as a series of steps but as a cyclical, iterative approach involving several cycles of evidence review, user engagement, development/design and testing (ideally with users). Incorporation of psychological theory may be useful as it can highlight which factors should be targeted in order to bring about behaviour change. However, it should be noted that behaviour change theories do not always predict future behaviour accurately, and may not be suited to all contexts (e.g. specific cultural contexts). Therefore a review of extant literature and extensive engagement with your target population is of critical importance and should always be used to supplement theoretical underpinnings.

- Intervention development is likely to involve a cyclical approach, iterating through different stages repeatedly to continuously refine the intervention as new insights emerge, with no fixed start and end point, and no prescribed order of the stages
- It is recommended to use available evidence as well as insights from relevant users and stakeholders to inform the development of initial ideas for the health app
- Ethical considerations during intervention development include whether there is potential for harm to users and how this can be mitigated, whether the intervention would be classed as a medical device, and who would own data produced by the app
- Frameworks and approaches like the person-based approach can provide a useful basis to guide intervention development
- Behaviour change theories may be useful to identify which factors need to be changed in order to change behaviour
- Translation of theory into practice can be facilitated by Behaviour Change Techniques (BCTs)
- Methods to facilitate the incorporation of user input include interviews, focus groups, paper prototyping, and Think Aloud
- During development, thought should be given to what constitutes the appropriate type and level of engagement that should lead to successful behaviour change
- It is useful to devise plans for evaluation early on so that the intervention and its component features is testable

3.12 Quiz

1. Which statement best describes the Behaviour Change Wheel?

   (a) A framework which postulates that policy factors, intervention functions and different sources of behaviour interact to change behaviour
   (b) A linear model which postulates that behaviour change interventions have to include certain components and policy categories
   (c) A linear model in which components within the behaviour system interact with each other as do the functions within the intervention layer and the categories within the policy layer.

2. Which of the following is crucial to the person-based approach for digital intervention development? Several may apply.

   (a) Qualitative research to elicit users' views
   (b) Review of available evidence
   (c) Rigorous testing of the intervention in a randomised controlled trial
   (d) Review of relevant behaviour change theories
   (e) User testing of the intervention

3. Which of the following statements is most accurate?

   (a) Health apps are classed as medical devices and are therefore subject to national regulatory frameworks for medical devices.
   (b) Health apps are not classed as medical devices and are therefore not subject to regulatory frameworks.
   (c) Health apps are not classed as medical devices but are nevertheless subject to certain regulations set out by the Medicines and Health-care products Regulatory Agency
   (d) Health apps may be classed as medical devices depending on their functions, features, and intended use, and therefore national regulatory frameworks for medical devices may apply

Answers to the quiz can be found in "Solutions to Quizzes".

3.13 Exercises

1. Match the elements of the MRC Framework for Developing and Evaluating Complex Interventions to their descriptions.

1. Development	a. Testing procedures and determining sample size
2. Implementation	b. Assessing effectiveness
3. Evaluation	c. Dissemination and long-term follow-up
4. Feasibility/piloting	d. Identifying theory and evidence

2. A study with focus groups of people with asthma has shown that a main reason why people do not comply with prescribed treatment is because they are not sure how to use their inhaler. Identify the relevant precursor of behaviour based on the behaviour change wheel, and list features that could be included in an app to address this problem.
3. Using the most up-to-date guidance, assess whether the following app would be considered a "medical device" in the UK: An app was developed to help patients with fibromyalgia track and monitor their symptoms, including pain, stiffness, fatigue, sleep problems, and cognitive problems. The app encourages users to use the app during consultations with their healthcare professionals to help inform treatment decisions.

Recommended Reading

1. Conner M, Norman P. Predicting and changing health behaviour: research and practice with social cognition models, 3rd edn. Berkshire: Open University Press; 2015.
2. Ogden J. Health psychology: a textbook. Berkshire: Open University Press; 2012.
3. Greenhalgh T. How to implement evidence-based healthcare. Hoboken: Wiley/Blackwell; 2018.
4. Michie S, Richardson M, Johnston M, Abraham C, Francis J, Hardeman W, · · · Wood CE. The behavior change technique taxonomy (v1) of 93 hierarchically clustered techniques: building an international consensus for the reporting of behavior change interventions. Annals of Behavioral Medicine?: A Publication of the Society of Behavioral Medicine, 2013;46(1):81–95. https://doi.org/10.1007/s12160-013-9486-6
5. Michie S, Atkins L, West R. The behavior change wheel: a guide to designing interventions. Silverback Publishing; 2014.
6. Michie S, Yardley L, West R, Patrick K, Greaves F. Developing and evaluating digital interventions to promote behavior change in health and health care: recommendations resulting from an international workshop. J Med Internet Res. 2017;19(6):e232. https://doi.org/10.2196/jmir.7126
7. Mueller J, Davies A, Jay C, Harper S, Blackhall F, Summers Y, Harle A, Todd C. Developing and testing a web-based intervention to encourage early help-seeking in people with symptoms associated with lung cancer. Br J Health Psychol. 2018;24:31–65. https://doi.org/10.1111/bjhp.12325
8. Yardley L, Morrison L, Bradbury K, Muller I. The person-based approach to intervention development: application to digital health-related behav-ior change interventions. J Med Internet Res. 2015;17(1):e30. https://doi.org/10.2196/jmir.4055
9. Davies A. Carrying out systematic literature reviews: an introduction. Br J Nurs. 2019;28(15):1008–14.

References

1. Australian Government – Department of Health – Therapeutic Goods Administration. Regulation of software as a medical device; 2018. https://www.tga.gov.au/regulation-software-medical-device
2. Cane J, Richardson M, Johnston M, Ladha R, Michie S. From lists of behaviour change techniques (BCTs) to structured hierarchies: comparison of two methods of developing a

hierarchy of BCTs. Br J Health Psychol. 2015;20(1):130–50. https://doi.org/10.1111/bjhp. 12102

3. Centre for Reviews and Dissemination. Systematic reviews: CRD's guidance for undertaking reviews in health care; 2009.

4. Conner M, Norman P. Predicting and changing health behaviour: research and practice with social cognition models, 3rd edn. Berkshire: Open University Press; 2015.

5. Connolly V, Unwin N, Sherriff P, Bilous R, Kelly W. Diabetes prevalence and socioeconomic status: a population based study showing increased prevalence of type 2 diabetes mellitus in deprived areas. J Epidemiol Community Health. 2000;54(3):173–7. https://doi.org/10.1136/ JECH.54.3.173

6. Crane D, Garnett C, Brown J, West R, Michie S. Factors influencing usability of a smartphone app to reduce excessive alcohol consumption: think aloud and interview studies. Front Public Health. 2017;5:39. https://doi.org/10.3389/fpubh.2017.00039

7. Davies A, Mueller J, Hennings J, Caress A-L, Jay C. Recommendations for developing support tools with people suffering from Chronic Obstructive Pulmonary Disease: co-design and pilot testing of a health prototype. JMIR Human Factors. 2020;7(2):e16289. https://doi.org/10.2196/ 16289

8. Davis SR, Peters D, Calvo RA, Sawyer SM, Foster JM, Smith L. Kiss myAsthma: using a participatory design approach to develop a self-management app with young people with asthma. J Asthma. 2018;55(9):1018–27. https://doi.org/10.1080/02770903.2017.1388391

9. Estacio EV, Whittle R, Protheroe J. The digital divide: examining socio-demographic factors associated with health literacy, access and use of internet to seek health information. J Health Psychol. 2019;24(12):1668–1675. https://doi.org/10.1177/1359105317695429

10. Federal Trade Commission. Mobile health apps interactive tool; 2016. https://www.ftc.gov/ tips-advice/business-center/guidance/mobile-health-apps-interactive-tool

11. Flores Mateo G, Granado-Font E, Ferré-Grau C, Montaña-Carreras X. Mobile phone apps to promote weight loss and increase physical activity: a systematic review and meta-analysis. J Med Internet Res. 2015;17(11):e253. https://doi.org/10.2196/jmir.4836

12. Greenhalgh T, Thorne S, Malterud K. Time to challenge the spurious hierarchy of systematic over narrative reviews? Eur J Clin Investig. 2018;48(6):e12931. https://doi.org/10.1111/eci. 12931

13. International Medical Device Regulators Forum. (n.d.). IMDRF technical documents. Retrieved December 11, 2019, http://www.imdrf.org/documents/documents.asp#technical

14. Jamshed S. Qualitative research method-interviewing and observation. J Basic Clin Pharm. 2014;5(4):87–8. https://doi.org/10.4103/0976-0105.141942

15. Kontos E, Blake KD, Sylvia Chou W-Y, Prestin A. Predictors of eHealth usage: insights on the digital divide from the Health Information National Trends Survey 2012. J Med Internet Res. 2014;16(7):e172. https://doi.org/10.2196/jmir.3117

16. Krebs P, Duncan DT. Health app use among US mobile phone owners: a national survey. JMIR mHealth uHealth. 2015;3(4):e101. https://doi.org/10.2196/mhealth.4924

17. Lyon D, Knowles J, Slater B, Kennedy R. Improving the early presentation of cancer symptoms in disadvantaged communities: putting local people in control. Br J Cancer. 2009;101(Suppl):S49–S54.

18. Medicines and Healthcare products Regulatory Agency. Guidance: medical device standalone software including apps (including IVDMDs); 2018. https://www.gov.uk/government/ publications/medical-devices-software-applications-apps

19. Michie S, Johnston M, Francis J, Hardeman W, Eccles M. From theory to intervention: mapping theoretically derived behavioural determinants to behaviour change techniques. Appl Psychol. 2008;57(4):660–80. https://doi.org/10.1111/j.1464-0597.2008.00341.x

20. Michie S, van Stralen MM, West R. The behaviour change wheel: a new method for characterising and designing behaviour change interventions. Implement Sci. 2011;6(1):42. https://doi.org/10.1186/1748-5908-6-42

21. Michie S, Atkins L, West R. The behaviour change wheel: a guide to designing interventions. London: Silverback Publishing; 2014. www.behaviourchangewheel.com

22. Michie S, Yardley L, West R, Patrick K, Greaves F. Developing and evaluating digital interventions to promote behavior change in health and health care: recommendations resulting from an international workshop. J Med Internet Res. 2017;19(6):e232. https://doi.org/10.2196/jmir.7126

23. Moher D. Preferred reporting items for systematic reviews and meta-analyses: the PRISMA statement. Ann Intern Med. 2009;151(4):264. https://doi.org/10.7326/0003-4819-151-4-200908180-00135

24. Moher D, Stewart L, Shekelle P. All in the family: systematic reviews, rapid reviews, scoping reviews, realist reviews, and more. Syst Rev. 2015;4(1):183. https://doi.org/10.1186/s13643-015-0163-7

25. Mueller J, Davies A, Jay C, Harper S, Blackhall F, Summers Y, Harle A, Todd C. Developing and testing a web-based intervention to encourage early help-seeking in people with symptoms associated with lung cancer. Br J Health Psychol. 2018;24:31–65. https://doi.org/10.1111/bjhp.12325

26. National Health Service. (n.d.). NHS Apps Library. Retrieved March 22, 2019. https://www.nhs.uk/apps-library/

27. Organisation for the Review of Care and Health Applications (ORCHA) www.orcha.co.uk, Feb 29, 2020

28. Poushter J. Smartphone ownership and Internet usage continues to climb in emerging economies. Technical report, Pew Research Center; 2016. http://s1.pulso.cl/wp-content/uploads/2016/02/2258581.pdf

29. Rabiee F. Focus-group interview and data analysis. Proc Nutr Soc. 2004;63(4):655–60. http://www.ncbi.nlm.nih.gov/pubmed/15831139

30. Rayment J, Lanlehin R, McCourt C, Husain SM. Involving seldom-heard groups in a PPI process to inform the design of a proposed trial on the use of probiotics to prevent preterm birth: a case study. Res Involvement Engagement. 2017;3(1):11. https://doi.org/10.1186/s40900-017-0061-3

31. Romeo A, Edney S, Plotnikoff R, Curtis R, Ryan J, Sanders I, Crozier A, Maher C. Can smartphone apps increase physical activity? Systematic review and meta-analysis. J Med Internet Res. 2019;21(3):e12053. https://doi.org/10.2196/12053

32. Sucala M, Cuijpers P, Muench F, Cardo R, Soflau R, Dobrean A, Achimas-Cadariu P, David D. Anxiety: there is an app for that. A systematic review of anxiety apps. Depress Anxiety. 2017;34(6):518–25. https://doi.org/10.1002/da.22654

33. Tricco AC, Antony J, Zarin W, Strifler L, Ghassemi M, Ivory J, Perrier L, Hutton B, Moher D, Straus SE. A scoping review of rapid review methods. BMC Med. 2015;13(1):224. https://doi.org/10.1186/s12916-015-0465-6

34. van Dijk J, Hacker K. The digital divide as a complex and dynamic phenomenon. Inf Soc. 2003;19(4):315–26. https://doi.org/10.1080/01972240309487

35. Webb TL, Joseph J, Yardley L, Michie S. Using the Internet to promote health behavior change: a systematic review and meta-analysis of the impact of theoretical basis, use of behavior change techniques, and mode of delivery on efficacy. J Med Internet Res. 2010;12(1):e4. https://doi.org/10.2196/jmir.1376

36. Williams G, Mueller J, Mbeledogu C, Spencer A, Parry-Harries E, Harrison A, Clough G, Greenhalgh C, Verma A. The impact of a volunteer-led community cancer awareness programme on knowledge of cancer risk factors and symptoms, screening, and barriers to seeking help. Patient Educ Couns. 2019;103:563–70. https://doi.org/10.1016/j.pec.2019.09.025

37. World Health Organization. (n.d.). International Classification of Health Interventions (ICHI). Retrieved March 8, 2019; https://www.who.int/classifications/ichi/en/

38. Yardley L, Morrison L, Bradbury K, Muller I. The person-based approach to intervention development: application to digital health-related behavior change interventions. J Med Internet Res. 2015;17(1):e30. https://doi.org/10.2196/jmir.4055

39. Yoon H, Jang Y, Vaughan PW, Garcia M. Older Adults' Internet use for health information: digital divide by race/ethnicity and socioeconomic status. J Appl Gerontol. 2020;39(1):105–110. https://doi.org/10.1177/0733464818770772

Chapter 4
Application Development and Testing

4.1 Introduction

This chapter focuses on the actual implementation of an mHealth application. Where the term development is used in this context, it refers to activities surrounding the application implementation itself. There have been entire books written about this aspect of development alone (e.g. [16, 25]) and it is beyond the scope of this book to cover this in depth. Frameworks and tools for developing mobile apps change so frequently that conveying such topics is challenging in the medium of a book. We recommend visiting the websites of the vendors of these tools directly to ensure that you are always using the most up-to-date versions and practices. There are usually many videos, blogs and tutorials that are invaluable in applying the latest methods of app development. This chapter will take an overview of the different choices that need to be made in order to transform your proposed intervention into an actual app. We will look at the kinds of technologies and options available with examples and case studies of their use. After reading this chapter, it is hoped that it would help to bridge the gap between the software developers and other members of the project team in terms of the different options available and what implementing them may entail.

In the first instance, following consideration of the broader issues around the general design of the proposed intervention and the methodology that will be adopted for its creation (see previous chapters), consideration then needs to be given to the actual app development process. This necessitates making certain decisions regarding what form this will take. As discussed in Chap. 2, the cost of a project increases the further along the development cycle we go. As we move into the production phase, the costs can be significant. Many of the decisions you make will be based on the goal of the intervention being produced and its target audience. The mobile app market more broadly is split essentially into apps that operate on two main operating systems, iOS and Android. The iOS is provided by Apple Inc. whereas Android was developed by Google following its acquisition of Android Inc.

© Springer Nature Switzerland AG 2020   111
A. Davies, J. Mueller, *Developing Medical Apps and mHealth Interventions*, Health Informatics, https://doi.org/10.1007/978-3-030-47499-7_4

in 2005. In 2018 Android made up around 69% of the market share (based on market shares) compared to iOS which had 29% [18]. The majority of apps produced are for one or both of theses platforms.

4.2   Choosing a Platform

As stated, the choice of platform(s) depends on the goal of the intervention and who you are trying to reach with your app. The mobile app market was worth 365 billion US dollars in 2018 and is projected to grow to 935 billion by 2023 [8]. The vast majority of app downloads are for free apps. This means that in order to monetise an app, one has to consider alternative revenue streams. These can include paid advertising promotions, subscriptions for services, selling on user data and sponsorship. Given the nature of health and medical apps and their potential for collecting personal and/or sensitive data, careful consideration should be given to the security aspects regarding keeping people's data safe. In some cases, third party components included in apps for commercial purposes can introduce security risks. These aspects are discussed in more detail in Chap. 5.

The most popular category of app downloaded across all platforms are games (22%) followed by business (10%) [9]. Health and fitness apps make up only 3.3% with medical app downloads even lower at 1.9% [9]. Commercialisation of an app may well come through other services and organisations of which the app forms a component. Apps are usually distributed via an 'app store' such as the Google Play store (Fig. 4.1) or a dedicated library, such as the UK's NHS Apps Library (Fig. 4.2).

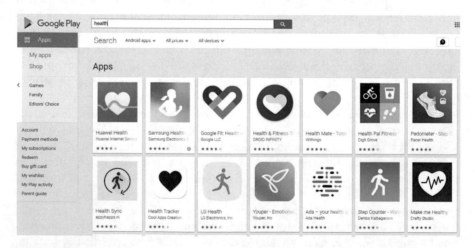

Fig. 4.1 Screenshot of Google Play store in category 'Health'. (Screenshot reproduced with permission). Google Play is a trademark of Google LLC

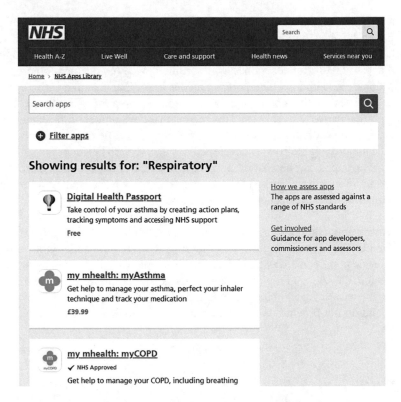

Fig. 4.2 NHS Apps Library, category 'respiratory'; https://www.nhs.uk/apps-library/. (Screenshot reproduced with permission)

The main two ways of coding (programming) mobile applications is to either embark on native app development or hybrid app development. The former involves writing code in a programming language(s) that is designed to work on a particular mobile operating system (OS). The main advantages of this are that apps tend to perform better. This is because, by writing them for a specific OS, they are optimized to leverage performance features of that OS. This can be especially useful if your app relies a lot on fast and efficient performance (e.g. uses a lot of processing power or requires lots of graphical features). The tool-kits for native development often include various templates and functionality that help the app look and feel like other apps on that platform, giving users a consistent user experience. This approach is also ideal if you know that you only want to target one specific OS. Even if you decide to develop natively for multiple operating systems, it can still be easier to fix bugs if you have two different code bases, one for each version, than a single shared code base. This may mean that despite higher up-front costs, the longer term maintainability of native apps may be less costly.

The alternative to this is to make a web app or a hybrid app (progressive web app). This option involves building the app using web technologies (e.g. HTML, CSS, JavaScript) as one would for a conventional web site. There are tools that bridge the hybrid app so that it can access hardware on the device (e.g. camera, microphone, notifications, etc.) although their performance is lower than that of a native app. The main advantages are that coding this type of app can be a lot easier than using the languages that native apps rely on. This means that development time can be much faster, which in turn reduces some of the up-front costs. The other main advantage is that the majority of the code is developed in the core web languages meaning that these types of apps can be written once and work on both iOS and Android with minimal additional extra work. This approach definitely has advantages for simple apps with minimal performance requirements.

These hybrid or Progressive Web Apps (PWA) are not to be confused with web apps. A web app requires an active internet connection and is essentially a web site optimized for use on a device. They are not able to access the underlying hardware on the device in the same way that PWA can. A simple web app is the fastest way to build an app, they do not require installation or downloading from an app store, and they are the easiest type to build, maintain and update. They do not however work offline, and do not provide the same functionality or look and feel as a native app or PWA.

4.2.1   iOS

In order to release your apps on iOS, you must first sign up for a developer account with Apple. Developer accounts can be set up by individuals or companies/organizations. For companies, a DUNS number (Data Universal Numbering System) for identifying unique companies is required. Another requirement is a public facing website. Once signed up, a developer can use what is known as a *provisioning profile*. This lets you link particular devices to the development team, allowing you to run and test the app on a device(s) (e.g. iPhone, iPad). As only signed (by Apple) apps can be installed on iOS devices, one cannot simply run their app on their device. In order to test the app on a device, the provisioning profile which is downloaded from your developer account is used. A provisioning profile is actually a collection of different entities that contain the ID of the individual app that you want to test, a development certificate (public key) and details of the authorised device (its ID). These are then linked to the development team's provisioning profile that contains details of the app ID's, certificates and authorised device IDs. To move from testing and development to release one has to switch from a development to a distribution profile. Subsequently the app can be submitted to the app store for checking and distribution.

4.2.2   Programming for iOS

The main programming languages used for developing code for iOS applications are
Objective-C and *Swift*. Objective-C is an object orientated language used for Mac
OS and iOS development. An example of the syntax can be seen in Listing 4.1.

```objectivec
#import "MainViewController.h"

@implementation MainViewController

- (id)initWithNibName:(NSString *)nibNameOrNil bundle:(NSBundle *)
    nibBundleOrNil
{
    self = [super initWithNibName:nibNameOrNil bundle:
    nibBundleOrNil];
    if (self) {
        // Custom initialization
    }
    return self;
}

- (void)didReceiveMemoryWarning
{
    // Releases the view if it doesn't have a superview.
    [super didReceiveMemoryWarning];

    // Release any cached data, images, etc that aren't in use.
}

#pragma mark — View lifecycle

- (void)viewWillAppear:(BOOL)animated
{
    // Set the main view to utilize the entire application frame
    space of the device.
    // Change this to suit your view's UI footprint needs in your
    application.

    UIView* rootView = [[[[UIApplication sharedApplication]
    keyWindow] rootViewController] view];
    CGRect webViewFrame = [[[rootView subviews] objectAtIndex:0]
    frame]; // first subview is the UIWebView

    if (CGRectEqualToRect(webViewFrame, CGRectZero)) { //
    UIWebView is sized according to its parent, here it hasn't
    been sized yet
        self.view.frame = [[UIScreen mainScreen] applicationFrame
    ]; // size UIWebView's parent according to application frame,
    which will in turn resize the UIWebView
    }

    [super viewWillAppear:animated];
}
```

```
38
39  - (void)viewDidLoad
40  {
41      [super viewDidLoad];
42      // Do any additional setup after loading the view from its
        nib.
43  }
44
45  - (void)viewDidUnload
46  {
47      [super viewDidUnload];
48      // Release any retained subviews of the main view.
49      // e.g. self.myOutlet = nil;
50  }
51
52  - (BOOL)shouldAutorotateToInterfaceOrientation:
53      (UIInterfaceOrientation)interfaceOrientation
54  {
55      // Return YES for supported orientations
56      return [super shouldAutorotateToInterfaceOrientation:
        interfaceOrientation];
57  }
58
59  ...
```

Listing 4.1 Snippet of Objective-C code form the 'mainViewController.m' file generated by Xcode. Available under the Apache License, Version 2.0 (http://www.apache.org/licenses/LICENSE-2.0)

Swift [4] is a language that supports development for iOS (also macOS, watchOS, tvOS). Both Swift and Objective-C can be used together and are interoperable. An example of a basic *Hello World* program written in Objective-C and Swift can be seen in Listings 4.2 and 4.3 respectively.

```
1  #import <Foundation/Foundation.h>
2
3  int main(int argc, const char *argv[]) {
4      @autoreleasepool {
5          NSLog(@"Hello, World!");
6      }
7      return 0;
8  }
```

Listing 4.2 Hello world program written in Objective-C

```
1  import Swift
2  print("Hello, World!")
```

Listing 4.3 Hello world program written in Swift

4.2.3 Tools for Health and Medical App Development

Apple provide some dedicated open source frameworks for health-related application development. These include *CareKit*, *HealthKit* and *ResearchKit*.

CareKit can be used for care plan development, symptom tracking and connecting individuals to teams that provide care by linking individual patients to care plans. Care plans contain contacts for the care providers and task entities. The tasks are activities the patient should carry out with an associated schedule (e.g. to take medication at a specific point in time). Tasks can also have associated outcomes and values [1].

The HealthKit can be integrated into apps to provide a central repository for fitness and health related data [2]. HealthKit apps can exchange data (with permission from the user) to provide a more seamless experience.

ResearchKit [3] has been used successfully for several app-based research projects. An example of its use is the first phase of the PRIDE study which used the ResearchKit to recruit over 18,000 participants and collect survey data from over 24,000 surveys [29]. Another app aimed at pregnant women in the US used the ResearchKit to gather survey and sensor data from over 2000 pregnant women [24].

4.2.4 Android

The Android app for fitness tracking is *Google Fit* [14]. Using sensor data from the device, Google Fit is able to track various user activities, such as walking, running etc. This can be linked to other vendor-made apps to display the users' data in one place. Developers can use this to upload various fitness data to a central repository for users to access [15]. This also allows developers to access data collected by others apps, store data from sensors and wearables as well allowing user data to persist when they decide to upgrade their various fitness devices [15]. There are a variety of APIs available as part of the Google Play services. These include APIs for sensors, recording/storing fitness data, history (to manage such data) and goals that allow tracking of the goals the user sets in the various apps.

4.2.5 Programming for Android

The main language used to develop Android apps is *Java*. Java is an object orientated programming language that is compiled to byte-code and then run on a java virtual machine (JVM). Another language growing in popularity is *Kotlin* [21], which works similarly to Java. It can also interact with Java and runs on the JVM. Kotlin is arguably simpler for beginners to learn than Java. A sample *Hello World* program can seen in both Java (Listing 4.4) and Kotlin (Listing 4.5).

```java
1  public class HelloWorld{
2      public static void main(String []args) {
3          System.out.println("Hello World!");
4      }
5  }
```

Listing 4.4 Hello world program in Java

```kotlin
1  fun main() {
2      println("Hello World!")
3  }
```

Listing 4.5 Hello world program in Kotlin

Other languages that are used for Android app development (although with less frequency than Java and Kotlin) include C++ and C# (pronounced C-sharp). An example of a simple Hello world program written C++ can be seen in Listing 4.6.

```cpp
1  #include <iostream>
2  using namespace std;
3
4  int main()
5  {
6      cout << "Hello world!" << endl;
7      return 0;
8  }
```

Listing 4.6 Hello world program in C++

It is also possible to write apps using Python. One such Python library for app development is called *Kivy* [20]. A sample program written using the Kivy library can be seen in Listing 4.7.

```python
1  import kivy
2  kivy.require('1.11.0')
3  from kivy.app import App
4  from kivy.uix.label import Label
5
6  class HelloWorldApp(App):
7      def build(self):
8          return Label(text='Hello world!')
9
10 if __name__ == '__main__':
11     HelloWorldApp().run()
```

Listing 4.7 Hello world program using the Python Kivy library

4.2.6   Progressive Web Apps (PWA)

Coding a PWA often requires creating a *WebView*. This is an embedded browser that the native app uses to display the web content. Lines 17 and 18 of Listing 4.8 show an example of how the folder and associated main app HTML page (the start page) are referenced in the Objective-C file that would launch the PWA on the device creating a WebView loading the *index.html* page.

```objc
- (BOOL)application:(UIApplication *)application
    didFinishLaunchingWithOptions:(NSDictionary *)launchOptions
{
    NSURL* url = [launchOptions objectForKey:
    UIApplicationLaunchOptionsURLKey];
    NSString* invokeString = nil;

    if (url && [url isKindOfClass:[NSURL class]]) {
        invokeString = [url absoluteString];
        NSLog(@"nighttimeExpress launchOptions = %@", url);
    }

    CGRect screenBounds = [[UIScreen mainScreen] bounds];
    self.window = [[[UIWindow alloc] initWithFrame:screenBounds]
    autorelease];
    self.window.autoresizesSubviews = YES;

    self.viewController = [[[MainViewController alloc] init]
    autorelease];
    self.viewController.useSplashScreen = YES;
    self.viewController.wwwFolderName = @"www";
    self.viewController.startPage = @"app/index.html";
    self.viewController.invokeString = invokeString;

    // NOTE: To control the view's frame size, override [self.
    viewController viewWillAppear:] in your view controller.

    // check whether the current orientation is supported: if it
    is, keep it, rather than forcing a rotation
    BOOL forceStartupRotation = YES;
    UIDeviceOrientation curDevOrientation = [[UIDevice
    currentDevice] orientation];

    if (UIDeviceOrientationUnknown == curDevOrientation) {
        // UIDevice isn't firing orientation notifications yet go
        look at the status bar
        curDevOrientation = (UIDeviceOrientation)[[UIApplication
        sharedApplication] statusBarOrientation];
    }

    if (UIDeviceOrientationIsValidInterfaceOrientation(
    curDevOrientation)) {
        if ([self.viewController supportsOrientation:
    curDevOrientation]) {
            forceStartupRotation = NO;
        }
    }

    if (forceStartupRotation) {
        UIInterfaceOrientation newOrient;
```

```
40       if ([self.viewController supportsOrientation:
     UIInterfaceOrientationPortrait]) {
41           newOrient = UIInterfaceOrientationPortrait;
42       } else if ([self.viewController supportsOrientation:
     UIInterfaceOrientationLandscapeLeft]) {
43           newOrient = UIInterfaceOrientationLandscapeLeft;
44       } else if ([self.viewController supportsOrientation:
     UIInterfaceOrientationLandscapeRight]) {
45           newOrient = UIInterfaceOrientationLandscapeRight;
46       } else {
47           newOrient = UIInterfaceOrientationPortraitUpsideDown;
48       }
49
50       NSLog(@"AppDelegate forcing status bar to: %d from: %d",
     newOrient, curDevOrientation);
51       [[UIApplication sharedApplication]
     setStatusBarOrientation:newOrient];
52       }
53
54       self.window.rootViewController = self.viewController;
55       [self.window makeKeyAndVisible];
56
57       return YES;
58 }
```

Listing 4.8 Snippet of Objective-C code form the 'AppDelegate.m' file generated by X-code. Available under the Apache License, Version 2.0 (http://www.apache.org/licenses/LICENSE-2.0)

4.2.7 PWA Frameworks

There are a few frameworks that can help with the design and construction of PWAs. These include Cordova (formally PhoneGap) [26]. Cordova provides web views for construction of PWAs using web technologies (JavaScript, CSS and HTML). This provides a wrapper for accessing native functionality on a device, such as the camera, accelerometer data, contacts and so on. Listing 4.9 show an example of a JavaScript function that uses the Cordova API to take a photo with the devices' camera using the *camera.getPicture* function. This then returns the image as a base64 encoded string.

```
1 function takePhoto() {
2     navigator.camera.getPicture(onSuccess, onFail, {
3         quality: 50,
4         destinationType: destinationType.DATA_URL
5     });
6 }
```

Listing 4.9 Example of JavaScript function for photo capture using Cordova API

Another popular framework is *Ionic* [17]. Ionic provides UI components that work across mobile platforms. It also provides access to plugins for native device functionality (camera access, geo-location etc.). An example section of code from an app made using Ionic can be seen in Listing 4.10.

```
import { Component } from '@angular/core';
import { Geolocation } from '@ionic-native/geolocation';
import { NavController, AlertController, LoadingController } from
    'ionic-angular';
import { Storage } from '@ionic/storage';
import { Http, Headers, RequestOptions } from '@angular/http';

import { Home } from '../home/home';

import * as moment from 'moment-timezone';

@Component({
  selector: 'page-symptoms',
  templateUrl: 'symptoms.html',
  providers: [Geolocation]
})
export class Symptoms {

  public symptoms = {
    howfeeling: 0,
    nose: 0,
    breathing: 0,
    eyes: 0,
    meds: 0,
    datetime: '',
    lat: 0.0,
    long: 0.0,
    rating: ['None', 'Mild', 'Moderate', 'Severe']
  }

  public page = {
    howfeeling: false,
    symptoms: true,
    thanks: true
  }
  ...
```

Listing 4.10 Example extract of code from Ionic mobile app for self-reporting of symptoms

Ionic also supports the use of *TypeScript* which is a superset of JavaScript. It was designed by Microsoft and supports static typing of variables, classes and interfaces (see box "what is an interface" for details). This can help with larger projects to make them more robust and reduce errors. Dynamic typing allows the creation of variables where the variable type is determined by its content. An example can be seen in Listing 4.11 where a variable named x is declared and assigned the value of 5. This is more flexible but can also allow a variable to subsequently change its type, leading to unexpected errors. In a statically typed language such as C this will generate an error (Listings 4.12 and 4.13).

```
1 x = 5
```

Listing 4.11 Python code showing variable declaration and assignment

```
1 #include <stdio.h>
2
3 void main(void);
4
5 void main(void)
6 {
7     x = 5;
8 }
```

Listing 4.12 C code showing variable assignment without defining the variables type prior to use

```
1 main.c: In function 'main':
2 main.c:15:5: error: 'x' undeclared (first use in this function)
3     x = 5;
4     ^
```

Listing 4.13 Compiler error message

To rectify this error in a statically typed language, the variables type needs to be defined before the variable can be used (Listing 4.14).

```
1 #include <stdio.h>
2
3 void main(void);
4
5 void main(void)
6 {
7     int x;
8     x = 5;
9 }
```

Listing 4.14 Defining the type of the variable before use. In this case an integer

Integrated development environments (IDEs) can also work with TypeScript to detect errors while you type. TypeScript is compiled into JavaScript and helps to scale JavaScript projects. Other popular mobile web development frameworks are summarised in Table 4.1.

PWAs can be developed using the development tools in modern web browsers. This lets us see what the layout looks like at different screen sizes and allows us to leverage web development tools like object inspectors and the console to help us debug the application (Fig. 4.3). It should be noted however that to test any interaction with the device's hardware such as cameras, sensors, contacts etc. we would need to use a simulator or build the code on the device itself.

Table 4.1 Some other web development frameworks for mobile app creation

Framework name	Description	Link
React Native	Created by Facebook. Allows JavaScript to use native components instead of web components like React to build native apps	https://reactnative.dev/
Appcelerator Titanium	Provides access to iOS and Android APIs and has a visual design interface	https://www.appcelerator.com/
Xamarin	Platform for building apps with .NET and C#	https://dotnet.microsoft.com/apps/xamarin
Flutter	Made by Google. An open sources UI SDK	https://flutter.dev/
jQuery Mobile	Described as a touch-optimised UI web framework	https://jquerymobile.com/

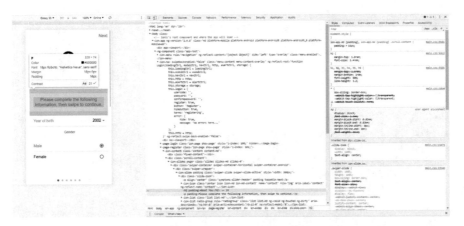

Fig. 4.3 Using web based development tools to debug a PWA and inspect its elements. Google Chrome Developer tools. Google Chrome is a trademark of Google LLC

What is an interface:

Interfaces provide another level of abstraction in Object Orientated Programming (OOP). They can be applied to a set of similar classes and follow a few conventions.

- The interface contains *function prototypes* which show the definition of an expected function(s)

(continued)

- They do not contain any variables or other code to implement the functions
- They are a description of possible actions rather than the actual implementation
- They enforce the correct use of a class, for example ensuring that they must have a particular function

Here is an example interface in Java for a set of Phone classes:

```java
interface Phone {
    public void checkProviderSignal();
    public float checkBatteryLevel();
}

class SmartPhoneXSeries implements Phone {

    float batteryLevelPC = 100;

    public void checkProviderSignal() {
        System.out.println("Checking provider signal!");
    }
    public float checkBatteryLevel(){
        System.out.println("Checking battery level");
        return(batteryLevelPC);
    }
}

public class InterfaceExample{
    public static void main(String [] args){
        SmartPhoneXSeries xseries = new SmartPhoneXSeries();
        xseries.checkProviderSignal();
        xseries.checkBatteryLevel();
    }
}
```

Here we have an interface for a set of Phone classes. The interface stipulates that the classes should include functions for checking the phone signal from the provider network and level of charge in the battery. All classes that use this interface must have implementations of these functions.

4.2.8 Coding Setup

Prior to starting development, some time should be factored in for setting up the development environment. This may not be necessary if one regularly produces apps using the same set of tools. Having the right setup configured correctly is essential for an individual or team that is considering app creation for the first time or maybe for a different operating system than usual.

It is important to have the required hardware and software for such tasks. One needs a well equipped workstation with a machine optimized for development. It would also be advantageous to have several physical devices (smartphones) for testing. There are many simulators that can be used to test the app on the machine it is being coded on. Although these simulators are extremely useful, especially in the earlier stages of development, nothing beats actually trying the app out on a device. We have at times found issues that were only present on the actual device but worked in the simulator. Obviously it is infeasible to have every single device you might want to deploy to given the plethora of different devices (especially for Android). Having 2 or 3 of the most widely used devices can be helpful. This is also useful for demonstrating the app to others (stakeholders, end users, developers).

Most programmers use an integrated development environment (IDE) to write code. This is the same for app developers. An IDE is software that provides several integrated features that are helpful for software development. This can include features like a code editor, a file browser to view files on the local system, an object browser that shows classes and related methods, a debugger for debugging code and often a console to view the output of code or execute commands directly. Some also come with version control integration. The code editor is usually the primary feature and does things like syntax highlighting to show keywords and other features of a particular language. Many will also allow auto completion and help with tasks like indenting blocks of code. Some IDEs are aimed at specific languages, while others support development in multiple languages. Table 4.2 provides some examples of commonly used IDEs. These features combine to make the task of software development easier and faster for the developer.

For native iOS projects, *Xcode* is the preferred IDE. This also supports features for app deployment onto the app store. For Android the main IDE is *Android Studio* and was designed specifically for app development purposes.

4.3 Design Patterns

When writing code, there are lots of ways that you could go about designing how your code will work. This is important because it can be easy to design the code in such a way that makes it difficult to respond to future changes or to maintain it. As this is quite a common issue, others have come up with a set of common ways of approaching the design of code that over time have been distilled into various

Table 4.2 List of some common Integrated Development Environments (IDEs)

IDE name	Description	Link
Android studio	Designed for Android app development	https://developer.android.com/studio
Eclipse	Mostly known for Java but supports other languages	https://www.eclipse.org/ide/
Xcode	For iOS development (Objective-C/Swift)	https://developer.apple.com/xcode/
Visual studio code	Multiple languages	https://code.visualstudio.com/
Atom	Multiple languages	https://ide.atom.io/
PyCharm	For Python	https://www.jetbrains.com/pycharm/
Spyder	Scientific Python/data science	https://www.spyder-ide.org/
NetBeans	Multiple languages	https://netbeans.org/

different design patterns. These patterns tend to fall into a main sub-category which include *behavioral*, *structural* and *creational* types. As seen in the box below, there are many different patterns to choose from:

List of design patterns:

- Singleton
- Command
- Composite
- Adapter
- State
- Template
- Factory
- Abstract factory
- Observer
- Strategy
- Iterator
- Decorator
- Facade
- Proxy

Adapted from [12]

Failing to use a design pattern and producing unstructured code can lead to problems like duplication of code and bloating of the code base [10]. This makes the code difficult to maintain and extend.

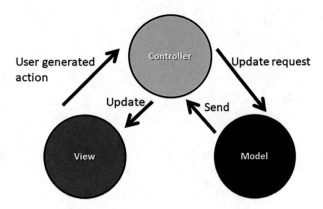

Fig. 4.4 Diagrammatic representation of Model-view-controller (MCV)

4.3.1 Model-View-Controller

The Model-view-controller or MCV is widely used in app development. It is used to separate out (decouple) the information representations between the three elements of *model*, *view* and *controller*. This has the effect of isolating the business logic from both the user interface and the data representation [10]. This type of design is often used with web development (and hence also applicable to web apps and PWA). It supports simultaneous development, as different developers can work on the different components simultaneously. This helps to organise code into related sections and can help to add structure to larger projects making them more manageable. The MCV pattern can also be extended to include other patterns (Fig. 4.4).

An example of the MVC can be seen in Listings 4.15 (models), 4.16 (controller) and 4.17 (views). This was for an information dashboard to present prescribing data written in Python.

```
from app import db

class PrescribingData(db.Model):
    """class for the prescription data table."""
    __tablename__ = 'practice_level_prescribing'
    id = db.Column(db.Integer, primary_key=True)
    SHA = db.Column(db.String(3))
    PCT = db.Column(db.String(3))
    practice = db.Column(db.String(6))
    BNF_code = db.Column("BNFCODE", db.String(15))
    BNF_name = db.Column("BNFNAME", db.String(40))
    items = db.Column(db.Integer)
    NIC = db.Column(db.Float)
    ACT_cost = db.Column("ACTCOST", db.Float)
    quantity = db.Column(db.Integer)
```

Listing 4.15 Models file showing representing the database tables as classes

```
 1 from sqlalchemy.sql import func
 2 from flask import Blueprint
 3
 4 from app import db
 5 from app.database.models import PrescribingData , PracticeData
 6
 7 database = Blueprint('dbutils', __name__, url_prefix='/dbutils')
 8
 9 class Database:
10     """Class for managing database queries."""
11     def get_total_number_items(self):
12         """Return the total number of prescribed items."""
13         return int(db.session.query(func.sum(PrescribingData.
    items).label('total_items')).first()[0])
14
15     def get_prescribed_items_per_pct(self):
16         """Return the total items per PCT."""
17         return db.session.query(func.sum(PrescribingData.items).
    label('item_sum')).group_by(PrescribingData.PCT).all()
18
19     def get_distinct_pcts(self):
20         """Return the distinct PCT codes."""
21         return db.session.query(PrescribingData.PCT).distinct().
    all()
22
23     def get_n_data_for_PCT(self, pct, n):
24         """Return all the data for a given PCT."""
25         return db.session.query(PrescribingData).filter(
    PrescribingData.PCT == pct).limit(n).all()
26
27     ...
```

Listing 4.16 The controller that queries the database using the models

```
 1 from flask import Blueprint, render_template, request
 2 from app.database.controllers import Database
 3
 4 views = Blueprint('dashboard', __name__, url_prefix='/dashboard')
 5
 6 # get the database class
 7 db_mod = Database()
 8
 9 # Set the route and accepted methods
10 @views.route('/home/', methods=['GET', 'POST'])
11 def home():
12     """Render the home page of the dashboard passing in data to
        populate dashboard."""
13     pcts = [r[0] for r in db_mod.get_distinct_pcts()]
14     if request.method == 'POST':
15         # if selecting PCT for table , update based on user choice
16         form = request.form
17         selected_pct_data = db_mod.get_n_data_for_PCT(str(form['
    pct-option']), 5)
18     else:
```

```
19        # pick a default PCT to show
20        selected_pct_data = db_mod.get_n_data_for_PCT(str(pcts
          [0]), 5)
21
22    # prepare data
23    bar_data = generate_barchart_data()
24    bar_values = bar_data[0]
25    bar_labels = bar_data[1]
26    title_data_items = generate_data_for_tiles()
27
28    # render the HTML page passing in relevant data
29    return render_template('dashboard/index.html', tile_data=
      title_data_items,
30                           pct={'data': bar_values, 'labels':
      bar_labels},
31                           pct_list=pcts, pct_data=
      selected_pct_data)
32
33    ...
```

Listing 4.17 The views that display the results and receive input from the users

We would recommend exploring different design patterns that best suit the type of app you are building and programming languages and frameworks you are building them with.

4.4 Sensors and the Internet of Things (IoT)

The following sections explore how sensors in-built into smartphone devices can be utilised in health apps, and how health apps can connect to everyday objects that have embedded computing devices.

4.4.1 Sensors

Modern smartphones have a plethora of sensors and other data streams (Fig. 4.5) that can be utilised for research and monitoring purposes. Data from these input streams can be used by an intervention to personalise the app or to generate behavioural insights.

Some of the most ubiquitously available sensors include:

- **Global Positioning Systems (GPS):** This calculates your geographical co-ordinates based on triangulation of your phone's position relative to various orbital satellites. This can provide very accurate and precise positioning of a device often using longitude and latitude positioning
- **Light sensors:** Can detect levels of ambient light

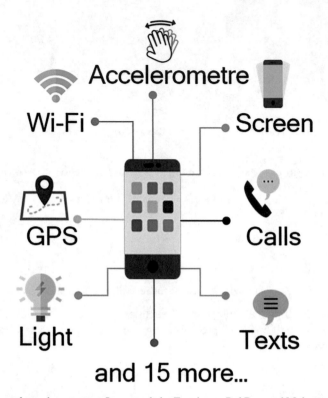

Fig. 4.5 Smartphone data streams. Icons made by Free icons, Raj Dev, and Muhammed Haq from www.freeicons.io. Icons are distributed under a Creative Commons (Attribution 3.0 Unported) license https://creativecommons.org/licenses/by/3.0/. (Image created by Julio Vega)

- **Accelerometer:** This shows the acceleration force caused by movement or gravity in 3D space. Most accelerometers provide the acceleration in terms of X, Y and Z as well as a timestamp.
- **Gyroscope:** This can be used to detect the orientation of the device and is often used in conjunction with the accelerometer.
- **Magnetometer:** Measures magnetic fields and can provides features like a compass. Often used with GPS and accelerometer for map applications
- **Barometer:** Can detect pressure in the air. This can be used to detect altitude.
- **Microphone:** For recording sounds
- **Touchscreen sensor:** Used to detect interaction with the device. Usually works by touch altering the electrical signals passing through the screen
- **Pedometer:** Used to count the number of steps taken. Often used in fitness applications

Other devices also have a range of additional sensors including heart rate sensors, ambient air and humidity sensors. Different makes of smartphone will have more or less sensors available. Some interventions may work with very specific sensors.

The quality and functionality of such sensors varies depending on the make of smartphone. Gathering data from these sensors can be challenging given the fact that devices do not generally support the same range of sensors or provide the same functionality. Some frameworks and tools exist for those that want to access context of use and sensor data. One such example is the AWARE framework [6].

Case study: Unobtrusive monitoring of Parkinson's disease
A project using the AWARE framework [11] aimed to gather smartphone data from patients diagnosed with Parkinson's disease in an unobtrusive way in order to identify patterns of potential disease progression from the data [30]. Many existing methods examine the tremor aspect of the condition and involve participants using sensors and other devices that are usually attached to their bodies. This can be obtrusive especially for longer term longitudinal studies. The project aimed to look for baseline patterns and then identify deviations from these patterns that might be indicative of a progression of the disease. Data were obtained from smartphones which participants used normally in their everyday lives, rather than having to use additional devices. The use of multiple data sources (n = 22) allowed for more accurate inferences concerning what the data may represent. The study looked at 7 participants in the early stages of the disease. These data were collected alongside 6 weekly validated clinical tests (MDS-UPDRS) along with the daily self-reporting of the severity of symptoms. The data were used to inform a Personal Prediction method that was able to derive a feature subset of smartphone sensor metrics that was able to track fluctuations in participants' self-reported symptoms (10 symptoms from 6 patients based on 14 location and 2 activity recognition metrics) [30].

4.4.2   Internet of Things (IoT)

The Internet of Things (IoT) refers to the interconnection of computing devices using the Internet, enabling devices to send and receive data within an IoT system. Such computing devices are often embedded within everyday objects. For example, "smart homes" now enable users to control the lights, fridge, washing machine, heating, security cameras and even locks on the doors via an app, because the different devices are interconnected via the Internet. This kind of technology is increasingly used in health care and health promotion. It can be used, for example, to enable remote monitoring of health parameters and to integrate information from multiple sources, thus enhancing system-related determinants of health. It can also facilitate data collection and recording. Importantly, IoT technology means that smartphone apps can be connected to and exchange data with other devices such as wearables or biosensors like digital glucose monitors.

In the following we explore several examples of how IoT has been used in health-related settings.

IoT Example 1: Using an IoT system for diabetes management
In Chang et al.'s study [7], diabetic patients took blood glucose readings at set intervals, and these data were analysed and fed back to health professionals and caregivers using an mHealth IoT system. Patients used an Android-based, two-way communication device to take blood glucose readings at set intervals. The device automatically uploaded these data to a cloud server, and analysed it to identify any abnormalities in the blood glucose readings. This information was then fed back to health professionals and family members/caregivers, appearing in an online wellness diary within a smartphone application. Depending on the severity of identified abnormalities, notifications appeared in either the health professionals' or the caregivers' application.

Example 2: Using an IoT system for heart attack monitoring
Wolgast et al. [31] developed a system to measure and monitor heart activity.

Participants in their study used an electrocardiogram (ECG) sensor to measure their heart activity. The data were processed by a microcontroller and forwarded via Bluetooth to participants' smartphones, where the data were further processed and displayed in an app. The author suggests this system could be used by patients and/or hospitals to measure heart activity and identify critical events early. However, there are several limitations:

- Users may attach electrodes incorrectly, leading to inaccurate data.
- Further software development is needed for the prediction of heart attacks. To date, human interpretation of ECG data is often superior to computerised algorithms. Algorithms often entail issues with specificity and sensitivity (they are very good at spotting myocardial infarction but also very often overstate that people are having one when they are not).

Example 3: IoT use in emergency services
The IoT is increasingly used to enhance communication between different infrastructures that form part of emergency response systems, including communication between vehicles and hospitals. This can improve the coordination

(continued)

of responses and reduce the risk of errors and delays. For example, IoT can be used to remotely check whether emergency vehicles are running smoothly, to prevent breakdowns during emergency situations.

IoT technology can also be used to improve the management of hospital beds, to prevent long waiting times and delays. For example, the "AutoBed" programme at Mt. Sinai Hospital in New York uses real-time location aware-ness devices like radio-frequency identification tags, infrared, and computer vision to identify which hospital beds are available [27]. The system then combines these data with information about the patient from electronic medical records to identify the best possible match between patients and available beds. The programme was found to decrease wait times among incoming emergency room patients [27].

Example 4: Using IoT technology to improve health record-keeping in rural India

The "Khushi-Baby" project in rural Udaipur in India addresses the problem of a lack of reliable health records, and the lack of awareness among mothers of the importance of antenatal care visits and vaccines [13]. It uses a system which integrates mobile health, wearable Near Field Communication (NFC) technology and cloud computing. Mothers are given a pendant to wear which uses NFC technology; this can then be scanned by a health worker using a smartphone, and the health workers can easily and quickly access the child's records and assess their vaccination needs. The acquired data are synced from the health worker's phone to a cloud-based dashboard.

This approach was evaluated in a cluster-randomised trial [13]. Three groups were compared: (i) mothers who were provided with the NFC necklace and who also received voice calls onto their mobile phones to remind them to attend the next immunization camp, (ii) mothers who received the necklace (no voice calls), and (iii) mothers who received an NFC sticker placed on the immunization card (control group).

The findings indicate that embedding a data collection tool within a culturally appropriate wearable proved to be a useful approach to data collection; the necklace was reportedly well liked among the mothers in the study and also generated discussion among mothers [13].

4.5   Testing

There have been many incidents in recent history involving software systems failing. This failure can have a critical impact depending on what the software was designed to do. This had led to costly consequences, both financially and in cost to human life. In the mid to late 1980s the *THERAC-25* radiation therapy machine gave several patients hundreds of times the required radiation doses leading to their death or serious injury. This was related to programming errors and the overconfidence of the engineers in their work. In the mid 1990s a China Airlines Airbus hit the ground on final approach killing hundreds on board. This was related to a software update that was not installed because it was deemed to be non-critical. A more recent example can be seen in the following case study about the Boeing 737 Max aircraft incidents.

Case study: Boeing 737 Max
An automated safety system called MCAS (Manoeuvring Characteristics Augmentation System) was fitted to Boeing 737 Max aircraft. The system was designed to prevent the aircraft from stalling in manual flight when making steep turns. This worked by pushing the nose of the plane down to reduce a stall. Two separate fatal incidents involving 737 Max planes crashing in Ethiopia and Indonesia were believed to be related to a software error in the system causing false readings to push the nose of the plane down even when it was flying level. This resulted in a tug of war between the pilots and the aircraft leading to the fatal incidents. This in turn led to the grounding of the fleet until a new software update could be implemented to allow the use of two sensors instead of one, as well as enabling the crew to override the system more easily if required.

Incidents like this serve to highlight the continuing need to test the software we produce. This is ever more important as we become increasingly reliant on software systems to carry out daily tasks. This is also becoming more and more relevant in healthcare with advances such as telemedicine, wearables/sensors, smartphone apps, virtual/augmented reality, artificial intelligence, robotics and gnomic technologies all impacting on the way in which healthcare is delivered and will be delivered in the future [28].

This should also be a primary consideration when developing mHealth interventions. Even if the system is not critical to safety, failures in the system and other software bugs may lead to people discontinuing use of the application and losing confidence in the company or institution that created the system. As such thought should be given as to how technical support and maintenance of such interventions will be implemented.

Many projects, especially those related to academic research, may not consider issues of maintainability owing to the nature of academic funding (block of funding for a finite time frame). This is a central issue to products arising from academic research as researchers and other staff tend to move to different projects once the funding for a project is spent and the project has run its course. This can be problematic for users of such systems if ongoing support and maintenance is not ensured. Ideally a support email should be included in-app. It is desirable that this email be checked regularly and if possible picked up by several people (e.g. Listserv). One way to ensure that testing is a core component of the development process rather than an afterthought is to use a process such as *test driven development*.

4.5.1 Test Driven Development

Test driven development, also known as TDD, is a method whereby the development of a software system is driven by the development of unit tests. Unit testing involves the testing of the smallest units/components of functionality in the software and validating that they perform as intended. They are commonly built up into test suites containing multiple individual unit tests (Fig. 4.6).

Suppose we wanted to create a simple function that converts the temperature in degrees Fahrenheit (T_f) to temperature degrees Celsius (T_c).

$$T_c = \frac{5}{9}(T_f - 32)$$

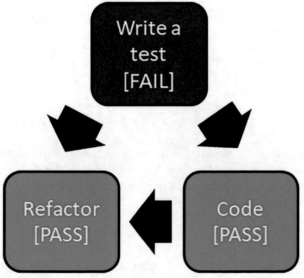

Fig. 4.6 Test driven development. Write a test that fails then add the minimal amount of code required to pass the test

```
In [1]:  import unittest

         class TestFahrenheitTocelsius(unittest.TestCase):
             def test_conversion(self):
                 self.assertAlmostEqual(fahrenheit_to_celsius(32), 0)
                 self.assertAlmostEqual(fahrenheit_to_celsius(104), 40)
```

```
In [2]:  if __name__ == '__main__':
             unittest.main(argv=['first-arg-is-ignored'], exit=False)
```

```
E
============================================================================
ERROR: test_conversion (__main__.TestFahrenheitTocelsius)
----------------------------------------------------------------------------
Traceback (most recent call last):
  File "<ipython-input-1-eb0b49fbc268>", line 5, in test_conversion
    self.assertAlmostEqual(fahrenheit_to_celsius(32), 0)
NameError: name 'fahrenheit_to_celsius' is not defined

----------------------------------------------------------------------------
Ran 1 test in 0.006s

FAILED (errors=1)
```

Fig. 4.7 First write the test

```
In [3]:  def fahrenheit_to_celsius(f):
             return (f-32)*5/9
```

```
In [4]:  import unittest

         class TestFahrenheitTocelsius(unittest.TestCase):
             def test_conversion(self):
                 self.assertAlmostEqual(fahrenheit_to_celsius(32), 0)
                 self.assertAlmostEqual(fahrenheit_to_celsius(104), 40)
```

```
In [5]:  if __name__ == '__main__':
             unittest.main(argv=['first-arg-is-ignored'], exit=False)
```

```
.
----------------------------------------------------------------------------
Ran 1 test in 0.001s

OK
```

Fig. 4.8 First write the function then test again

We could use TDD to accomplish this. First, as counter-intuitive as this sounds, you start by writing your test knowing that it will fail. Figure 4.7 shows an example of this process in Python. First we import the *unittest* module and build a test class for our function. We start by testing it with a few values.

As you can see the test fails as expected informing us that the function *fahrenheit_to_celsius* does not exist. So in order to pass the test we write the minimum amount of code required (Fig. 4.8).

This time the test passes and we are informed that 1 test was run in 0.001 s. We can now write some more tests, this time to deal with unexpected inputs. To convert the temperature correctly we require that the function receives either an integer or floating point value as a parameter. We can write some test to test for different types.

```
In [1]:  def fahrenheit_to_celsius(f):
             return (f-32)*5/9
```

```
In [2]:  import unittest

         class TestFahrenheitTocelsius(unittest.TestCase):
             def test_conversion(self):
                 self.assertAlmostEqual(fahrenheit_to_celsius(32), 0)
                 self.assertAlmostEqual(fahrenheit_to_celsius(104), 40)

             def test_types(self):
                 self.assertRaises(TypeError, fahrenheit_to_celsius, True)
                 self.assertRaises(TypeError, fahrenheit_to_celsius, "A string")
                 self.assertRaises(TypeError, fahrenheit_to_celsius, 5+4j)
```

```
In [3]:  if __name__ == '__main__':
             unittest.main(argv=['first-arg-is-ignored'], exit=False)

         .F
         ======================================================================
         FAIL: test_types (__main__.TestFahrenheitTocelsius)
         ----------------------------------------------------------------------
         Traceback (most recent call last):
           File "<ipython-input-2-7c932b86cc4e>", line 9, in test_types
             self.assertRaises(TypeError, fahrenheit_to_celsius, True)
         AssertionError: TypeError not raised by fahrenheit_to_celsius


         ----------------------------------------------------------------------
         Ran 2 tests in 0.007s

         FAILED (failures=1)
```

Fig. 4.9 Testing for a type error when passed unexpected input types

This should raise a *TypeError*. We add another function to the test class to test for Boolean input, a character string and a complex number (Fig. 4.9). When we run the test it again fails.

And again we write the minimum amount of code required to pass the test (Fig. 4.10).

We added more code to the function to deal with type errors. This process would continue to add functionality to the program by incrementally improving the code base. Additionally as the code is being developed you are also creating a test suite. This process puts testing at the heart of development and leads to robust code. It must however be noted that not all code lends itself to test driven development.

Example: Using TDD to enhance clinical adoption and adaptation of innovative technologies

Kannan et al. [19] evaluated how different agile co-development practices can be implemented within the constraints of working with busy clinicians. The approaches they evaluated were:

- user stories

(continued)

- time-boxed development
- automated acceptance test driven development
- monitoring how clinicians interact with the product after implementation, for continuous adaptation and improvement of the product.

The evaluation was undertaken with clinicians working in hospitals or clinics affiliated with the University of Texas Southwestern.

Automated acceptance test driven development was implemented by arranging acceptance tests in table format, listing all system inputs in one column, and the corresponding accepted system outputs in another column. The tables were written up in plain language/lay terms, avoiding technical jargon, to ensure they could be assessed meaningfully by clinicians. Tests based on the table were then implemented in FitNesse, a fully integrated acceptance testing framework. Tests were designed to fail before development of the feature had commenced, and to pass when the feature was fully developed. Once a feature had been released, the test was added to an automated regression test suite for the production environment, in order to test features in production. This ensures continuous testing (as stipulated by the agile method), and helps test features under changing conditions during production, e.g. when the application experiences high traffic, or when users frequently change data.

The authors conclude that automated acceptance tests serve the following four useful purposes [19]:

1. The process of writing and setting up the tests prior to commencement of development helps specify what features need to be built and how they need to function
2. The automated tests highlight when features have been successfully built (and when further work is required)
3. The automated regression test suite helps identify problems occurring during production and thus identify any unintended changes in a timely manner
4. It facilitates documentation of the design process

Overall, the authors conclude that the four agile methods they tested – including automated acceptance test-driven development – can feasibly be implemented in healthcare settings that involve working with busy clinicians. They were able to successfully engage with clinicians and obtain their feedback iteratively. These methods helped promote clinicians' acceptance and adoption of the newly developed technologies and helped augment value in practice.

```
In [8]: def fahrenheit_to_celsius(f):
            if type(f) not in [int, float]:
                raise TypeError("Error, expecting an int or float")
            return (f-32)*5/9
```

```
In [9]: import unittest

        class TestFahrenheitTocelsius(unittest.TestCase):
            def test_conversion(self):
                self.assertAlmostEqual(fahrenheit_to_celsius(32), 0)
                self.assertAlmostEqual(fahrenheit_to_celsius(104), 40)

            def test_types(self):
                self.assertRaises(TypeError, fahrenheit_to_celsius, True)
                self.assertRaises(TypeError, fahrenheit_to_celsius, "A string")
                self.assertRaises(TypeError, fahrenheit_to_celsius, 5+4j)
```

```
In [10]: if __name__ == '__main__':
             unittest.main(argv=['first-arg-is-ignored'], exit=False)

         ..
         ----------------------------------------------------------------
         Ran 2 tests in 0.005s

         OK
```

Fig. 4.10 Test now passes and handles type error

4.5.1.1 Advantages and Disadvantages of Test Driven Development

There are several advantages to using test driven development in software development projects. These include the building of an intrinsic test suite by default as part of the process. This improves confidence in the code because we know there are a large number of tests underpinning our code. This large number of tests helps to identify and remove defects in the code. Thinking hard about what tests to write can inspire robust design and delivery of features and the test suite can act as a form of documentation about how the software works. The main disadvantages are that more code is written. Writing and maintaining all of these tests takes time and effort. Not all things lend themselves to unit testing (for example UI components). Finally TDD requires management to buy-in to the concept and support it. If they believe that too much time is being 'wasted' writing tests and don't support the initiative, it is unlikely to be successful.

4.5.1.2 Coverage

Another important area of testing is test coverage. This refers to the percentage of code that is actually being tested. Ideally you want to have tests that test as much of your code-base as possible. This can best be explained with an example. If we were

```
  tdd_example.py  ☒    tests.py  ☒
▲1 import coverage
 2
 3 def fahrenheit_to_celsius(f):
 4     if type(f) not in [int, float]:
 5         raise TypeError("Error, expecting an int or float")
 6     return (f-32)*5/9
 7
 8
```

```
  tdd_example.py  ☒    tests.py  ☒
 1 import unittest
 2 from tdd_example import fahrenheit_to_celsius
 3
 4 class TestFahrenheitTocelsius(unittest.TestCase):
 5     def test_conversion(self):
 6         self.assertAlmostEqual(fahrenheit_to_celsius(32), 0)
 7         self.assertAlmostEqual(fahrenheit_to_celsius(104), 40)
 8
 9 if __name__ == '__main__':
10     unittest.main()
11
```

Fig. 4.11 Top: Fahrenheit conversion function in file tdd_example.py, Bottom: test suite (tests.py) that imports the function for testing

```
(base) C:\Users\Alan_Davies>dir *.py
 Volume in drive C has no label.
 Volume Serial Number is 402B-4C57

 Directory of C:\Users\Alan_Davies

19-Mar-19  10:57 PM                176 tdd_example.py
22-Mar-19  11:02 AM                336 tests.py
               2 File(s)          512 bytes
               0 Dir(s)  790,267,875,328 bytes free

(base) C:\Users\Alan_Davies>coverage run tests.py
.
----------------------------------------------------------------------
Ran 1 test in 0.000s

OK
```

Fig. 4.12 Running coverage on the test suite

to place our *fahrenheit_to_celsius* function into its own file and create a separate file for the test suite (Fig. 4.11), and if we now remove the second test for checking the input types there would be some code in our function that wouldn't get tested.

If we check our test coverage using a module designed for such things (i.e. coverage.py) as shown in Fig. 4.12 we can create a report to see how much of the code is being tested (Fig. 4.13).

Here we can see a report consisting of the modules and the number of programmatic statements (a command written by a programmer). We can also see in *missing* how many of these statements are not being tested and the amount of code being tested as a percentage in the coverage column. In this case only 80% of

Coverage report: 92%

Module ↓	statements	missing	excluded	coverage
tdd_example.py	5	1	0	80%
tests.py	8	0	0	100%
Total	**13**	**1**	**0**	**92%**

coverage.py v4.5.3, created at 2019-03-22 11:07

Fig. 4.13 HTML based coverage report generated by the coverage.py module

Coverage for **tdd   example.py** : 80%

5 statements | 4 run | | 1 missing | | 0 excluded |

```
1  import coverage
2
3  def fahrenheit_to_celsius(f):
4      if type(f) not in [int, float]:
5          raise TypeError("Error, expecting an int or float")
6      return (f-32)*5/9
7
8
```

« index   coverage.py v4.5.3, created at 2019-03-22 11:07

Fig. 4.14 Report highlights which bits of the code are not being tested in red

our *tdd_example.py* file is being tested. We can examine the module further to see which parts are not being tested (Fig. 4.14).

This is because we are not performing any tests that trigger this part of the code. If we add back in our original second set of tests for testing the input type and run coverage again we can see that we now have 100% coverage and no missing statements (Fig. 4.15). Optimally we would like out tests to test as much of our code as possible and aim for 100% test coverage.

4.6   Types of Software Test

Apart from the unit testing discussed previously, there are also several other types of testing that are performed in a software system (Fig. 4.16).

The next level up from unit testing is *integration testing*. This involves combining smaller components together and testing how they interact with one another as a group. An example of the concept can be seen in Fig. 4.17. On the left we see a light fitting that has undergone the equivalent of functional unit testing. The light unit works, electricity supply is present, it switches on and off and lights a fitted light bulb. The middle image shows a door that also works functionally. The door opens

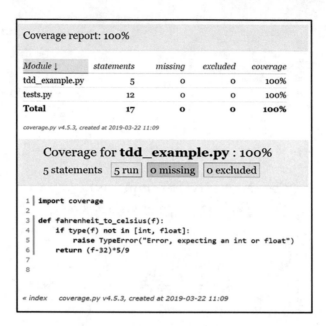

Fig. 4.15 Now the tests are testing all the statements in the code and the coverage is 100%

and closes properly and locks correctly. The image on the right however shows that when tested together these items do not work. The door would shatter a light bulb when opened suddenly, alternatively the door can't be opened wide enough to enter or exit without risking damage to a light bulb. This illustrates the dangers of overconfidence in unit testing. Failure to test the interaction of components that in themselves work correctly can have detrimental effects to a larger system. Following on from this we then have *system testing* where the entire system and all of its sub-components are tested together and we verify that the system meets the specified functional requirements as a whole. Finally we have *acceptance testing*, where we test to see if the system is acceptable and complies with the business requirements/needs and is ready for delivery/deployment. Above these levels of software testing we also have *usability testing*, which is discussed in more detail in Chap. 7.

Once an intervention is ready for wider testing, one could consider using *Beta testing*. This is a form of acceptance testing carried out with the desired end user. This can help us to evaluate levels of customer satisfaction. Any issues can be fed back to improve the design. Customers are also more likely to be forgiving of problems if a product is promoted as being in Beta testing, especially for early adopters that want to try out a new product or feature early on. This also helps to identity issues with various platforms or devices etc. Beta testing is carried out after initial (alpha) testing and before the app is released onto the market in its final form (and before it is promoted with advertising/marketing campaigns). There are also tools to support Beta testing, such as Apple's *TestFlight* [5] that allows for beta

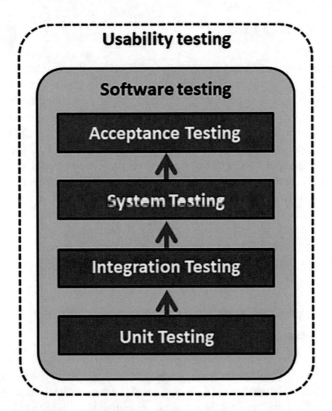

Fig. 4.16 Levels of testing applied to software systems

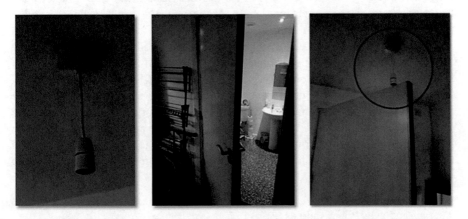

Fig. 4.17 Left: light fitting, Middle: door, Right: problem identified when using items together

testing of apps before release onto the App Store. The ORCHA organisation also provides a pre-launch review aimed specifically at health apps [22].

4.7 App Maintenance

A common assumption is that the process of developing and releasing the app is the endpoint. Instead this should be seen as an ongoing process. Each time an OS receives an upgrade, this could have implications for your intervention. You may need to consider providing updates of your app to account for this as well as things like patches for security issues and bug fixes. According to ORCHA, 65% of apps designed for specific conditions had not been updated for over a year and a half [23]. This ongoing maintenance adds costs to the project and needs to be resourced. This is perhaps easier with a dedicated software development team, but is often not accounted for in research projects. Once the funding runs out and the papers have been written, the app is no longer supported. One also needs to consider risk to patients in the case of apps that some may have come to rely on (for example medication management or mental health interventions). It is recommended that this is made clear to patients and participants upfront, or that a plan to phase out the app is put into place to ease the transition.

4.8 Summary of Key Points

After the initial design of the intervention has been completed considerations should be given to the implementation of the app itself. This is as important as the wider design because this is the vehicle required to realise your intervention and make it a manifest entity in the real world. To map your design into a tangible product that meets its design requirements, one must consider the target audience and the platforms and devices the app will be developed to support. Careful consideration should be given to the type of app that will be developed and that this app type supports the project's objectives, timescales and the skill set of the project team. A formal development methodology should be applied (see Chap. 2 for details) as well as the use of an appropriate design pattern. Following these steps will allow for the rapid construction and maintainability of your intervention. Testing should also be considered throughout the development process to ensure a high-quality and robust product. Finally consideration should be given to the longer-term maintenance and support of the intervention to ensure that sufficient resources can be allocated to this.

- Choose the type of app (native, PWA, web) that is most suitable for the project's goals and available resources
- Consider using a formal design pattern to improve production quality and ongoing maintenance
- Make sure that testing is considered throughout the development process to ensure the production of a robust product
- Consider and plan for the longer-term maintenance of your intervention

- Consider the setup requirements for a new project, such as workstation, setup of frameworks and environments and account for this in planning
- Determine the best programming language and frameworks to use that suit the needs of your project and take into account the target platform and developer experience

4.9   Quiz

1. When applying test driven development (TDD), we first...

    (a) Write our implementation function
    (b) Start by writing a test
    (c) Run coverage on the code base

2. Which of the following is **not** a commonly included sensor included in most mobile smartphones

    (a) Global positioning system (GPS)
    (b) Radiation detector
    (c) Accelerometer

3. The MVC pattern is commonly used with web development projects

    (a) True
    (b) False

4. The main development languages for iOS development include

    (a) Java, Kotlin and Python
    (b) Objective-C and Swift
    (c) C++, C# and Ruby

5. Basic web apps are able to interface easily with the hardware components of a mobile device

    (a) True
    (b) False

6. The most commonly downloaded apps are...

    (a) Health apps
    (b) Business apps
    (c) Games

Answers to the quiz can be found in "Solutions to Quizzes".

4.10 Exercises

1. Using test driven development in a language of your choice:

    (a) Write a function to convert seconds into milliseconds (seconds $\times$ 1000)
    (b) Write a function to output a message stating if a given number is a prime number or not

2. Visit NHS Digital https://digital.nhs.uk/services/nhs-apps-library/guidance-for-health-app-developers-commissioners-and-assessors/how-we-assess-health-apps-and-digital-tools#how-the-assessment-works to see the requirements for publishing an app on the NHS Apps Library in the UK.

    (a) Either see how your proposed intervention meets these criteria or
    (b) Read through the criteria and consider how a speculative intervention might be designed to meet these requirements

3. Consider the following project proposals. Which type of app do you think would be most suitable for each and why?

    (a) Requirement to build an app for iPhone users that would allow them to take a photo of a rash and save this securely on their device.
    (b) A plan to create an app that connects users to trusted website information sources about heart disease and allows them to view these resources on their phone via a main menu
    (c) A symptom logging app that works on both Android and iOS to transmit data securely to a database on a university research server

Recommended Reading

1. Freeman E, Freeman E. Head first: design patterns. Beijing: O'Reilly; 2004.
2. Radin J et al. The healthy pregnancy research program: transforming pregnancy research through a ResearchKit app. NPJ Digit Med. 2018;1(1):1–45. https://doi.org/10.1038/s41746-018-0052-2
3. Majumder S, Jamal Deen M. Smartphone sensors for health monitoring and diagnosis. Sensors. 2019;19:1–45.

References

1. Apple Inc. Apple developer; 2020. https://developer.apple.com/carekit/
2. Apple Inc. Apple developer; 2020. https://developer.apple.com/healthkit/
3. Apple Inc. Apple developer; 2020. https://developer.apple.com/researchkit/
4. Apple Inc. Swift – Apple developer; 2020. https://developer.apple.com/swift/
5. Apple Inc. TestFlight – Apple developer; 2020. https://developer.apple.com/testflight/

6. AWARE. AWARE – open-source context instrumentation framework for everyone; 2020. https://awareframework.com/
7. Chang S-H, Chiang R-D, Wu S-J, Chang W-T. A context-aware, interactive M-health system for diabetics. IT Prof. 2016;18(3):14–22. https://doi.org/10.1109/MITP.2016.48
8. Clement J. Statista; 2019. https://www.statista.com/statistics/269025/worldwide-mobile-app-revenue-forecast/
9. Clement J. Statista, 2019. https://www.statista.com/statistics/270291/popular-categories-in-the-app-store/
10. Ezlina Shahbudin F. Design patterns for developing high efficiency mobile application. J Inf Technol Softw Eng. 2013;3(3):1–9. https://doi.org/10.4172/2165-7866.1000122
11. Ferreira D, Kostakos V, Dey AK. AWARE: mobile context instrumentation framework. Front ICT. 2015;2:1–9. https://doi.org/10.3389/fict.2015.00006
12. Freeman E, Freeman E. Head first: design patterns. Beijing: O'Reilly; 2004.
13. Ganesh Venkat P. Intermediate assessment of the Khushi baby cRCT: implementation of a novel mHealth solution for vaccination record keeping in rural Udaipur, Rajasthan, India. Ph.D. thesis, Yale University; 2016. https://elischolar.library.yale.edu/cgi/viewcontent.cgi?article=1299&context=ysphtdl
14. Google. Google fit; 2020. https://www.google.com/fit/
15. Google. Google fit | Google developers; 2020. https://developers.google.com/fit
16. Horton J. Android programming with Kotlin for beginners. Birmingham: Packt Publishing; 2019.
17. Ionic. Ionic – cross-platform mobile app development; 2019. https://ionicframework.com/
18. Jabangwe R, Edison H, Duc AN. Software engineering process models for mobile app development: a systematic literature review. J Syst Softw. 2018;145:98–111. https://doi.org/10.1016/j.jss.2018.08.028
19. Kannan V, Basit MA, Youngblood JE, Bryson TD, Toomay SM, Fish JS, Willett DL. Agile co-development for clinical adoption and adaptation of innovative technologies. In: 2017 IEEE healthcare innovations and point of care technologies (HI-POCT), vol. 2018. IEEE; Nov 2017. p. 56–9. http://www.ncbi.nlm.nih.gov/pubmed/30364762; http://www.pubmedcentral.nih.gov/articlerender.fcgi?artid=PMC6197812; http://ieeexplore.ieee.org/document/8227583/
20. Kivy. Kivy; 2020. https://kivy.org/#home
21. Kotlin Foundation. Kotlin; 2020. https://kotlinlang.org/docs/reference/android-overview.html
22. ORCHA. ORCHA; 2018. https://www.orcha.co.uk/who-we-help/developers/#0
23. ORCHA. ORCHA; 2018. https://www.orcha.co.uk/the-challenge/
24. Radin JM, Steinhubl SR, Su AI, Bhargava H, Greenberg B, Bot BM, Doerr M, Topol EJ. The healthy pregnancy research program: transforming pregnancy research through a ResearchKit app. NPJ Digit Med. 2018;1(1):1–7. https://doi.org/10.1038/s41746-018-0052-2
25. Ray J. iPhone application development, 2nd edn. Indianapolis: Sams; 2011.
26. The Apache Software Foundation. Overview – Apache Cordova; 2015. https://cordova.apache.org/docs/en/3.1.0/guide/overview/index.html
27. Thomas BG, Bollapragada S, Akbay K, Toledano D, Katlic P, Dulgeroglu O, Yang D. Automated bed assignments in a complex and dynamic hospital environment. Interfaces. 2013;43(5):435–48. https://doi.org/10.1287/inte.2013.0701
28. Topol E. The topol review – preparing the healthcare workforce to deliver the digital future. Technical report February, Health Education England; 2019. https://topol.hee.nhs.uk/
29. Using mobile technology to engage sexual and gender minorities in clinical research. PLoS One. 2019;14(5):1–19. https://doi.org/10.1371/journal.pone.0216282
30. Vega Hernandez JE. Unobtrusive and personalised monitoring of Parkinson'S disease using smartphones. Ph.D. thesis, The University of Manchester; 2019. https://www.researchgate.net/profile/Julio_Vega7/publication/333675748_Unobtrusive_and_Personalised_Monitoring_of_Parkinson%27s_Disease_Using_Smartphones/links/5cfe6aff4585157d15a1e65d/Unobtrusive-and-Personalised-Monitoring-of-Parkinsons-Disease-Using-Sm
31. Wolgast G, Ehrenborg C, Israelsson A, Helander J, Johansson E, Manefjord H. Wireless body area network for heart attack detection [Education Corner]. IEEE Antennas Propag Mag. 2016;58(5):84–92. https://doi.org/10.1109/MAP.2016.2594004

Chapter 5
Data Collection, Storage and Security

5.1 Introduction

An intervention that collects and processes data presents challenges, both in terms of technical issues (storage and security) and in terms of data custodianship. This can be even more complex if the intervention is deployed in multiple countries or regions, or the data are transmitted/stored in different locations. Projects that operate internationally, or have some element of the project that is based or shared with partners in another country can be complex to manage from a regulatory perspective, as they may have to comply with legislation that differs in different areas. Further to this the storage and transmission of the data themselves requires careful implementation in order to protect them from malicious exploitation. When interventions are designed, a lot of thought (usually) goes into the design of the intervention itself.

From a personal perspective having worked as a researcher, app developer and Research Software Engineer (RSE), it always surprised me when I met with people to discuss building an intervention that they had rarely considered the 'back end' of the system. By this we mean the server or data storage platform that would store the data that their intervention inevitably relied on. Although interventions can use local storage on a device, many have the requirement of storing data or retrieving data from some back end system. This is often overlooked, especially as planning and development time mostly focuses around the app itself. The requirement to build a storage platform or set up a server for the intervention can add considerable development overhead and requires specific skills. Naive approaches to data processing can open you and your team up to potential litigation as well as reputational damage. What data you collect and store, and where and how you store them are all potentially difficult challenges to overcome depending on the exact nature of your requirements. Rather than leaving these important decisions as an afterthought, we would recommend that due consideration is given to such matters and that they are addressed formally early on in the project, with appropriate time built into the project to consider and implement them. This chapter serves to highlight some of the important and often overlooked aspects of the storage, transmission and security issues surrounding data collection and processing. It also discusses the legal and technical challenges surrounding the implementation of mHealth interventions.

5.2   Data Storage

We may need to store the data that are produced by the intervention or entered into the intervention by a user. This can be for research purposes where we might want to aggregate data at a population level to determine the effect of an intervention on a desired group or population. We may also need to collect data for processing. For example we may have a complex machine learning algorithm that we need to run on the users' data. Perhaps this takes too long, or is inefficient to carry out on the device itself. In such a case we may transmit the data somewhere for processing and return some result to the user's device based on this process.

5.2.1   Local Storage

The most straightforward solution is to store data on the device itself. This can be further protected using a pin or passcode that can restrict access to the app and its data in the case that the user loses their device or leaves it unattended. Security of the data becomes more problematic when the data collected need to be sent somewhere for storage or further processing. Often such systems require the use of a *back end*.

5.2.2   The Back End

By 'back end' we are referring to part of the system that the user does not directly interact with as opposed to the 'front end' which is the software system that the user directly interacts with (including the user interface). The back end is usually a computer system that stores and processes data. Typically this consists of a *server*, an *application*, and a *database*. The server is the part of the system that manages access to resources stored remotely.

5.2.3 Cloud Storage

One way to store and manage the data that are produced by your intervention is to use "cloud services". If you belong to a large organisation, such as a university or large company, you may have an IT department that can do things like set up servers and manage data storage for you. A newer way of overcoming these requirements for smaller organisations or individuals is to use cloud computing. In this case the servers and maintenance are provided for you, without you having to worry about buying or renting servers. This can also be faster than waiting for an internal IT department to approve requests for hosting. Cloud solutions provide more than just servers. As well as a more flexible and agile infrastructure that can expand and contract based on your needs, cloud services also provide platforms (i.e. Java, Peal, etc.) and applications (Fig. 5.1). Some organisations may have deals in place with a cloud service provider thus facilitating access to such resources.

Cloud services can be public, private or a hybrid and provide several different types of services, such as software, platform and infrastructure as a service (SaaS, PaaS and IaaS). Cloud services can be billed per hour or for a set duration, meaning that you only pay for the resources that you use. Furthermore these resources can be scaled up and down to deliver the required amount of resources for your project(s). The two main market leaders are Microsoft's Azure and Amazon's AWS (Amazon Web Services). If you want to maintain full control over your data and their management, or for some other reason cannot use cloud services, you might want or need to create your own solutions for the management and storage of the data you collect. The usual way to do this would be to set up a server with database support to store the data that the intervention produces. To this end there are several main types of database that are commonly used, *structured* and *unstructured* databases.

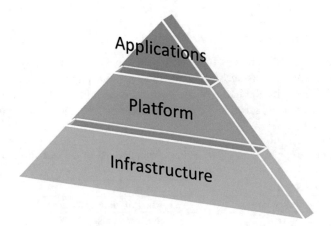

Fig. 5.1 Cloud service components

5.2.4 Structured Databases

A structured database is a database where the data are stored in a structured way in the form of tables. Each table is usually semantically derived. If for example you created an online shopping service, you could have a *customers* table with information about your customers and a *stock* table with product information (Table 5.1). In such a system each row represents a single record and each column represents a field (feature).

A *Relational Database* will allow for connections (relationships) to be made between different tables in the database. This is useful because it allows for data to be organised and stored in tables that relate in someway to what is being stored, which makes logical sense for users of the database. In addition it prevents having to replicate data. You probably wouldn't want to store your customer information, supplier information and stock data all in one giant table. This would make searching the database slower and would be generally inefficient. *Relational Database Management Systems* (RDBMS) exist for managing such databases and include:

- MySQL
- SQLite
- PostgreSQL
- MS SQL

The SQL part of these systems refers to Structured Query Language. This is a query language that is used to carry out interactions with a database. This allows simple commands to be written. For example if we had some data on people's heart rates and blood pressures stored in a table (Table 5.2) we could retrieve the data using an SQL query (Listing 5.1).

```
SELECT * FROM med_data;
```

Listing 5.1 SQLite query to retrieve all the data in table 'med_data'

There are slight differences in syntax between the different SQL versions. In these examples we are using SQLite. In the example above we use the *SELECT* command followed by the name of the column or columns separated by commas. The asterisk (star) indicates that we want all columns. We then have to indicate the

Table 5.1 Example of a basic 'stock' table. Each column is a field and each row is a record in the database

Id	Stock code	Stock item	Description	Price ($)
1	124246	Roller blades	A pair of inline skates	45
2	754543	Bicycle	Men's road bike	246.55
3	468537	Karate belt (blue)	A blue Karate belt (child size)	3.00
4	765657	Tent	2 person 1 room dome tent	13.95
5	965775	Horse saddle	Jumping saddle	790.50

Table 5.2 Database table of blood pressure and heart rate data called 'med_data'

Id	Name	Age	Sex	Blood pressure	heart rate
1	Alan Smith	25	M	120/70	78
2	Maureen Skipper	87	F	156/82	82
3	Adam Blythe	55	M	132/73	72
4	Darren Sanders	34	M	120/70	67
5	Sally-Ann Joyce	19	F	121/72	65

Table 5.3 Results of the query to find males with heart rate above 70 beats per minute

Id	Name	Heart rate	Sex
1	Alan Smith	78	M
3	Adam Blythe	72	M

table that we want the data from. We use the *FROM* keyword followed by the name of the table (in this case med_data). This would retrieve the entire table as seen in Table 5.2.

> Although not necessary, it is common practice to capitalise SQL commands.

More advanced queries can be made using conditional statements to select certain data based on it meeting a specific requirement. For example in Listing 5.2 we retrieve data from the columns *Name, Heart rate* and *sex* only if the *Heart rate* is higher than 70 and the *sex* is male. The query would produce the result seen in Table 5.3.

```
SELECT "Name", "Heart rate", "Sex" FROM med_data WHERE "Heart
    rate" > 70 AND "Sex" = "M";
```

Listing 5.2 SQLite query to retrieve columns based on a condition

As mentioned previously, the main advantage of such a system is the ability to store semantically related data in separate tables and link these tables together using relationships. There are three types of such relationships:

1. *One-to-One*
2. *One-to-Many/Many-to-One*
3. *Many-to-Many.*

In the One-to-One case, a table row can have a single matching row in another table and the other way around. A One-to-Many or Many-to-One relationship is where a row in one table can have multiple matching rows in another. This is the most commonly encountered relationship type. Finally a Many-to-Many relationship is where rows can have multiple matching rows in both tables. When a database is created, a database *schema* is defined. This specifies how the data are

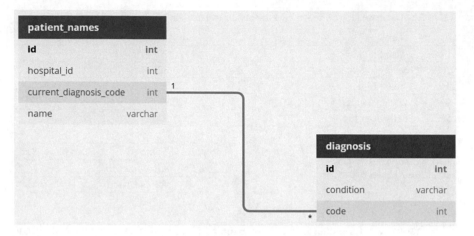

Fig. 5.2 Schematic diagram showing One-to-Many relationship between two tables

Table 5.4 (Left) the patient_names table, (right) the diagnosis table

Hospital_id	Name	Current_daignosis_code	Condition	Code
123456	Mike Chong	24	Diabctes	24
342244	Darren Hay	12	Ischemic heart disease	12
433242	Julie Mueller	15	Lupus	15
453821	Julio Vameera	29	Parkinsons	29
975783	Glen Osborne	36	Lung cancer	36

Table 5.5 Results of query to display patient name and condition description

Name	Condition
Mike Chong	Diabetes
Darren Hay	Ischemic heart disease
Julie Mueller	Lupus
Julio Vameera	Parkinsons
Glen Osborne	Lung cancer

organised and what the relationships are. Each table in a database has a *primary key* which is a column containing a unique value for each row in the database. This gives each record a unique ID. A *foreign* key is a column in a table that refers to the primary key of another table. Let's say we had a table in a database called *patient_names* containing details of their name, hospital ID and a code relating to a diagnosis. In a separate table we could then store a description of the condition in question. Figure 5.2 shows a representation of the two tables and their relationship.

The code in Listing 5.3 shows the creation of the two tables in SQL. In Listing 5.4 we add some data to the tables (Table 5.4). And finally we can create a query that returns all the patients' names and a description of the patients' conditions by using the diagnosis code. Note that we type the name of the table followed by a period (dot) and the name of the column (field). This produces the result seen in Table 5.5.

```
 1  DROP TABLE IF EXISTS patient_names;
 2  CREATE TABLE patient_names (
 3       hospital_id int,
 4       name varchar(255),
 5       current_diagnosis_code int
 6  );
 7
 8  DROP TABLE IF EXISTS diagnosis;
 9  CREATE TABLE diagnosis (
10       condition varchar(255),
11       code int,
12       FOREIGN KEY(code) REFERENCES patient_names(
         current_diagnosis_code)
13  );
```

Listing 5.3   Create the patient_names and diagnosis tables

```
 1  INSERT INTO patient_names VALUES(123456, "Mike Chong", 24);
 2  INSERT INTO patient_names VALUES(342244, "Darren Hay", 12);
 3  INSERT INTO patient_names VALUES(433242, "Julie Mueller", 15);
 4  INSERT INTO patient_names VALUES(453821, "Julio Vameera", 29);
 5  INSERT INTO patient_names VALUES(975783, "Glen Osborne", 36);
 6
 7  INSERT INTO diagnosis VALUES("Diabetes", 24);
 8  INSERT INTO diagnosis VALUES("Ischemic heart disease", 12);
 9  INSERT INTO diagnosis VALUES("Lupus", 15);
10  INSERT INTO diagnosis VALUES("Parkinsons", 29);
11  INSERT INTO diagnosis VALUES("Lung cancer", 36);
```

Listing 5.4   Populate both tables with data

```
 1  SELECT patient_names.name, diagnosis.condition FROM patient_names
    , diagnosis WHERE patient_names.current_diagnosis_code =
    diagnosis.code;
```

Listing 5.5   Query to return the names and descriptions of conditions by diagnosis code

5.2.4.1   Joins

When we want to combine data from several columns we can use a *join*. This
essentially refers to combining columns from one or more tables into a single set.
Appending rows to the bottom of a table is called a *union*. Using joins allows us to
combine data in different ways. The most common types of join include; inner, left,
right and full joins. An inner join returns records from table A and B where the join
condition is satisfied. A left join returns all records from table A and ones from B
that meet the join condition. Right join returns all records from B and records form
A that meet the join condition. Finally the full join returns all records from A and
all records from B regardless of join condition. This can be seen visually in Fig. 5.3.
  This chapter does not aim to provide an exhaustive guide to SQL and relational
databases, but rather an introduction to some of the key concepts. Many interven-

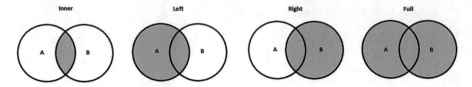

Fig. 5.3 Venn diagrams illustrating some common relational database table join types

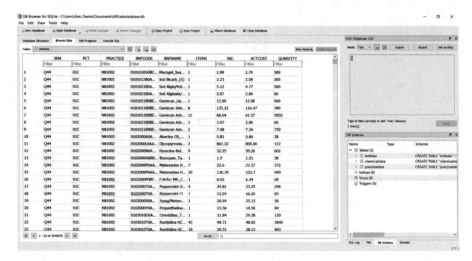

Fig. 5.4 A screenshot showing a structured SQLite database viewed using the DB Browser for SQlite tool

tions may collect and store data in such a relational database. Data can be exported and analysed in the traditional way or analysis pipelines can be set up to query the data directly using SQL for data sub-setting prior to analysis. There are many useful tools available for working with structured databases. The DB Browser for SQLite (Fig. 5.4), which is free to download and use at the time of writing this book allows for the inspection of SQLite databases. The figure shows the browser viewing a table in a database showing UK prescribing data. The window in the bottom right shows the database schema. SQL commands can be typed in to run various queries on the data directly.

5.2.4.2 Object Relational Mapping

One issue with using such structured databases is how to interact efficiently with them when your software is written in a different language. One technique that can help with this is *Object Relational Mapping* or ORM. This uses Object-Oriented Programming (OOP) to convert data into objects that can be used in programs. A modified example can be seen below from a web based intervention aimed at

encouraging early help seeking behaviour for people with symptoms of lung cancer
[13]. The intervention used the Python Flask microframework and ORM to map
an SQLite database. The code in Listing 5.7 shows how simple Python functions
can be used to access data in the database without having to write SQL statements.
This has the advantage of keeping all the code written in the Python language and
avoiding multiple languages being used. The Listing 5.6 shows how we can map
data from the database using a class *StoreConditionData*. We can see the table name
conditions that has an ID column that is the primary key and a column containing
data about conditions. We can essentially use this to load data from the SQL
database into the Python object, which is easier to use and interact with in the Python
environment.

```python
import os
from flask import Flask, session
from flask.ext.sqlalchemy import SQLAlchemy

basedir = os.path.abspath(os.path.dirname(__file__))
app = Flask(__name__)

app.config['SQLALCHEMY_DATABASE_URI'] = 'sqlite:///' + os.path.
    join(basedir, 'webdata.db')
app.config['SQLALCHEMY_COMMIT_ON_TEARDOWN'] = True

# create db instance
db = SQLAlchemy(app)

# import database class models
from models import *

def get_conditions():
    conditions = db.session.query(StoreConditionData).all()
    if not containsAny('1234', str(conditions)):
        return False
    else:
        return conditions

def update_conditions(conditions_list):
    conditions = ','.join(conditions_list)
    db_cond = db.session.query(StoreConditionData).order_by(
    StoreConditionData.id.desc()).first()
    db_cond.conditions = conditions
    db.session.commit()

...

if __name__ == '__main__':
    app.run(debug=True)
```

Listing 5.6 *views.py* sample excerpt form Python Flask app

```
from  app  import  db

class  StoreConditionData(db.Model):
    __tablename__  =  'conditions'
    id  =  db.Column('id',  db.Integer,  primary_key  =  True)
    conditions  =  db.Column('conditions',  db.String(8))

    # initialize  fields
    def  __init__(self,  conditions):
        self.conditions  =  conditions

    # define  how  the  object  is  output  as  a  string
    def  __repr__(self):
        return  '%r'  %  self.conditions
```

Listing 5.7 *models.py* excerpt from the database models file

5.2.5   Migrations

Problems arise with structured databases if you decide to add/remove fields in the schema once you have started using the database to store data. To make such changes in the past it would have been necessary to delete the data from the table, modify the schema and start collecting new data. Alternatively you could add a new table with the altered features. Now most popular frameworks come with libraries to carry out schema migration. There is also standalone software for this. Migration allows the database schema to be modified without affecting the data already stored. Another way around this and other issues of relational databases is to use a *NoSQL* database instead.

5.2.6   NoSQL Databases

Aside from relational databases using SQL there are also document databases or "NoSQL" databases that do not use SQL and are not relational. An example of this is *MongoDB*. Instead of using tables they use *collections* of documents with data stored in a binary version of JSON (JavaScript Object Notation) called BSON. The notation is fairly straightforward. Curly braces represent objects. Data are stored in key/value pairs separated by a colon with data separated with commas. Arrays are represented by square brackets. The format is the same as JavaScript objects, which is where the JSON name comes from. The code in Listing 5.8 shows how to create a database in MongoDB.

```
use  medicalData
```

Listing 5.8 Create a new database called medicalData

Once created, we can create a collection called *medData*, which will work in a similar way to the table of the same name used in the previous SQL example. We can then add records, either one by one (Listing 5.9) or in batches as seen in Listings 5.10 and 5.11.

```
db.medData.insert({"Name": "Alan Smith", "Age": 25, "Sex": "M", "
    Blood pressure": "120/70", "Heart rate": 78},)
```

Listing 5.9 Insert data into the new database

```
db.medData.insertMany([{}, {}, {}, {}])
```

Listing 5.10 Format of multiple item insert into the database

```
db.medData.insertMany([{"Name": "Maureen Skinner", "Age": 87, "
    Sex": "F", "Blood pressure": "156/82", "Heart rate": 82}, {"
    Name": "Adam Blythe", "Age": 55, "Sex": "M", "Blood pressure"
    : "132/73", "Heart rate": 72}, {"Name": "Darren Sanders", "
    Age": 34, "Sex": "M", "Blood pressure": "120/70", "Heart rate
    ": 67}, {"Name": "Sally-Ann Joyce", "Age": 19, "Sex": "F", "
    Blood pressure": "121/72", "Heart rate": 65}])
```

Listing 5.11 Example of multiple data insertion

To view the collection we can use the query function *find()* and style the output to make it more readable with the *pretty()* function. This shows the results seen in Listing 5.12. Also note that an *_id* has been added to uniquely identify each document in a collection.

```
db.medData.find().pretty()
{
    "_id" : ObjectId("5cf636773ec8a0a14875e33"),
    "Name" : "Alan Smith",
    "Age" : 25,
    "Sex": "M",
    "Blood pressure" : "120/70",
    "Heart rate" : 78
}
{
    "_id" : ObjectId("5cf638700d49e10463047acf"),
    "Name" : "Maureen Skinner",
    "Age" : 87,
    "Sex": "F",
    "Blood pressure" : "156/82",
    "Heart rate" : 82
}
{
    "_id" : ObjectId("5cf639f8455882efa5b614d7"),
    "Name" : "Adam Blythe",
    "Age" : 55,
    "Sex": "M",
    "Blood pressure" : "132/73",
    "Heart rate" : 72
}
```

```
26  {
27      "_id" : ObjectId("5cf639f8455882efa5b614d8"),
28      "Name" : "Darren Sanders",
29      "Age" : 34,
30      "Sex": "M",
31      "Blood pressure" : "120/70",
32      "Heart rate" : 67
33  }
34  {
35      "_id" : ObjectId("5cf639f8455882efa5b614d9"),
36      "Name" : "Sally-Ann Joyce",
37      "Age" : 19,
38      "Sex": "F",
39      "Blood pressure" : "121/72",
40      "Heart rate" : 65
41  }
```

Listing 5.12 Command to view the collection and resulting output

We can also carry out queries of the data in much the same way as with SQL. The example in Listing 5.13 shows how to retrieve all the males from the collection.

```
1  db.medData.find({Sex:"M"})
2  { "_id" : ObjectId("5cf636773ec8a0a14875e33"), "Name" : "Alan
       Smith", "Age" : 25, "Sex": "M", "Blood pressure" : "120/70",
       "Heart rate" : 78 }
3  { "_id" : ObjectId("5cf639f8455882efa5b614d7"), "Name" : "Adam
       Blythe", "Age" : 55, "Sex": "M", "Blood pressure" : "132/73",
       "Heart rate" : 72 }
4  "_id" : ObjectId("5cf639f8455882efa5b614d8"), "Name" : "Darren
       Sanders", "Age" : 34, "Sex": "M", "Blood pressure" : "120/70"
       , "Heart rate" : 67 }
```

Listing 5.13 Query to select all the males from the collection and resulting output

There are many comparison query operators available for selecting data from a collection. Table 5.6 provides an overview.

So far you might be asking yourself what the point of using such a system would be, or what advantages it has over using an SQL based database system. The choice of database depends very much on the task you are trying to accomplish and

Table 5.6 Comparison and matching operators

Operator	Description
$eq	Finds equal matches
$gt	Greater than
$gte	Greater than or equal to
$lt	Less than
$lte	Less than or equal to
$in	Matches any values in an array
$ne	Matches not equal to a value
$nin	Matches no values in array

the tools you have at your disposal. There are however some specific advantages of using a system like MongoDB. These include having a dynamic schema. This means that we can change the structure of the data as we go without having to have different versions of the database or having to use migration. For example say we want to add another patient to our database but for this one we want to add some extra information like a DNR (Do Not Resuscitate) status to indicate that no cardiopulmonary resuscitation should be attempted on this patient. We could simply add this extra data to the database (Listing 5.14).

```
1  db.medData.insert({"Name": "Mary Allen", "Age": 95, "Sex": "F", "
       Blood pressure": "183/75", "Heart rate": 101}, "DNR": true)
2  db.medData.find({Name:"Mary Allen"}).pretty()
3  {
4      "_id"  :  ObjectId("5cf67a583c2cfbd2177e64b"),
5      "Name"  :  "Mary Allen",
6      "Age"  :  95,
7      "Sex"  :  "F",
8      "Blood pressure"  :  "183/75",
9      "Heart rate":  101,
10     "DNR"  :  true
11 }
```

Listing 5.14 Example of dynamic schema support

This has obvious advantages in terms of maintenance and performance. Another advantage is that the documents are essentially objects and correspond to data types in other languages, such as JavaScript and Python, making working with database data more seamless. Another big advantage is the ability to store embedded/nested documents in another document. This makes it easy to store multiple and complex data together in one place reducing the need to carry out table joins. For example lets say we wanted to add some test results to a patient's data. Listing 5.15 shows how we can use MongoDB to add these data by embedding documents. Here we are storing some results, which include a link to an ECG (electrocardiogram) image, and some data on cardiac enzymes that can show damage to the heart muscle; creatine kinase (CK), Troponin I (TROP) and Aspartate aminotransferase (AST). Here we have an array of tests stored within results, with a further array of key/value pairs for the name of the blood test and the result. This offers a very powerful way of storing complex data without having duplication or requiring complex table joins.

```
1  db.medData.insert({"Name": "Karen Baker", "Age": 34, "Sex": "F",
       "Blood pressure": "130/73", "Heart rate": 68, "Results": [{"
       ECG": "\scans\ECGs\ecg00023.png"}, {"BIOCHEM": [{"AST": 37},
       {"CK": 180}, {"TROP": 0.03}]}]})
2  db.medData.find({Name:"Karen Baker"}).pretty()
3  {
4      "_id"  :  ObjectId("5cf67ec9a45e13dec84f6cd1"),
5      "Name"  :  "Karen Baker",
6      "Age"  :  34,
7      "Sex"  :  "F",
8      "Blood pressure"  :  "130/73",
9      "Heart rate":  68,
```

```
10    "Results" : [
11        {
12            "ECG" : "\scans\ECGs\ecg00023.png"
13        },
14        {
15            "BIOCHEM" : [
16                {
17                    "AST" : 37
18                },
19                {
20                    "CK" : 180
21                },
22                {
23                    "TROP" : 0.03
24                }
25            ]
26        }
27    ]
28 }
```

Listing 5.15 Example of nested data

5.2.7   Graph Databases

Another (NoSQL) method of storing and querying data is to use a graph database. Graph databases have performance advantages over relational databases and add value when the structure and relationships of the data items are as important as the data themselves. This is often used to improve the performance of machine learning pipelines by including this information about the data structure in the analysis. Often when using relational databases, data are normalised by removing duplicates and separating out information into separate tables. This process is then often undone somewhat by engaging in denormalisation to improve the efficiency of running queries and maintaining flexible dynamic schemata. Graph databases are also good for data modelling as they are said to be "whiteboard friendly". This refers to the fact that people often intuitively draw data and relationships using a graph in the planning stages, and then turn these images into data tables or other structures. With graph databases the graphical design is replicated in the implementation of the database itself. The graphs are made of nodes, represented by circles and relationships (arrows) that connect the nodes. The graphs are labelled property graphs that allow us to add labels to the nodes and relationships. Relationships also have a direction. Unlike the temporary nature of joins in SQL databases that connect data in the various tables, the relationships between nodes are persistent in a graph database and of equal importance to the node data.

Figure 5.5 shows two nodes that represent people, *Jeff* and *Ann*. The arrow shows a relationship between them. This shows that the relationship *Loves* is a one way relationship and that Jeff 'Loves' Ann but Ann does not love Jeff back.

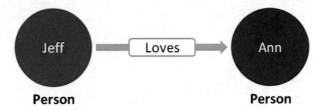

Fig. 5.5 Example relationship between 2 people nodes

Fig. 5.6 Example node in
neo4j

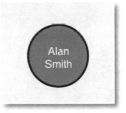

One of the most popular tools for graph databases is *neo4j*. This uses the graph query language called *Cypher*. Cypher uses ASCI art. So the image seen in Fig. 5.5 would be represented like this:

$$(Jeff) - [: LOVES] - > (Ann)$$

Nodes are represented by round brackets (parenthesis), and relationships in square brackets with lines and arrows $-[]- >$. We can create a node in neo4j using Cypher like so:

```
CREATE (: Person {})
```

Listing 5.16 creating a node in Cypher

We can add additional labels using comma separated key values pairs in the same way we do in MongoDB. For example let's make a node for a person and give them a name and some associated data, including their age, sex, blood pressure (bp) and heart rate (hr).

```
CREATE (: Person {name:"Alan Smith", age:24, sex:"M", bp:"120/70",
    hr:78})
```

Listing 5.17 Adding data labels to the node

We can then return the graph by typing:

```
MATCH (n) RETURN n
```

Listing 5.18 View the database

This now allows us to view our single Person node (Fig. 5.6).

We can also add a label to demarcate individual nodes. For example we can use *p* for person, or write the name *alan* in-front of the colon.

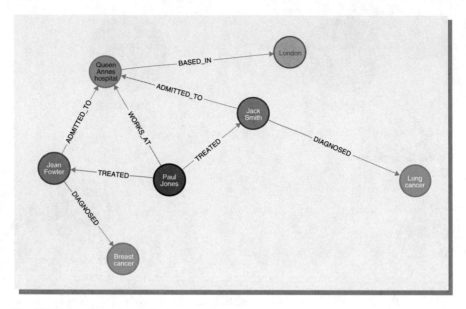

Fig. 5.7 Example graph, neo4j

```
1 CREATE (alan:Person {name:"Alan Smith", age:24, sex:"M", bp:"
     120/70", hr:78})
2 MATCH (alan) RETURN alan.name
```

Listing 5.19 Label individual nodes and return specific data (e.g. name)

Here is a small example to generate some nodes and relationships. The resulting graph can be seen in Fig. 5.7.

```
1  CREATE (jack:Patient {name:'Jack Smith'}),
2  (cancer:Condition {name:'Lung cancer', type:'small cell'}),
3  (jack) -[:DIAGNOSED {year:1999}]->(cancer),
4  (paul:Doctor {name:'Paul Jones'}),
5  (paul) -[:TREATED {year:1999}]->(jack),
6  (london:Place {name:'London', type:'City', country:'UK'}),
7  (queenannes:Hospital {name:'Queen Annes hospital'}) -[:BASED_IN
     ]->(london),
8  (paul) -[:WORKS_AT]->(queenannes),
9  (jack) -[:ADMITTED_TO {date:'12/04/1999',ward:'Seagul'}]->(
     queenannes),
10 (jean:Patient {name:'Jean Fowler'}),
11 (bcancer:Condition {name:'Breast cancer', type:'ductal carcinoma'
     }),
12 (jean) -[:DIAGNOSED {year:2004}]->(bcancer),
13 (paul) -[:TREATED {year:2004}]->(jean),
14 (jean) -[:ADMITTED_TO {date:'07/08/2004',ward:'Dolphin'}]->(
     queenannes)
```

Listing 5.20 Cypher code to generate example graph

The graph generated shows a doctor (Paul Jones) that works in a hospital called St. Anne's that is based in London. We can also see that he treated 2 patients (Jack and Jean) for cancer. We can encode extra information in the nodes and relationships. For example we have details of the cancer type (e.g. small cell lung cancer) stored in the nodes. In the relationships, such as *DIAGNOSED* we can see the year of diagnosis and for *ADMITTED*, we can see the ward name and date of admission. We can then write queries to extract sub-graphs of information or individual properties from the data similar to those we would write using SQL. The following are some examples of queries you could run on these data.

```
MATCH (p:Patient) WHERE p.name="Jack Smith" RETURN p
```

Listing 5.21 Query the node where the name is *Jack Smith*

This could also be written like this:

```
MATCH (p:Patient {name:"Jack Smith"}) RETURN p
```

Listing 5.22 Query the node where the name is *Jack Smith* alternative method

We can also query on relationships. For example find the doctor that treated the patient with the name *Jack Smith*.

```
MATCH (d:Doctor)-[TREATED]->(p:Patient) WHERE p.name="Jack Smith"
    RETURN d
```

Listing 5.23 Returns the doctor (Paul Jones node) that treated the patient *Jack Smith*

Or all the patients treated at Queen Anne's hospital.

```
MATCH (p:Patient)-[TREATED]->(h:Hospital)
WHERE h.name="Queen Annes Hospital"
RETURN p
```

Listing 5.24 Returns the patient nodes (Jack and Jean)

This often leads to more intuitive and less complex queries that are traditionally generated with SQL. There are also considerable performance gains over SQL queries. These features along with the flexibility of data schema and the flexibility for adaption are leading lots of companies to move toward graph database solutions in place of more traditional relational database options. We would recommend that you engage in data modelling prior to implementation, regardless of the system used to store your data. This will help identify logical and technical errors and reduce subsequent development time and cost.

5.3 Legal Aspects

After considering the technical issues and solutions for storing our data, we must also consider the legality of doing so. The collection and storage of data is governed by certain legal principles. Different territories operate under different legislative systems. A detailed examination of the legislation concerning data regulations is beyond the scope of this text. We will however mention some of the key aspects concerning this topic and discuss some details regarding relevant legislation in the United States (US) and the European Union (EU).

5.3.1 European Union/European Economic Area (EU/EEA)

In the case of the EU and European Economic Area (EEA) the *General Data Protection Regulation* (GDPR) was adopted in 2016 (and became enforceable in May 2018) succeeding the previous Data Protection Directive.[2] The principle of the regulation is to give individuals more control over their personal data, including how and why they are used and by whom. Previous data protection rules came about before the internet was as ubiquitous as it is currently. It has taken some time for legislation to catch up with the rapid changes in technology. These regulations have triggered big alterations for companies and organisations that store and process personal data in the EU/EEA as well as other countries that carry out data transactions with the EU. Each member country will integrate this into their legal system. For example the UK's Data Protection Act[3] covers GDPR which is managed by the Information Commissioner's Office (ICO) [1] that acts as the statutory authority for the UK.

Many items of data come under the expansive definition of personal data. Examples include things like an individual's name, date of birth, address, medical information and computer's IP address [3]. From a research perspective, the majority of researchers will apply the *task in public interest* option as the legal basis for processing these data [3]. Many researchers will use pseudonymised data as they are interested in pooling data for analysis rather than individual information. Pseudonymisation is carried out by removing identifying records and replacing them with either a pseudonym or a unique identifier. For example the name "Mary Jones" could be replaced with "P1F". This unique identification is however linked to other records that include identifying information. For example, you might store some survey data in one location using unique identifiers. In a separate location, you might store survey participants' names and addresses using the same unique identifier. Under the scope of GDPR, pseudonymised data are still considered personal data [3], as there is a potential for the data to be linked to other information that could be used to re-identify the participant. In the UK, the NHS Health Research Authority (HRA) has published guidance for researchers on GDPR and other relevant legislation [4].

---

[1] General Data Protection Regulation (EU) 2016/679.
[2] Data Protection Directive 95/46/EC.
[3] Data Protection Act 2018.

5.3.2   USA

The situation in the US is somewhat different with state level and national guidelines on data protection. Specific federal statutes address certain sectors. The common law element of right to privacy also covers some aspects of data protection.

The Health Insurance Portability and Accountability Act (HIPPA) sets the national standards for the protection of sensitive patient data. HIPAA Compliance requires that all people with personal health information access using computer systems are compliant.

As part of HIPAA, the Privacy Rule, which covers the governance of individually identifiable health information, was developed. It was published in its final form in 2002. The Privacy Rule covers any entity that transmits health information electronically. This includes [19]:

- Health care providers
- Health plans (e.g. insurance companies and government-sponsored health plans, health maintenance organizations. . .)
- Health Care Clearinghouses (i.e. entities that receive data from other entities and process it from nonstandard into standard format, e.g. billing services, repricing companies)
- Business associates (i.e. entities that provide services to, or perform certain functions for, a covered entity, without being part of the covered entity's workforce, e.g. entities that perform data analysis or process claims for a covered entity); in such cases the covered entity must impose a Business Associate Contract to stipulate how the individually identifiable health information is to be used by the business associate

The Privacy Rule protects all individually identifiable health information in any form of media. This includes the following types of information (unless it is fully anonymised) [19]:

- Information about an individual's health
- Information about the health care an individual has received information about payment for health care received by an individual

Full anonymisation can be achieved by either approval of a qualified statistician, or by removing certain identifiers from the data to the extent that the remaining information could not be combined with other information to re-identify the individual [19]. For example, if a dataset shows that only five individuals in a certain geographic area have a certain health condition, and further information such as age and gender is provided, this information could easily be combined to re-identify the individuals. This is a relatively simple example for illustration purposes; in practice much more complex combinations of data for re-identification are possible and therefore anonymisation requires careful consideration.

5.3.3   Regulatory Compliance

Guidelines are set out by the British Standards Institution and Innovate UK in the Publicly Available Specification (PAS) 277:2015 [18] for quality criteria related to health and wellness apps. These guidelines make several suggestions aimed at software/app developers regarding both documentation and quality criteria. These include ensuring the app meets any regulatory and legal requirements, functionality (meeting need), addressing User Experience (UX) and accessibility issues, safety, security and performance (being reliable and stable). In relation to documentation, the recommendations include keeping a 'risk register' to document any potential risks associated with the app. This can include details such as the type of risk, the risk itself and related consequences. An example given for a medication reminder app with the risk category 'safety' is the risk of developers ceasing to support the app (thus ceasing to carry out updates and bug-fixes), which could lead to users no longer receiving medication reminders. This could in turn lead to missed medication doses. This could have a potentially greater impact if for example the app was a mental health intervention that was suddenly withdrawn or no longer supported.

Public Health England has also produced some guidance on the criteria for health app assessment, which states that the purpose of the app must be clear, and the app should be built using the latest evidence-based knowledge. Demonstration of clinical effectiveness is required for an app to achieve evaluated status from NICE [16]. In the UK, if the app meets the definition of a medical device, it must be registered with the Medicines and Healthcare Products Regulatory Agency (MHRA) and have a CE mark [16]. The CE mark informs consumers that the product was assessed for safety as well as environmental and health protection requirements [6]. Health apps have to demonstrate the following: evidence of their effectiveness, regulatory approval, clinical safety, privacy and confidentiality, security, usability and accessibility, interoperability and technical stability [16].

The European Commission highlights in its green paper that mHealth apps should include security features, such as the use of encryption for patient data and methods of authentication [5]. They also highlight the issues surrounding the slow-going introduction of international interoperability standards caused by individuals and SMEs lacking legal knowledge and resources to carry this out [5]. This means that the apps may not be compatible or able to deal with data sharing with other systems.

Many health and medical apps directly collect and store individuals' health data as shown in Fig. 5.8, where details concerning blood pressure, weight, glucose levels and mood are collected.

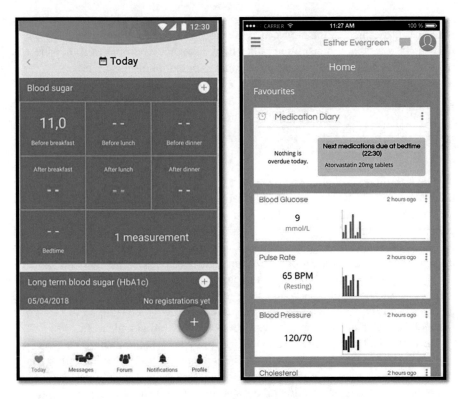

Fig. 5.8 A selection of apps from the UK's NHS Apps Library [2]. (Apps from left to right: ©
Liva Healthcare, from https://www.nhs.uk/apps-library/liva-uk/ © Evergreen Life, from https://
www.nhs.uk/apps-library/evergreen-life/. Screenshots reproduced with permission)

5.4 Geo-Location

Many interventions may require the collection of location data to make use of
various features. Where the data are stored and transmitted to a server there exists
a potential to compromise the individual's rights to privacy. In addition to simply
knowing where an individual is at a given time, this information can be used to
determine certain patterns relating to where the individual spends their time. A
picture could be constructed of work, leisure and social patterns. This information
may be intentionally sought to produce interactions that deal with some aspect of
measuring social interaction or other activities of daily living, as was the intention
in a longitudinal study that used such features among others for the unobtrusive
monitoring of Parkinson's disease [21]. Specific consent should be sought and the
intended use of these data should be clearly explained to participants where these
data are sought for research purposes or for use with a feature of an intervention.
Another question to ask when considering the collection of location data is what
level of granularity you actually need. The intervention may need to know for

example what country/town/city a user is in, or even which zip code area. If this is the case, the precise location can be used to derive this information, which in turn can be stored and transmitted rather than the exact co-ordinates if they are not required. This will make the app more robust to potential disclosure issues.

> Ideally, store location data at the highest level of granularity required to protect users' confidentially and privacy.

The technique of *abbreviation* can be used to remove records from areas where there is a low population count [11]. The 'Britain Breathing' app [22], which uses experience sampling to collect data about seasonal allergy symptoms also collected geospatial data. The data was intended to be open access and included location information from participants. The method used worked by generating an approximation of the number of participants in a postcode (zipcode) area in the UK. It worked by using a combination of the participants' year of birth and gender. This meant that all people of a certain gender born in a particular year would be classed as a single entity. Although less accurate, it was generally considered to be a good trade off between accuracy and the risk of identifying individuals [22].

Recommendations for preventing disclosure by geo-spatial data include deliberately reducing spatial and temporal precision (especially if not required), training members of the project team in location privacy threats, and storing data safely and removing them from devices. Identifiers should be removed from the data to prevent individuals being identified [11]. Stored datasets should also be anonymised or have access to them restricted [11].

5.5   Information Governance (IG) and Data Management Plans (DMP)

Many funders and university or medical ethics panels will want to know how you intend on managing the data you will collect and use. One way to lay this out formally is in a document called a Data Management Plan (DMP) which gives an overview of the type of data you are collecting, how it stored (including its security) and who else has access to it and how. One such tool that can be used to create and share DMPs is *DMPOnline* (https://dmponline.dcc.ac.uk/), as seen in Fig. 5.9.

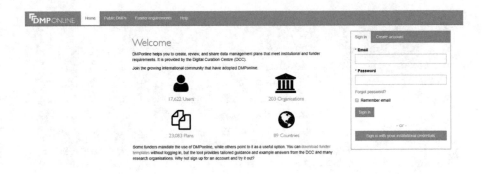

Fig. 5.9 DMPOnline – a tool for creating and sharing data management plans. (https://dmponline. dcc.ac.uk/ Screenshot reproduced with permission)

5.6 Data Security

If an mHealth application needs to collect and store users' data but does not require that data are sent to a server, either for storage or for processing then the simplest way of protecting these data is to store the data on the device itself. The app can be set up to require the user to enter a password or pin to access the app and its associated data. This way if the user leaves their device unattended or it is lost or stolen, the data will be more secure. Additional encryption can also be added to the data. Data security becomes a more complex challenge if the app does require that the data are transmitted and stored/processed on a remote sever. In this instance if the data are lost or stolen they could constitute a *data breach* which brings with it associated legal and financial implications for those charged with controlling the data.

There have been many high profile data leaks including Yahoo, Facebook, Uber, Microsoft Office 365 and PlayStation among many other well known companies. As technology and practices evolve to overcome security vulnerabilities, those carrying out these attacks also improve their methods of attack. These attacks can be carried out by hackers, hackavists (people hacking for social or political reasons), terrorists/rogue states, or employees carrying out inside jobs (e.g. because they are disgruntled or for the purpose of industrial espionage).

Case study: Ashley Madison

Ashley Madison was an online dating and social network service originating in Canada. The site was aimed at customers who were in a relationship including marriage and who wanted to have an affair. In 2015 the service was attacked by a group calling itself 'The Impact Team' and the resulting data breach saw more than 60 GB of customers' data released. The data included information on customers' sexual preferences, email and physical addresses and partial credit card details. This allegedly led to a series of additional crimes including extortion following threats to expose members. Additionally, according to France24, there were a number of Saudi Arabian emails leaked. Adultery can be punishable with the death penalty in Saudi Arabia. The BBC in the UK also reported that there were 2 suicides related to the hack. Poor security practices, such as hard coding credentials (including database passwords) were discovered by security researchers following the incident.

A data breach can be a costly issue to deal with regardless of whether it occurs through a malicious attack or by some error caused by people or technology. If the type of data you process is personal and/or sensitive then the impact could be even higher, as highlighted in the Ashley Madison case study. If your intervention stores user data in some way, it could be vulnerable to data breaches. Some of these vulnerabilities can be rectified through training and awareness of how to process data, who you can and can't share it with and the regulations surrounding these issues. Apart from these factors there is also a technical aspect to data security that is directly linked to how you choose to implement the part of your intervention that processes data. The following sections detail some of the technical aspects that you should have some awareness of. In the UK, the previous maximum fine for a data breach was £500,000. Now under the new GDPR the maximum fine is €20 million. Data are potentially vulnerable not just when stored in a database but during transmission to and from a server as well.

5.6.1   HTTP and HTTPS

Hypertext Transfer Protocol or (HTTP) is a protocol for internet data transmission. It is mainly concerned with the presentation of information to end users (i.e. in the form of HTML pages). Information sent using HTTP can be potentially intercepted by third parties leading to potential security breaches in web based software or software that transmit data via the web. HTTP was extended and combined with an additional protocol called Secure Sockets Layer (SSL) to become HTTPS. This extended version uses SSL to encrypt information sent over the web and improve security. The Transport Layer Security (TLS) has more recently replaced SSL as a more secure method.

These protocols provide advantages for mobile security relating to the transmission of personal and medical information via mHealth interventions. The main disadvantages are that server speed can be reduced due to the need to encode information being sent. Additionally using SSL requires the issuing of a certificate which is a monetised service.

5.6.2   GET and POST Requests

The HTTP protocol also supports several methods to transfer data between a client and a server. Essentially the client makes a request and the server provides a response. The two most commonly used methods of the HTTP methods are *GET* and *POST*. GET requests pass parameters inside the URL (Uniform Resource Locator) as key value pairs (e.g. /mywebpage/myform.php?name1=value1&name2=value2). This means that these parameters are stored in the server logs/browser history and are potentially accessible by third parties, precisely because GET requests can be cached and stored in browser history etc. There is also a limit to the length of data they can transfer ($\approx$2000 characters). They are fast and very usable. It is recommended that GET is used for safe actions only. More sensitive data should be transferred using POST requests that store the data in the message body. Additionally they are never cached, bookmarked, stored in browser history and have no limit on the length of the data sent.

Listing 5.25 shows an example of some code from an Ionic health app that transmits data using a HTTP POST request to a database on a server.

```
import { Http, Headers, RequestOptions } from '@angular/http';

...

this.http.post(apiURL, messageString, options).map(res => res.
    json()).subscribe(data => {
    // success
    if (data.Code < 200) {
      // show thanks page
      loading.dismiss();
      self.showThanksPage();
    }
    else {
        loading.dismiss();
        let alert = this.alertCtrl.create({
            title: 'Error Sending Data',
            subTitle: data.Message,
            buttons: ['OK']
        });
        alert.present();
    }
```

```
21    }, error => {
22        // something went wrong
23        loading.dismiss();
24        let alert = this.alertCtrl.create({
25            title: 'Error Sending Data',
26            subTitle: 'Your data could not be sent at this time.
     Please check your connection and try again.',
27            buttons: ['OK']
28        });
29        alert.present();
30    });
```

Listing 5.25 Code snipet from an Ionic app showing HTTP POST request

5.6.3   TCP/IP

The Transmission Control Protocol and Internet Protocol are responsible for actually transmitting the data (TCP) to a given internet address (IP) by breaking down data into smaller packets for transmission. These packets are also assigned a *port* for the type of application that should process the data (Table 5.7).

Apps that transmit data may use one or more of the protocols mentioned above to transmit the data. Data are at risk of interception during transit. One way to add further security to such data is to use *encryption* .

5.6.4   Encryption

Encryption is a process of encoding information such that it can only be decoded by someone with a corresponding decryption key (essentially an algorithm). There are several types of encryption that can be applied. *Symmetric* encryption uses a key to encrypt and decrypt information. The principle drawback of this approach is that both sender and receiver of information require access to the key and this could be potentially intercepted by a third party. This situation is improved by using *asymmetric* encryption (public-key encryption). This works by using both a *public*

Table 5.7 Commonly used TCP ports

Port number	Used by	Purpose
20	File Transfer Protocol (FTP)	Transmission and receiving of files
21	File Transfer Protocol (FTP)	Transmission and receiving of files
22	Secure Shell (SSH)	Logging in securely
25	Simple Mail Transfer Protocol (SMTP)	Email
80	Hypertext Transfer Protocol (HTTP)	Web pages

and *private* key (called a key-pair). Because a cipher can produce a near infinite quantity of potential outputs they can be publicly shared without risk that a third party can use them effectively. The encryption key itself is in essence a string of zeros and ones (bits). Longer keys are less prone to brute force attacks and relatively small key lengths can produce many values: 2^n, where n is the key's length. Using this system the private key should never be shared but the public key can be given to as many people as required. There exist public key servers that can distribute public keys. The asymmetric method is slower than the symmetric encryption. There is an even faster method available called *elliptic curve* encryption that works by using a curve whose points satisfy an equation for 2 variables. The geometric qualities of these curves make them difficult to compute and therefore more robust than older systems that used factoring such as Rivest-Shamir-Adleman (RSA) and Diffie-Hellman algorithms that underpinned public-key encryption.

5.6.5   Password Management

Some interventions may require you to collect and store users' passwords. You should not collect and store this information without real need. Many people will use their passwords in multiple places and users are trusting you and your software to keep this information secure. Therefore only collect and store this information if there is no other solution. If there is an existing system (Google, Facebook etc.) that you can use to handle the passwords and logging in for you and that takes responsibility for security, then this would be the preferable option. The *OAuth* (Open Authentication) method was originally designed for Twitter. This uses a token to authorize access and acts as an intermediary without the user having to share their passwords. OAuth can be used to integrate Google sign-in into your web apps [7]. If you do however have to implement a system for password management then you should aim to use existing and recommended solutions rather than attempting to build such a system from the ground up.

> A strong password is typically long and preferably made up of non-dictionary words with upper/lowercase text, numbers and punctuation all used. Sometimes people also use a series of words together in an unusual phrase.

Passwords in plain text should never be stored in a database/file in raw text form. Instead the password input provided when a user tries to login should be *hashed* and compared to their stored hashed password. A *hash* is a function that converts data to fixed length hash values. Hashing a password is a good idea, but if the same input is used, i.e. several users choose the same password then the hash will be the same for all of these users. If a hacker can determine such a hashed password they would be potentially able to access all users' information where the same password was used. Many people also use the same passwords on multiple sites and programs. If a hacker is able to obtain this information from your program, they could potentially compromise the same user's accounts for multiple different applications and websites. Weak passwords can be cracked more easily and therefore should be avoided.

> **Case study: The Adobe hack**
> Adobe incorporated is an American multinational software company that is behind software such as Photoshop and the Portable Document Format (PDF). In 2013 Adobe suffered a hack which impacted around 150 million customers. The data accessed included credit and debit card numbers, email addresses, passwords and password hints. The data were widely circulated on the internet in a compressed file. Experts reviewing the file were able to analyse the data and found that many of the passwords used were weak. These included passwords like *password, 1234, qwerty* and *00000*. Adobe was also criticised for using weak encryption that was easy to break.

Salting hashes comes from the field of cryptography and refers to making the hash unique by adding some extra random information to it. This means that each hashed password will be unique for every user. This requires a new random salt to be added each time for each user.

> Even with salting and hashing, weak passwords can be broken with relative ease.

The random data used in a salt should not be generated with the typical random function of a programming language. Instead a Cryptographically Secure Pseudo-Random Number Generator (CSPRNG) should be used. *Key-stretching* algorithms (i.e. PBKDF2, bcrypt, scrypt) can be used to deliberately slow down the hashing function to mitigate against certain forms of attack (i.e. brute force).

When users are entering their data for the first time (i.e. a registration process), you should avoid informing the user that their password is not unique as this can be very useful information for a hacker, as can telling them if it was the password or the username that was inputted incorrectly. The code shown in Listing 5.26 gives an example of hashing a password. Please note that the code examples used here are for illustrative purposes only. Do not use this code to create a password system. As software security is a rapidly changing field you are advised to consult a recent tutorial for implementing a password storage system in the language and framework that you are developing in.

```
1  import hashlib
2
3  def register_password():
4      pw = input("Please register a password: ")
5      pw_hashed = str(hashlib.sha256(pw.encode('utf-8')).hexdigest
       ())
6      return pw_hashed
7
8  print(register_password())
```

Listing 5.26 Example of hashing a password

The code takes the password entered by the user and hashes it. If we run the code twice and enter the same password i.e. *bunnyboiler79* we get the result shown below.

```
1  Please register a password: bunnyboiler79
2  c37374bf558eb26ce8cff59c85e975957bc6572f4d56278158429aa91b0488b0
3  Please register a password: bunnyboiler79
4  c37374bf558eb26ce8cff59c85e975957bc6572f4d56278158429aa91b0488b0
```

Listing 5.27 Program output

As mentioned previously, this is a problem if multiple users share the same password. In the next listing (5.28) we add the salting to the hashed passwords to make them unique. Note we are using the *os.urandom()* function for random generation as it is a Cryptographically Secure Pseudo-Random Number Generator as opposed to Python's *rand()* function.

```
1  import hashlib, os
2
3  def register_password():
4      pw = input("Please register a password: ")
5      pw_hashed = str(hashlib.sha256(pw.encode('utf-8')).hexdigest
       ())
6      salt = str(hashlib.sha256(os.urandom(60)).hexdigest().encode(
       'utf-8'))
7      salted_hash = salt + pw_hashed
8      return salted_hash
9
10 print(register_password())
```

Listing 5.28 Example of salting and hashing a password

Again if we run the code twice with the same password as before we get:

```
1  Please register a password: bunnyboiler79
2  b'33ea6f002db14afbd714582b0c44d22985f9fbd67c1dfa042dd6daa45
3
4  Please register a password: bunnyboiler79
5  b'7e5c2aa6d05105579f909de7f0009eb3dab16d7876a602d98b5732c68
```

Listing 5.29 Program output (hashes shortened for readability)

We now have a unique hash for each user, even if they use the same password. Finally the code shown in Listing 5.30 shows an implementation in Python using the *bcrypt* password hashing function that can be used to hash and salt passwords as well as check a password's validity. In a real example the salt and hash would be stored and retrieved form a database before being compared with the inputted password at login.

```
import bcrypt

def salt_hash_password(password):
    return bcrypt.hashpw(password, bcrypt.gensalt())

def validate_password(password, hashed_password):
    return bcrypt.checkpw(password, hashed_password)

def register_password():
    pw = input("Enter password to register: ")
    return salt_hash_password(pw.encode('utf-8'))

def login(registered_password):
    pw = input("Enter password to login: ")
    if validate_password(pw.encode('utf-8'), registered_password):
        print("Logged in")
    else:
        print("Incorrect details entered")

# register a password and login with it
registered_password = register_password()
login(registered_password)
```

Listing 5.30   Example of salting and hashing a password using bcrypt

- Ideally use a system that manages passwords and logging in for you
- Otherwise consult an up to date tutorial in your chosen development language/framework

5.6.5.1   Multi-factor Authentication

This refers to a system where more than one item of information is required to authenticate a user. Two-factor authentication is an example where 2 pieces of information are required. This is usually the user's password and some temporary value that is sent to their mobile phone.

5.6.6   Cyberattacks

There are many potential ways that people or groups may steal, damage, destroy or attempt to gain control of a software system. The reasons behind this are also varied and can include financial gain, notoriety and can even be carried out by nation states for the purposes of cyberterrorism or cyberwarfare. They can also be perpetrated by experts to test a system's vulnerabilities to potential attacks, so that these vulnerabilities can be removed or reduced.

If your app is intending to use passwords then they should enforce the use of strong passwords. Attacks such as *brute force*, where a machine will sequentially try combinations of values until it is successful or *dictionary attacks* which use words and other references are very good at breaking weaker passwords. Another option to reduce the risk of such attacks is to restrict the number of attempts a user has at logging in and then blocking their account when this limit is reached.

Another common type of attack is known as *SQL injection* which is one of the most common web attacks given that SQL databases are very commonly used. This technique involves adding SQL code to a web form, for example a text box on a form that is sent to the server. This can then execute SQL code on your database and retrieve data or delete tables and cause damage to the data. Figure 5.10 shows how a simple trick with a single quote can be used to access data. It could be translated to an SQL statement like that seen in Listing 5.31 where as 1 does equal 1 the id will be returned from the database.

```
SELECT id FROM usersdata WHERE username='uname' AND password='
    pword' OR 1=1'
```

Listing 5.31 Possible server query run with SQL injection

One can mitigate this sort of attack by validating input (checking the input prior to submission), avoiding the use of dynamic SQL by using stored queries and not using string concatenation (joining strings of text together) to form queries. A lot of web frameworks now also provide functions to help with this as well as parameterized queries which are a form of prepared SQL command that are supplied with parameters (variables) to prevent additional commands being added to the query.

Some attacks are mostly technical in nature like SQL injection, whereas others are *social engineering attacks* that involve obtaining information to steal personal information that can be used to access other accounts. The Open Web Application Security Project (OWASP) based in the US is an international charity that aims to

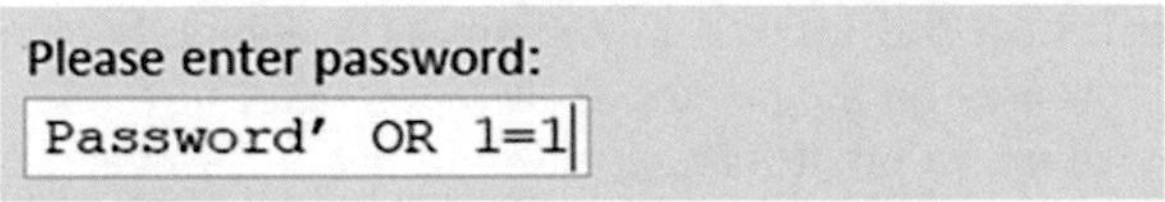

> Please enter password:
> `Password' OR 1=1`

Fig. 5.10 SQL injection being carried out on an input box on a web form

promote best practice in software security [14]. The organisation produces a top 10 list of current application security risks and is a useful source of information for keeping up to date with the latest digital security threats. Another obvious but important consideration relating to data security is regularly backing up data and archiving data (if required). This way if data are stolen, damaged or destroyed, they can be restored thus minimizing the potential impact. Ideally data should be backed up regularly and stored in a safe location separate to the original location in case it becomes compromised. This could include remote or offsite backups. This sort of service can be provided by various companies, alternatively one could back up data to a Cloud service.

5.6.7 The State of Data Security in mHealth Apps

A study about the security and privacy of mHealth applications highlighted serious concerns about the current state of practice in relation to security and protection of private data [15]. The study included an analysis of 20 mHealth apps that were free, with English content, had $\geq$100,000 downloads with minimum 2.5 out of 5 star rating. The apps also had to require the entry of personal and/or health data which would be transmitted to a remote host [15]. Most of the apps used in the study did not meet security/privacy standards. The main issues observed were:

- Requiring permission to access devices (i.e. camera, microphone, Blue-tooth) beyond the app's scope
- Storing data in web server log files (potentially exposing the data to unauthorised access)
- Sending geo-location or postal addresses using HTTP
- Transmitting passwords and doing so insecurely (i.e. using GET requests)

Adapted from Papageorgiou (2019) [15].

Another issue was related to a poor standard of privacy policies. 5% had broken links to policy details, a further 5% were not written in English, despite the app content being presented in English. Finally others were of poor quality and did not meet expected standards [15]. The lack of security was found to be due to poor design and inappropriate implementation [15]. The recommendations of PAS 277:2015 include a detailed product description and a privacy statement concerning how data are collected and handled by the app [18], which is often not included in health apps currently on the market. If the app is part of a research project we would recommend including the participant information sheet and consent form in the app itself. Ideally the user can refer back to this information at any point. The information would include the purpose of the study, the users' rights and details of what data will be collected and how they will processed. Apart from issues like those described by Papageorgiou (2019) [15] that are in the hands of the developers to a larger extent, the Android platform's security model itself falls short of completely protecting user data privacy and security [9].

5.7   Users' Access to their Own Data

An online survey concerning the use of personal health data that was carried out with both researchers ($n = 134$) and individuals ($n = 465$) found that the majority of individuals wanted to either own (75%) or at least share ownership (30%) of their data with the companies and organisations collecting their data [1]. The study also found that many people falsely believed that they did in fact already own the data they inputted into the app [1]. Given this desire of users to own and share these data with healthcare providers, friends and family, those building interventions that collect users' data should give some thought to whether or not to allow access to these data to the user and how this will be technically achieved. This may also provide extra work for the developers of such projects. Some of the ways in which users can access this information include the use of *APIs*, *platforms* or direct *file downloads* [10].

APIs (Application Programming Interfaces) involve being able to code (program) to make use of the API, which is beyond the scope of most users. This is a good option however if you want other researchers or organisations to access the data. To do this an API has to be well documented and tested.

Specific health platforms that users can log into and view and share their data are useful for users who may lack technical skills. There is again an overhead in creating such a platform unless existing platforms are used.

Finally a direct download option may exist for the data. The main issue here is the format that the data is downloaded as. Users may have difficulties in opening or sharing these data, especially if it is in a format like JSON. Interoperability is an ongoing issue in this area. Many software developers and companies are creating their own standards rather than using a system that offers compatibility for sharing and viewing data such as the Open mHealth standard [8]. Given the needs of various stakeholders, including researchers, developers, healthcare providers and patients themselves, getting access to the data collected should be considered an important component of the design process [10]. In terms of GDPR, which relates to EU countries, this is not just a courtesy but a requirement to give users the right to data portability [3]. This includes the right of the user who has personal data processed to obtain a copy of such data in a commonly used and structured format [3]. Hert et al. also highlight the potential of competitive market practices by allowing users to switch providers and move their data between them [3]. Another (less ideal) option

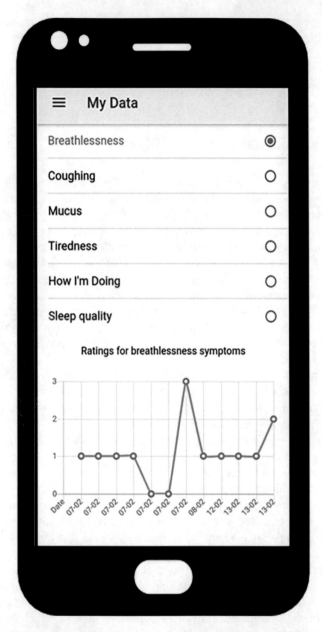

Fig. 5.11 Screenshot from an app that collects user data for aggregate analysis but also allows the user to view their own data in graphical form in the app itself. App created by the authors

is to at least display the users' data to them through the app itself. Figure 5.11 shows an app that collects data for research purposes and aggregates those data for analysis.

The user can also view their own individual data on the app itself. Although they cannot download or access the data in a portable form, they can at least view this in the app. When developing such apps, one should consider the impact of no longer supporting the app. This could happen when a research project finishes (or runs out of money), a company closes down, or no longer wishes to support a certain product line. In such cases what happens to the users' data? And how can they access this at a point after the app is no longer supported? In the case of time limited research projects, this should at least be communicated to users in the terms and conditions so that they are aware the app may only operate and be supported for a limited period of time. This way they can make a more informed choice about whether or not to use the app. Ideally app developers and healthcare workers should communicate and work together to create standards and ensure these standards are upheld in order to foster trust between users of these apps and the people involved in making them [17]. One technology that is showing promise for both the security and access issues to data is *Blockchain*, which has been widely used in cryptocurrencies (a digital encrypted currency) such as Bitcoin.

5.8 Blockchain

Blockchain as the name implies is a chain of blocks. Each of these blocks consists of 3 main features, some data that the block contains, a hash that is calculated based on the block's data, and a link to the previous hash. The first block in a blockchain is called the *genesis block* and doesn't point to a previous hash. In the context of a blockchain a hash is some function that converts an alphanumeric input into an encrypted output of a certain fixed length. For a blockchain, they act like a digital signature for each block (Fig. 5.12).

As each hash is unique like a fingerprint and is generated based on the data contained within the block, any attempt to tamper with the data will alter the block's hash. Of course with modern computing power, one could simply use brute force to recalculate the hashes. To overcome this, blockchain also utilises *proof-of-work*,

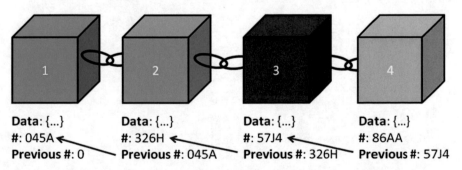

Fig. 5.12 A visual representation of a blockchain consisting of 4 blocks (# = hash)

which enforces a time limit to slow the creation of new blocks. To make it even more secure blockchains use a distributed peer-to-peer network to provide everyone in the network with a copy of the complete chain. Each new block is sent to everyone in the network to gain consensus, with each network node checking the validity of the new block. A malicious entity would have to gain control of 51% of the network in order to compromise it.

A good way to understand some of these concepts is with an example. The code below (Listing 5.32) shows how a simple blockchain might be constructed in Python. The code shows the creation of a class to represent a single block in a blockchain. The class constructor (init) takes as parameters an index value, a date/time stamp, some data (in this case a simple text string) and a previous hash. The *generate_hash()* function creates a hash value based on the values input to the Block class constructor. The *outputBlockInfo()* function displays the values of the block index, hash and previous hash.

```
1  class Block:
2      def __init__(self, index, time_stamp, data, previous_hash):
3          self.index = index
4          self.time_stamp = time_stamp
5          self.data = data
6          self.previous_hash = previous_hash
7          self.hash = self.generate_hash()
8
9      def generate_hash(self):
10         sha = hasher.sha256()
11         str_hash = (str(self.index) + str(self.time_stamp) + str(
    self.data) + str(self.previous_hash)).encode('utf-8')
12         sha.update(str_hash)
13         return str(sha.hexdigest())
14
15     def outputBlockInfo(self):
16         print("Block:", self.index, "Hash:", self.hash, "Previous
    hash:", self.previous_hash)
```

Listing 5.32 The Block class

Once we have made a Block class we can now make a class to manage the entire chain (Listing 5.33).

```
1  class BlockChain:
2      def __init__(self):
3          self.chain = [self.makeGenesisBlock()]
4          self.chain[0].outputBlockInfo()
5
6      def makeGenesisBlock(self):
7          return Block(0, date.datetime.now(), "Genesis block", "0"
    )
8
9      def getMostRecentBlock(self):
10         return self.chain[len(self.chain) - 1]
11
12     def addNewBlock(self, new_block):
```

```
13    new_block.previous_hash = self.getMostRecentBlock().hash
14    new_block.hash = new_block.generate_hash()
15    self.chain.append(new_block)
16    new_block.outputBlockInfo()
```

Listing 5.33 The Blockchain class

The constructor of the Blockchain class creates a list of blocks. The first item (block) added to the chain is the special *genesis block*. This block has no previous hash and is set to zero. We then add a few helper functions; one to return the most recent block in the chain and one to add new blocks to the chain. We can then implement these classes to create a rudimentary blockchain (Listing 5.34).

```
1  import datetime as date
2  import hashlib as hasher
3
4  myBlockChain = BlockChain()
5  myBlockChain.addNewBlock(Block(1, date.datetime.now(), "Some data
       ", "0"))
6  myBlockChain.addNewBlock(Block(2, date.datetime.now(), "Some more
       data", "0"))
```

Listing 5.34 Implementing the chain

This produces an output like that seen in Listing 5.35.

```
1  Block: 0 Hash: dd3b33dcb Previous hash: 0
2  Block: 1 Hash: 9b99ea5ec Previous hash: dd3b33dcb
3  Block: 2 Hash: 8f49cbcfa Previous hash: 9b99ea5ec
```

Listing 5.35 Program output (hashes shortened to aid readability)

5.8.1 Applying Blockchain to Health Data

Given the security features of blockchain, there is presently a growing excitement about using this technology to manage Electronic Health Records (EHRs). If these records were stored on the cloud, blockchain could be used to maintain the privacy and security of these records whilst also improving interoperability and conforming to data protection regulations [20].

Software scripts (termed 'smart contracts') can be added to blocks to provide additional conditions for data processing. These contracts combined with the other security features of blockchain make them potentially suitable for health applications as they can help to provide customized consent for certain parties to access data, security for transferring and sharing data between health institutions, as well as the ability to store multiple and complex information, such as genomic data and medical imaging [20]. Some of the key benefits to administration of health systems, to the health of the patient and to research are highlighted in Table 5.8.

Blockchain has the potential to meet GDPR requirements well although there may be some exceptions that are harder to manage such as the right to be

Table 5.8 Some of the potential benefits of using blockchain for health data. (Adapted from [20])

Administration
1. Reduced cost
2. Improved interoperability
3. Reduce admin delays
4. High security and regulatory compliance
Health
1. Rapid access to patient data (remove delays waiting for previous test results)
2. Personalised treatment plans
3. Add data from wearables and other health tracking tools
Research
1. Patients can consent to take part in research studies (choosing who accesses their data; consent is ensured by the system)
2.Would make research more accessible giving potential access to rich and up to date health/medical data

forgotten and have data removed. This may be potentially overcome by the use of dynamic consent management [4]. Additional advantages of blockchain include decentralized data management, collaboration between healthcare stakeholders, auditing, security & privacy and data preservation [4]. They are also useful for providing data provenance (origin and changes made to data over time) [4]. This makes blockchain suitable for the management of critical assets, such as patient consent records [12]. Given the various potential advantages of blockchain for medical record management and research, this technology is likely to become a feature of digital healthcare systems, including mHealth interventions, in the future.

To realize the full potential of mHealth apps, users must be satisfied that their data are stored safely, correctly and that their relevant rights pertaining to their data are being upheld. Although the current state of security in the domain of mHealth is worrying, we must bear in mind that this is still a relatively new technology in a world of ever changing technological advancements, new and emerging threats and evolving regulations trying to keep pace with technological advances. An awareness of these challenges coupled with a team approach between developers, designers, law makers and healthcare providers can help to overcome these issues and increase users' trust in mHealth.

5.9 Summary of Key Points

Many current health apps are falling short of applying the required standards of security and data protection. Failing to secure users data appropriately can result in large fines. In addition to this it erodes the public trust in mobile health solutions. To improve users confidence and to comply with relevant regulations, designers and developers of interventions should aim to determine the relevant regulations for the type of app they are developing and ensure that the best practices in data security are met and reviewed on a regular basis. This is even more important if the intervention collects and stores data, especially if these data are of a sensitive or personal nature.

- Only collect the information that you need for your intervention to work, and at the highest resolution you can
- Be aware of any legal and regulatory requirements that may apply to your intervention in the geographical area(s) you intend to deploy it
- If possible try to avoid implementing your own security solutions and use existing systems that have been tried and tested. This is both faster and more secure
- If a back end server is required by your intervention, allow enough time in the project to research and implement options
- The choice of database type should be based on the nature of the project
- Consider how you will allow users access to their own data if requested and how long you will provide this service
- Blockchain has the potential to improve security and democratize access to health data

5.10 Quiz

1. When designing an app to collect and use geo-spatial data, it is preferred that:

   (a) We collect as much detailed and specific information as we can
   (b) We collect only the level of information that is absolutely necessary
   (c) We do not collect geo-spatial data at all

2. Apart from the first block, the hash in a block chain block. . .

   (a) points to the hash of the previous block
   (b) is set to NULL
   (c) stores protocol data in a peer-to-peer network

3. The first block in a blockchain is called the

   (a) generator block
   (b) genesis block

4. The most secure protocol for sending data to a server is with the

   (a) HTTPS
   (b) HTTP

5. Under the GDPR pseudonymised data is still considered to be personal data.

   (a) True
   (b) False

6. MongoDB is an example of...

   (a) a structured database
   (b) an unstructured database

7. SQL queries should ideally be made by joining strings together (concatenation).

   (a) True
   (b) False

8. Public keys should never be shared.

   (a) True
   (b) False

Answers to the quiz can be found in "Solutions to Quizzes".

5.11   Exercises

1. With regard to the data in the *diabetes_data* table (Table 5.9):

   (a) What data records would you expect the following SQL query to return?

   ```
   SELECT * FROM diabetes_data WHERE sex = "F" AND age < 70;
   ```

   (b) Write a query in SQL or MongoDb to extract all people with Type I diabetes from the table
   (c) Write a query in SQL or MongoDb to extract all males with a HbA1c between 7.5 and 8.5

Table 5.9 Table *diabetes_data* containing data from diabetic patients including type of diabetes and hemoglobin A1c (HbA1c)

Name	Sex	Age	Hospital_id	HbA1c	Diabetes_type
Daniel Green	M	62	143729	7.8	Type II
Sam Jones	M	73	459833	7.7	Type II
Sarah Smith	F	81	534989	8.3	Type II
John James	M	57	349829	6.7	Type II
Laura Howe	F	26	984322	8.8	Type I
Lucy Lane	F	17	093292	7.2	Type I
Pauline Brown	F	45	848382	6.9	Type II

2. Download 2 or 3 mHealth apps from one of the app stores that collects health/medical data. Did they have clear policies about what happens to your data and your rights surrounding it? What was the quality of the policies like? Did they miss any important details?
3. Go to the OWASP site https://www.owasp.org/index.php/Category:Attack and pick an attack from the list that you haven't heard of before. Read about the attack.
4. Go to DMPOnline https://dmponline.dcc.ac.uk/public_plans and view some of the publicly available plans. Then have a go writing your own plan for an intervention you are developing/considering developing (or make one up).
5. Go to SSL Report https://www.ssllabs.com/ssltest/index.html and paste in a URL from your web server if you have one. Otherwise you can pick a random website. View the security report about the site. What rating did it get? Were there any ways it could be improved?

Recommended Reading

1. Kounadi O, Resch B. A geoprivacy by design guideline for research cam-paigns that use participatory sensing data. J Empir Res Hum Re-search Ethics. 2018;13(3):203–22.
2. SOPHOS. Security Center Definitions. 2019. https://home.sophos.com/en-us/security-center/definitions.aspx. Accessed 09 July 2019.
3. Medicines & Healthcare products Regulatory Agency Medical devices: software applications (apps). 2018. https://www.gov.uk/government/publications/medical-devices-software-applications-apps. Accessed 21 Aug 2019.
4. De Hert P, Papakonstantinou V, Malgieri G, Beslay L, Sanchez I. The right to data portability in the GDPR: towards user-centric interoperability of digital services. Comput Law Secur Rep. 2018;342:193–202.

References

1. Bietz MJ, Bloss CS, Calvert S, Godino JG, Gregory J, Claffey MP, Sheehan J, Patrick K. Opportunities and challenges in the use of personal health data for health research. J Am Med Inform Assoc. 2016;23(e1):1–7. https://doi.org/10.1093/jamia/ocv118
2. Crown. NHS Apps Library; 2019. https://www.nhs.uk/apps-library/
3. De Hert P, Papakonstantinou V, Malgieri G, Beslay L, Sanchez I. The right to data portability in the GDPR: Towards user-centric interoperability of digital services. Comput Law Secur Rev. 2018;34(2):193–203. https://doi.org/10.1016/j.clsr.2017.10.003
4. Dimitrov DV. Blockchain applications for healthcare data management. Healthc Inf Res. 2019;25(1):51–6. https://doi.org/10.4258/hir.2019.25.1.51
5. European Commission. Green paper on mobile Health ("mHealth"). Technical report, European Commission, Brussels; 2014. https://en.calameo.com/read/002621988e1943d41ce07
6. European Commission. CE marking; 2019. https://ec.europa.eu/growth/single-market/ce-marking_en
7. Google. Integrating Google Sign-In into your web app; 2019. https://developers.google.com/identity/sign-in/web/sign-in

8. Haddad D, Sim I, Farrugia E, Carini S, Estrin D. Open mHealth; 2015. http://www.openmhealth.org/
9. Hussain M, Zaidan AA, Zidan BB, Iqbal S, Ahmed MM, Albahri OS, Albahri AS. Conceptual framework for the security of mobile health applications on Android platform. Telematics Inform. 2018;35(5):1335–54. https://doi.org/10.1016/j.tele.2018.03.005
10. Kim Y, Lee B, Choe EK. Investigating data accessibility of personal health apps. J Am Med Inform Assoc. 2019;26:412–9. https://doi.org/10.1093/jamia/ocz003
11. Kounadi O, Resch B. A geoprivacy by design guideline for research campaigns that use participatory sensing data. J Empir Res Hum Res Ethics. 2018;13(3):203–22. https://doi.org/10.1177/1556264618759877
12. Kuo TT, Kim HE, Ohno-Machado L. Blockchain distributed ledger technologies for biomedical and health care applications. J Am Med Inform Assoc. 2017;24(6):1211–20. https://doi.org/10.1093/jamia/ocx068
13. Mueller J, Davies A, Jay C, Harper S, Blackhall F, Summers Y, Harle A, Todd C. Developing and testing a web-based intervention to encourage early help-seeking in people with symptoms associated with lung cancer. Br J Health Psychol. 2019;24(1):31–65. https://doi.org/10.1111/bjhp.12325
14. OWASP Foundation. OWASP; 2019. https://www.owasp.org/
15. Papageorgiou A, Strigkos M, Politou E, Alepis E, Solanas A, Patsakis C. Security and privacy analysis of mobile health applications: the alarming state of practice. IEEE Access. 2018;6:9390–403. https://doi.org/10.1109/ACCESS.2018.2799522
16. Public Health England. Criteria for health app assessment; 2017. https://www.gov.uk/government/publications/health-app-assessment-criteria/criteria-for-health-app-assessment
17. Sampat BH, Prabhakar B. Privacy risks and security threats in mHealth apps. J Int Technol Inf Manage. 2017;26(4):153.
18. The British Standards Institution. Health and wellness apps – quality criteria across the life cycle – Code of practice. Technical report, The British Standards Institution; 2015.
19. US Department of Health & Human Services. Summary of the HIPAA Privacy Rule. 2020. https://www.hhs.gov/hipaa/for-professionals/privacy/laws-regulations/index.html
20. Vazirani AA, O'Donoghue O, Brindley D, Meinert E. Implementing blockchains for efficient health care: systematic review. J Med Internet Res. 2019;21(2):e12439. https://doi.org/10.2196/12439
21. Vega J, Jay C, Vigo M, Harper S. Unobtrusive monitoring of parkinson's disease based on digital biomarkers of human behaviour. In: ASSETS'17, number Oct. ACM – Association for Computing Machinery, Baltimore; 2017. p. 351–2. https://doi.org/10.1145/3132525.3134782
22. Vigo M, Hassan L, Vance W, Jay C, Brass A, Cruickshank S. Britain breathing: using the experience sampling method to collect the seasonal allergy symptoms of a country. J Am Med Inform Assoc. 2018;25(1):88–92. https://doi.org/10.1093/jamia/ocx148

Chapter 6
Feeding Back Information to Patients and Users with Visualisations

6.1 Introduction

It is often said "a picture is worth a thousand words". This is based on a quote said to originate from Fred R. Barnard to encourage the use of images for advertising in the trade journal called *Printer's ink*. This relates to the fact that visualisations are known to reduce complex information into simpler and easier to interpret displays [19] which can aid in comprehension. This is perhaps one of the main reasons that humans like to communicate information visually. Humans are known to have superior abilities for the processing of visual information in comparison to numerical and tabular data [20] as well possessing an ability to identify patterns. When visualisations are used effectively, they can reduce cognitive load and draw users to salient information. When used incorrectly however they can obscure relevant information and mislead people into making incorrect interpretations [19].

Producing effective visualisations to convey required information can be challenging to get right and requires an awareness of good visualisation practices. Complexity is dramatically increased when we move to displaying visualisations via different digital devices. Consider the variety of different devices that interact with a single Electronic Health Record (EHR) system [18]. Added to this is the requirement for such a system to offer different views of the data based on who is viewing it (e.g. patient, doctor, etc.) This means that the visualisations must provide these differing interfaces across a multitude of different devices for a range of users [18].

Visualisation can be a powerful tool for conveying information concisely, but how sure are we that the visualisations we use in our apps are interpreted correctly by our target population? Getting this right is important if the visualisation is used for decision making or to promote behavioural change as a direct intention of an intervention. In this chapter we look at the different types of visualisation that can be used to convey information ranging from the less formal like infographics to more scientific and specialised visualisations. We look at some examples of good and bad

© Springer Nature Switzerland AG 2020
A. Davies, J. Mueller, *Developing Medical Apps and mHealth Interventions*, Health Informatics, https://doi.org/10.1007/978-3-030-47499-7_6

visualisations along with some of the principles of visual design and composition that can be used to improve the design of visualisations. We will also examine some of the visualisation frameworks and libraries that can be used to create visualisations in our apps. Finally we provide some examples of how we can work with end users to improve the comprehension of the visualisations we produce in our interventions.

6.2   Visualisations

The primary use of a visualisation is for representation of some underlying data or information. This can be for initial exploration of data to gain insights into its structure and identify any interesting/useful patterns in those data. Visualisations can also be used to communicate information to different audiences. This can be for tasks for such as education, evaluation/monitoring, summarising of information and for decision making purposes. We have been using visualisations for hundreds of years to convey information. Early examples include a simple plot produced by an astronomer in 1644 that shows the longitude between Toledo and Rome (2 places in Italy) and the *Rose chart* created by the English nurse Florence Nightingale in the Crimean war. The chart shows several years of the war split into monthly segments showing the effect of the sanitary commissions work (send by British government) on the army's mortality rate. Another excellent example of an early visualisation is that of Napoleon Bonaparte's Russian campaign in 1812 created by Charles Joseph Minard. The visualisation (Fig. 6.1) conveys a surprisingly large amount of information.

This includes temporal and geographical information, temperature, and amount of troops at each point. The width of the large beige line shows the amount of troops

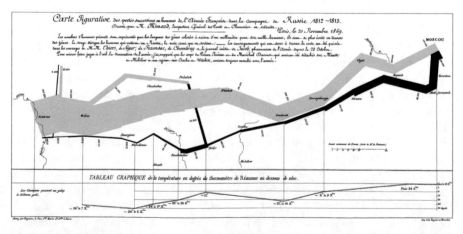

Fig. 6.1 Napoleon's 1812 Russian campaign from https://commons.wikimedia.org/wiki/File: Minard.png by Charles Minard (1781–1870) [Public domain] {{PD-US}}

at the start of the campaign. We can see the number of troops remaining as we
follow the line across through the various location names until we end up in Moscow
(Moscou). The black line shows the return journey. The information at the bottom
displays the temperature at various points. This visualisation shows how devastating
the campaign was for Napoleon. This early visualisation contains a large volume of
information about the campaign that is expressed visually. Modern visualisations
and infographics also aim to convey information in a concise way to their intended
audiences. There are different types of visualisation that can be used for different
applications depending on the target audience.

6.3   Types of Visualisations

There are many different types of visualisation available to suit different situations.
These range from the familiar scientific types that are commonly referred to as plots,
graphs or charts. These include bar charts, scatter plots, line plots, box and whisker
plots etc. They are often used to represent certain types of data. For example a bar
chart is often used to display categorical data to compare different groups, whereas a
line plot can be used for time series data. In addition to these, we also have medical
visualisations, such as X-rays, ECGs and other specialist medical and scientific
imaging. These types of image/visualisation tend to be for expert audiences that
are specially trained to interpret them (e.g. the ECG/EKG) and would be difficult
for lay people to interpret without first receiving training. There are also artistic
impressions that are usually more abstract in nature, these can be used to enhance
our understanding of various entities. Figure 6.2 gives an example of this with an

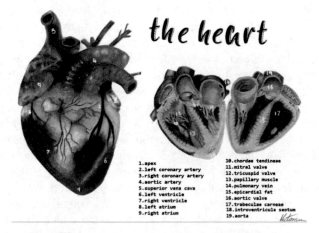

Fig. 6.2 Drawing of the human heart. (Reproduced with kind permission from Victoria Golaś)

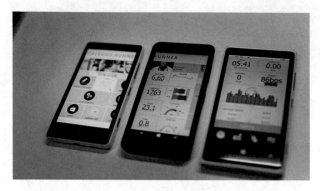

Fig. 6.3 Example of infographics used to display health data back to a patient/user. (Source: https://www.flickr.com/photos/15216811@N06/14504964841, reproduced under a CC BY 2.0 license https://creativecommons.org/licenses/by/2.0/)

artistic impression of the human heart. Such images can be used for educational purposes, such as learning anatomy.

Something perhaps more inbetween a more precise scientific visualisation and an artistic impression is the infographic. These can be used to display information to people in a more informal way than a traditional scientific visualisation by trying to make the information clearer and more accessible to its target audience (e.g. Fig. 6.3).

6.4   The Importance of Visualisations

The American statistician Francis Anscombe highlighted in his paper that many of the textbooks that teach statistical methods placed more emphasis on numerical calculations than graphing the data [4], and that there was a virtue in carrying out intricate calculations in comparison to "cheating" by looking at the data [4]. This led Anscombe to create the 4 simple datasets that can be seen in Table 6.1.

The descriptive statistics for these datasets are almost identical including the means of the X and Y variables, the regression coefficient, R^2 and the residual sum of squares. When we plot the data however we get the plots seen in Fig. 6.4. Here we can see that the datasets look very different when plotted. The results for the 4th dataset for example would be impacted greatly by the removal of the outlier point to the upper right of the plot [4]. Anscombe suggested that such results could contain a note about the importance of that single observation when reported on [4].

This goes to show that there is real value in visualising data, especially for the initial data exploration that may occur when presented with a new dataset. Many data scientists and statisticians start their analysis by plotting the data to look for relationships in the data and to see the structure and distribution of the underlying data (see Chap. 9 for more information). This is also helpful for outlier detection.

Table 6.1 Anscombe's quartet made up of 4 data sets (1–4). (Adapted from Anscombe (1973) [4], published by Taylor & Francis Ltd. www.tandfonline.com)

1		2		3		4	
X_1	Y_1	X_2	Y_2	X_3	Y_3	X_4	Y_4
10.0	8.04	10.0	9.14	10.0	7.46	8.0	6.58
8.0	6.95	8.0	8.14	8.0	6.77	8.0	5.76
13.0	7.58	13.0	8.74	13.0	12.74	8.0	7.71
9.0	8.81	9.0	8.77	9.0	7.11	8.0	8.84
11.0	8.33	11.0	9.26	11.0	7.81	8.0	8.47
14.0	9.96	14.0	8.10	14.0	8.84	8.0	7.04
6.0	7.24	6.0	6.13	6.0	6.08	8.0	5.25
4.0	4.26	4.0	3.10	4.0	5.39	19.0	12.50
12.0	10.84	12.0	9.13	12.0	8.15	8.0	5.56
7.0	4.82	7.0	7.26	7.0	6.42	8.0	7.91

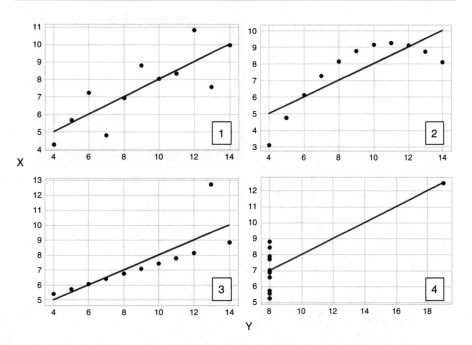

Fig. 6.4 Plots of each of the 4 datasets in Anscombe's quartet. (Adapted from Anscombe (1973) [4], published by Taylor & Francis Ltd. www.tandfonline.com)

6.5   Dynamic Visualisations

Dynamic visualisations are very useful for data exploration and allow one to drill down into the data by applying filters to data. Due to the dynamic nature of such visualisations they are often used less and poorly defined in certain work flows

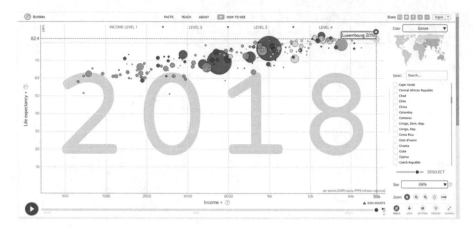

Fig. 6.5 Showing a free visualization from GAPMINDER.ORG, CC-BY license [13]. This bubble chart plots the income of countries (per person GDP/capita) against life expectancy in years. The plot can be animated to show changes over time and countries and regions filtered and individually selected

such as official reports [5]. This is often to do with the static print medium of books, papers and journals that do not lend themselves to the dynamic exploration of data, hence their main use being for data exploration and public engagement. One such example is the "Gapminder" project that aims to dispel misconceptions about global development [13]. Their website allows people to explore data for themselves freely. An example of this can be seen in Fig. 6.5 showing an interactive bubble chart visualisation that compares the life expectancy of countries against their level of wealth income which can be animated to show changes over years as well as supporting the filtering and selection of various data. The use of dynamic visualisation can also help to reduce information overload [9]. It can be difficult to reproduce dynamic visualisations without knowledge of the prior filtering, rotation, zooming and other actions applied to it.

6.6 Design Principles

When designing visualisations, there are many different design principles that can be applied to increase the effectiveness of the visualisation for communicating its main message and improving user comprehension. Here we discuss a few of the main principles that can be applied.

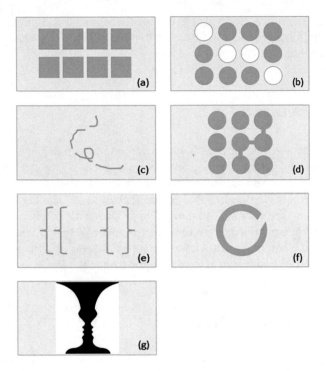

Fig. 6.6 Gestalt principles (**a**) proximity, (**b**) Similarity, (**c**) Continuity, (**d**) Connectedness, (**e**) Symmetry, (**f**) closure and (**g**) figure and ground

6.6.1   Gestalt Principles

The word Gestalt comes from the German meaning a unified whole. The Gestalt principles derive from the field of psychology. These principles concern laws surrounding the construction processes in visual perception and begins with laws that describe grouping in perception [8]. The principles are applied to many modern day logos and designs. The sub-figures in Fig. 6.6 show visual examples of these rules where objects presented in these ways are perceived to be grouped or associated in some way. This starts with *proximity* where the distance between objects makes us perceive them as grouped if they are close enough together. If there were several such blocks of 8 blocks where the 2 larger blocks were separated by some space, they would be perceived as 2 separate groups. In the second example, *similarity*, items are considered grouped if they are similar in some way, in this case a different colour. *Continuity* pertains to the fact that the eye will follow the line despite the breaks. This concept can be used to drive the eye in a specific direction along a path. The *connectedness* principle groups items that are perceived to be connected physically in some way. *Closure* is often used in logos where missing parts are essentially 'filled in' by the brain so it perceives a whole. The principle of *figure and ground* uses negative space and works in a similar way to the closure principle. The brain can distinguish between a background and foreground which can both contain images in some cases like that seen in Fig. 6.6g where we see two faces and a chalice.

6.6.2 Design Layout

There are different layouts that can help to arrange information in a way that makes it easier to read and access. This includes the *grid* layout where items are arranged in rows and columns surrounded by margins to add padding to the items. The Z layout is also frequently used. This is often applied to the landing pages on web sites and refers to the pattern of eye movement following a Z pattern from top left to right and then bottom left to bottom right tracing a letter Z type pattern. Placing key content along this route can help viewers to rapidly access information, often with a so-called call to action button at the end of the path (e.g. submit, sign up etc.).

6.6.3 Preattentive Attributes

There are certain visual properties that humans can notice very easily with minimal effort. These properties include:

- Colour (the intensity and hue)
- Positioning (the spatial location of items)
- Movement (motion)
- Form (this includes shape, orientation, width of lines, amount of curvature etc.)

An example can be seen in Fig. 6.7 where the leftmost sub-figure contains circles of the same size, colour and shape. The red circle in the middle image and square in the image on the right are easily and rapidly distinguishable form the other circles. We can use *visual mapping* to apply these attributes to elements of our

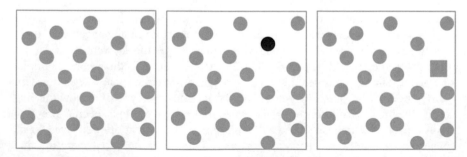

Fig. 6.7 Examples of pre-attentive attributes of colour and form

visualisations, e.g. by highlighting the colour of a single bar on a bar chart to focus attention there. We may also use them to display extra dimensions of data such as the size of the bubbles in a bubble plot representing population size while their colour represents a country or other sub group for example.

An example of a prize winning research poster that applies some of these techniques, including composition and layout and use of preattentive attributes can be seen in Fig. 6.8.

6.7   Visualisation for Decision Making

Complex data can be presented in the form of a visualisation that can then be used to promote decision making. This can range from a simple graph showing weight gain or loss that can be used to modify diet and exercise routines to more complex bespoke scientific plots for monitoring patients in clinical trials or allocating national resources based on need.

> **Case study: Decision making in clinical trials with biomarker data visualisations**
> This study looked at how people use data visualisations of various biomarker data to inform decision making for clinical trials. Interviews were carried out with experts (n = 18) and analysed with inductive thematic analysis [5]. The study found, among other things, that the use of labels and context for a visualisation helped with its interpretation. An example of this is using percentages to report findings but not including the raw numbers to give context to the percentages [5]. The work highlighted the importance of including provenance information related to the nature of changes to the underlying data that led to the final visualisation. This was deemed important for both reproducibility and to increase trust in decisions made based off the data/visualisation [5].

Information dashboards are increasingly being used to present data visualisations for decision-making in health. The purpose of dashboards can span a range of activities from decision support to communication and learning [23]. We do however need to consider the numerical and graph literacy of people using such dashboards for clinical decision making as well as the formats used to present such information [10, 23] which will impact on their subsequent design.

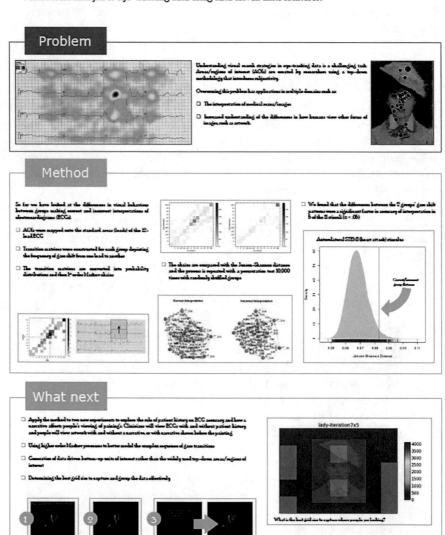

Fig. 6.8 Example of a research poster that applied principles of good visualisation and won award for best poster at the University of Manchester's research symposium in the school of Computer Science

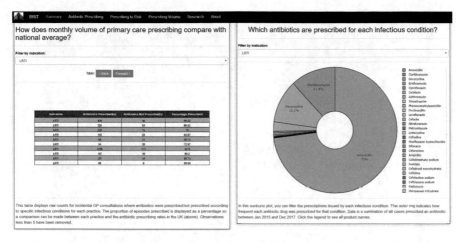

Fig. 6.9 Example visualisations from the dashboard showing data in tabular and doughnut chart form

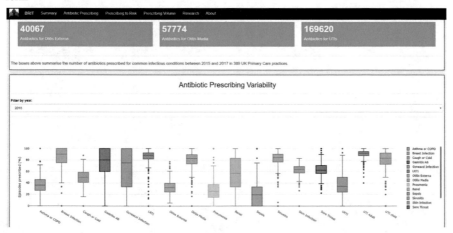

Fig. 6.10 Boxplot showing the variability of prescribing across different infection categories

Case study: The BRIT dashboard

The Building Rapid Interventions to reduce antibiotic resisTance (BRIT) project was designed to optimise the prescription of antibiotics in primary care in the UK [25]. The data are presented in the form of an information dashboard (Figs. 6.9 and 6.10). BRIT is an example of a *learning health system* (LHS). A LHS helps to improve care by generating knowledge which is then embedded in the daily activities of health care professionals, in this

(continued)

instance reducing the over prescribing of antibiotics which is leading to antibiotic resistant bacteria development.

The interactive plots that such dashboards present allow for the exploration of data which can be used for subsequent decision making such as targeting education around specific infections that are receiving sub optimal prescribing. An example can be seen in Fig. 6.11 where the infection group LRTI (lower respiratory track infections) prescribing rate is compared against the target for different risk categories. Here we see that the prescribing rate is too high for people in the low risk category but conversely too low for the very high risk group.

Accessing data in this way can be a powerful tool for decision-making allowing for resource allocation to be directed efficiently and for the results to be monitored.

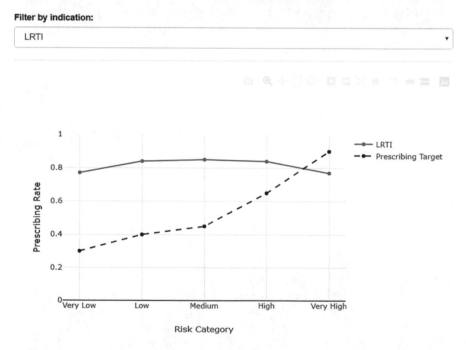

Fig. 6.11 Plot showing prescribing rate vs risk category for lower respiratory track infection (LRTI)

6.7.1 *Probabilistic Reasoning*

People find decision making difficult when presented with a decision between several outcomes where there is some amount of uncertainly as this involves using probabilistic reasoning [16]. Studies have shown that the application of *Bayesian inference* to solve such problems is often applied incorrectly [16]. Bayes' theorem was discovered by an English Reverend called Thomas Bayes in the 1700s. This was a form of probabilistic reasoning that takes into account knowledge of past events. It is represented thus:

$$P(A|B) = \frac{P(B|A)P(A)}{P(B)}$$

And is read as the likelihood of event A happening given that event B is true. The $P(A|B)$ and $P(B|A)$ are conditional probabilities, whereas $P(A)$ and $P(B)$ are marginal probabilities (derived from summing the margins of a table).

One of the classic examples of applying this theorem to medicine is known as the *mammography problem* that was presented by Eddy in 1982 [11]. In this example we see this reasoning applied to a test for breast cancer (mammography) where we are given some information about the situation: 1% of women have breast cancer, 80% of mammograms can detect that cancer but some mammograms (9.6%) detect cancer when there is none there (called a false positive) (Table 6.2).

Many people overestimate the likelihood that a woman has cancer given that they receive a positive test result. In the 1982 study, a large proportion of participants with medical training (95%) thought that the chance was somewhere between 70% to 80% [11]. What hopefully strikes you when looking at the information in the table (Table 6.2) is that although there is an 80% likelihood of the test correctly detecting cancer, the cancer is only present in 1% of the population, which is a small proportion overall. People tend to find these sorts of reasoning problems difficult. To determine the chance of actually having cancer given a positive test result in this scenario we can consider this in terms of true and false positives (Table 6.3).

Essentially we can divide the true positives by the chance of any positives using the Bayes formula:

Table 6.2 Probability table for mammogram breast cancer detection test

	Has cancer (1%)	No cancer (99%)
Positive test	80%	9.6%
Negative test	20%	90.4%

Table 6.3 True and false positives for the test

	Has cancer	No cancer
Positive test	TRUE POSITIVE	FALSE POSITIVE
Negative test	FALSE NEGATIVE	TRUE NEGATIVE

$$P(A|B) = \frac{P(B|A)P(A)}{P(B|A)P(A) + P(B|\neg A)P(\neg A)}$$

$$P(A|B) = \frac{(80 \times 1)}{(80 \times 1) + (9.6 \times 99)} = 0.0769 \times 100 = 7.76\%$$

This means that the real chance of having cancer given a positive a test result is much lower than usually estimated, at around 8%. You can imagine the effect incorrect reasoning might have on decision making. So would visualising such problems make them easier to interpret? To answer this question we created a tool (Fig. 6.12) to generate different visualisations and used this to present the classic mammography problem using several of these visualisation types, including Venn diagrams, tree diagram and icon arrays.

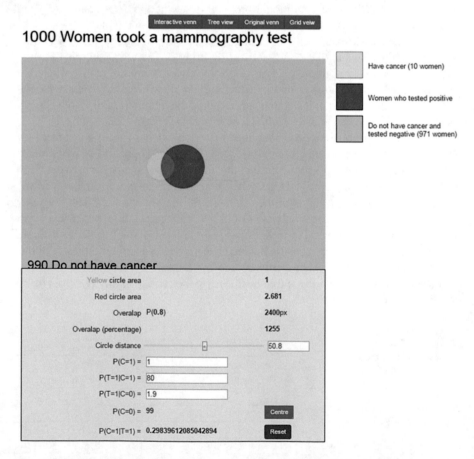

Fig. 6.12 Tool created to produce different visualisation types based on probability values

We also added a dynamic Venn diagram where the area of the circles would represent the population sizes. We were able to approximate the intersection of the circles where d is the distance between the centre points of the circles and r and R represent the radius of the circles respectively:

$$\text{Area} = r^2 \cos^{-1}\left(\frac{d^2 + r^2 - R^2}{2dr}\right) + R^2 \cos^{-1}\left(\frac{d^2 + R^2 - r^2}{2dR}\right)$$

$$-\frac{1}{2}\sqrt{(-d + r + R)(d + r - R)(d - r + R)(d + r + R)}$$

We found that for task performance the standard Venn and tree diagrams were equal but people found tree diagrams easier to interpret [21]. The icon arrays that are often used for presenting data involving risk were inefficient for conveying information concerning conditional probability [21]. In further work, we found that when the data presented were reflective of people's lived experience their accuracy improved [22]. Further to this, the reasoning process is different for people when provided with data using natural frequencies compared to percentages [22]. The prior experience of individuals was shown to influence their reasoning about uncertainty considerably [22]. This goes to show that it isn't just the format of the data visualisation presented but also the type of data used that affects interpretation accuracy.

6.8 Feeding Back Complex Data to Patients

We have so far discussed displaying relatively simple information in the form of visualisations using standardized plots and graphs and infographic-style information. While this may work well for cases like health tracking with metrics that are understood fairly well by the end user (e.g. weight monitoring or blood pressure monitoring), this is far more challenging with medical monitoring. This is especially true if the visualisation types require medical training in order to be interpreted. In some previous work we looked at the possibility of presenting such information back to the patient for self medical monitoring with a condition that was identifiable on the electrocardiogram (ECG) called drug-induced long QT syndrome (LQTS). The QT interval as seen in Fig. 6.13 can become prolonged. This in turn can lead to a dangerous arrhythmia called Torsades de pointes (TdP) which can be life threatening. Patients prescribed certain drugs, such as antiarrhythmic drugs, antibiotics, antiemetic (anti-nausea), antihistamines, some calcium-channel blockers and some opiates (e.g. Methadone) [15] can be at risk of developing drug-induced LQTS. Identifying LQTS is difficult even for medically trained personnel and even those who routinely interpret ECGs. Added to this is the further issue in the variation of the criteria for diagnosing LQTS between the sexes and the phenomenon

Fig. 6.13 Image identifying the QT interval from start of Q wave to end of T wave on the ECG. (Reprinted by permission from Springer Nature Customer Service Centre GmbH: Springer Nature, *Starting to Read ECGs: The Basics* by Alan Davies and Alwyn Scott, © Springer-Verlag London (2014) [7])

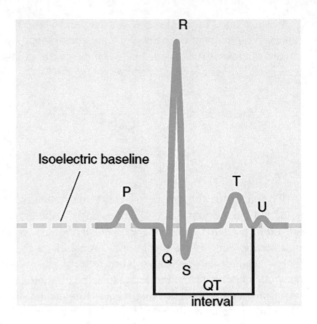

that increases in the patients' heart rate has an inverse exponential relationship with the QT-interval. We can see that the condition is challenging to identify.

Rather than take the approach of remote monitoring and relying on a clinician to access the data, we instead opted to explore the possibility of patients themselves being able to monitor their own ECG. Firstly they are not required to understand all aspects and conditions that can present on an ECG but only increases in the QT interval. In addition they also only need concern themselves with any deviation from their own baseline ECG trace. To investigate this possibility, experiments were carried out initially with lay participants with no prior ECG experience (n = 30). The experiment used psychophysical methods and eye-tracking and presented participants with a baseline and prolonged QT interval ECG in several different ways (single complex ECG signals aligned, not-aligned and rhythm strip) [3]. The initial study demonstrated that it was possible to rapidly train lay people to identify changes in their QT interval [3]. A further study with lay people (n = 42) experimented with the presentation format of the ECG for this purpose and found that the use of colour significantly improved the accuracy of participants in identifying the prolonged QT interval. Pseudo-colouring was used to alter the hue and intensity of colour in the area under the QT interval waveform (Fig. 6.14). The most effective presentation for improving accuracy in LQT detection was found to be colour with a polar (circular) representation of the ECG (Fig. 6.15) opposed to the traditional Cartesian layout commonly seen [2].

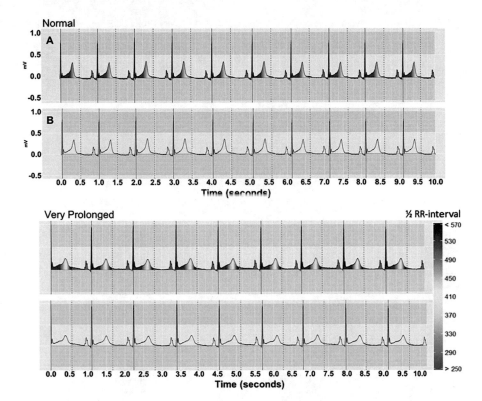

Fig. 6.14 Cartesian layout with normal (top) and prolonged QT interval (bottom). (Source: Alahmadi et al. [2]. Reproduced with permission)

6.8.1   Graph Literacy

One may ask how one can assess the end users' ability to interpret graphical data. This is especially useful if your intervention relies on the end user making decisions based off that information. For health applications there may be different intended demographics that the intervention may be targeted at. Those with lower levels of education and experience in interpreting graphical information may find it difficult to interpret the information provided in a visualisation even if the visualisation was created using the best practices. One way to quantify users' level of 'graph literacy' is to use a validated survey to score users. This can be applied to a sample representative of your intended demographic. The types of visualisations used and complexity can then be adjusted accordingly. One such validated tool is the tool developed by Galesic and Garcia-Retamero [12]. The scale was developed with participants from the USA (n = 492) and Germany (n = 495). The scale was designed for patients using visual aids. The scale uses standard visualisation types (pie charts, bar chart and line charts) to ask a series of questions about each visualisation based on levels 1 to 3. The first level is the ability to read data from the presented

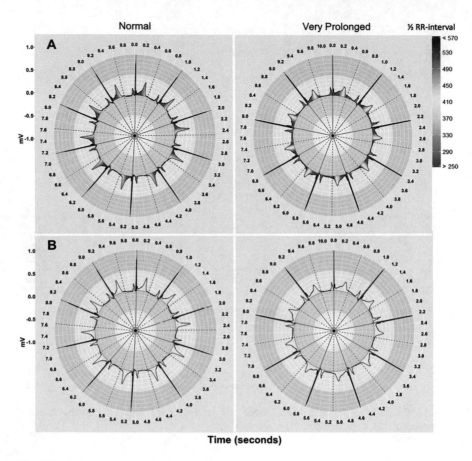

Fig. 6.15 Polar representation with pseudo-colouring on top row (left normal QT, right prolonged QT). Bottom row polar representation with no colour for normal and prolonged QT interval. (Source: Alahmadi et al. [2]. Reproduced with permission)

visualisation. The second is to read between data (e.g. a value between 2 data points) and the third level pertains to the ability to read beyond the data (e.g. project a trend line into the future) [12].

6.9   Creating Visualisations

It might at first seem like a relatively simple task to create a visualisation. There are however many considerations when producing a visualisation. Ideally you want to clearly and accurately display the data drawing a reader's eye to the salient points you are trying to convey without distorting the data and misleading people into drawing potentially untrue conclusions from your visualisation. This is especially important if the visualisation is to be used to make subsequent decisions. Consider

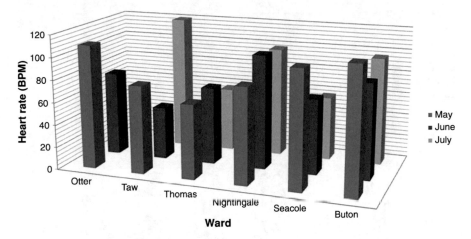

Fig. 6.16 An example of a poor visualisation. The value for the ward *Otter* for the month of July is 45 bpm. It is impossible to see this in the plot because it is hidden by the bars in the foreground

the 3D bar chart shown in Fig. 6.16. Here we see a bad example of a bar chart. The axis marks are small and difficult to read, as is the legend.

Bar charts are often used to help people make comparisons between categorical data. This plot shows us patients' heart rates recorded over a 3 month period from a number of hospital wards. It is difficult to see which numbers the bars on the right of the plot represent. The result for the month of July for the *Otter* ward is hidden behind the bars in the foreground of the plot. Figure 6.17 shows the same plot redesigned in two dimensions with the bars side by side. The values are now clearly readable and the previously hidden value from Otter ward is now also clearly visible. The axis labels and marks and the legend are now also easier to see and read. It is now also clear that the heart rate is an average. This second plot is much better for comparing the data between wards and months.

In Fig. 6.18 we see another bad example, this time of a pie chart. It is known that people find it hard to estimate angles, especially when they are narrow. Additionally three dimensional pie charts also add to this difficulty by adding an incline. Pie charts should ideally be used when there are a few categories of data that are clearly discernible. In this example there are far too many categories to provide any meaning. The angles are extremely hard to discern and the similar colours also add to the visual complexity.

Another example of poor practice relates to the scale used for the axis on graphs. Figure 6.19 shows the comparison between 2 drugs (A and B) and the percentage of patients that recovered from some illness as a result of taking either drug. For drug A this is 60% and for drug B 42%. The plot on the left of Fig. 6.19 shows a y-axis from 0 to 60% incremented in steps of 10. The plot on the right was re-scaled from 0 to 200%. In the second plot the difference between the bars appears to be smaller than the one on the left. This is an example of how perception can be altered based on changing the features of the visualisation. Unscrupulous people may use such

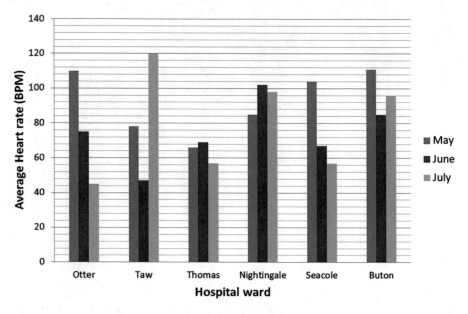

Fig. 6.17 Example of a better version of the previous bar chart

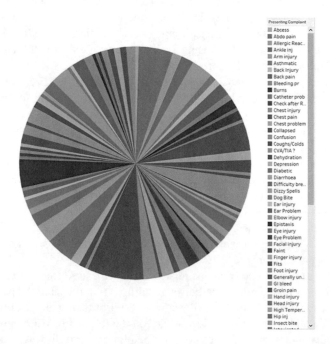

Fig. 6.18 Another example of a poor visualisation. There are too many categories for the pie chart to be meaningful

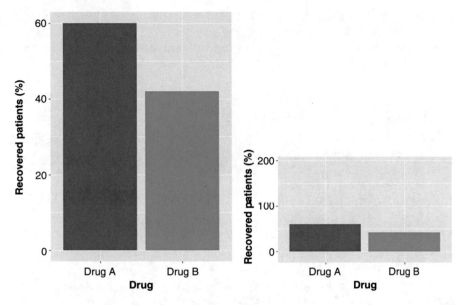

Fig. 6.19 Two bar charts generated with the same data showing how changing the scale can impact on perception of differences between the categories being compared

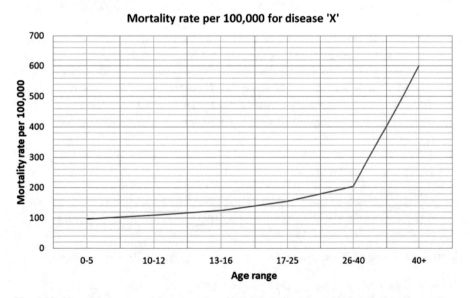

Fig. 6.20 Unequal range groupings can also affect the appearance and interpretation of a graph

methods to deliberately distort the impression the viewer has of the data represented by the visualisation.

Figure 6.20 provides an example of how uneven bins (ranges to group data) can affect the subsequent appearance of the plotted data. This could for example look like there is a sharp rise or sudden fall where this would possibly appear to be smoother with equal sized grouping and ranges. This also highlights the importance of how we collect the data, as this will limit its subsequent presentation and interpretation (Fig. 6.21).

Edward Tufte's principles of graphical excellence (Tufte, 2001) [26]

- Show the data
- Induce the viewer to think about the substance
- Avoid distorting what the data have to say
- Present many numbers in a small space
- Make large data sets coherent
- Encourage the eye to compare different pieces of data
- Reveal the data at several levels of detail (broad overview to the fine structure)
- Serve a reasonably clear purpose (description, exploration, ...)
- Be closely integrated with the statistical and verbal descriptions of a data set

There are different methods for creating visualisations in different software tools. One of the most elegant is that of the *ggplot2* library for R (there is also now a Python version) that was created by Hadley Wickham [29]. This package works with the concept of *aesthetics*. This describes how the data relate to the plot and can be added in layers. The code in listings 6.1 to 6.4 shows how a plot can be built up in stages by adding additional detail. This code corresponds to the sub images in Fig. 6.22 that shows how we can build up a bar plot by adding features in layers using the *plus* to add additional layers and styling information, resulting in the final image shown in Fig. 6.23.

```
library(ggplot2)
annual_spending <- c(1320, 920)
hospitals <- c("All Saints", "Lost Hope")
df <- data.frame(hospitals, annual_spending)
```

Listing 6.1 Create some fake data about 2 fictitious hospitals and load the ggplot2 library

```
plot <- ggplot(data=df, aes(x=hospitals, y=annual_spending))
print(plot)
```

Listing 6.2 Generate the plot using the data frame as a data source. The aes function applies the aesthetic where we add the x and y values to the plot

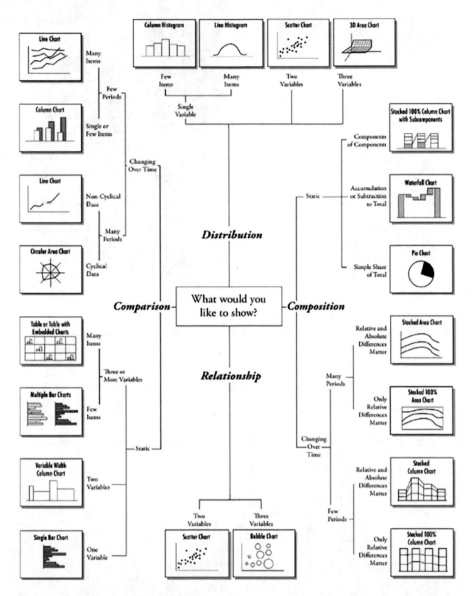

Fig. 6.21 Choosing the right chart type. (Reproduced with permission. Source: Abela [1]. © John Wiley and Sons, 2013. All Rights Reserved)

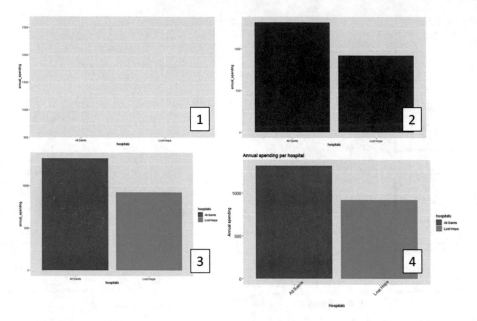

Fig. 6.22 Plots generated with the ggplot library from 1 to 4 showing the effect of adding additional layers to the plot

```
plot <- ggplot(data=df, aes(x=hospitals, y=annual_spending)) +
                geom_bar(stat="identity")
print(plot)
```

Listing 6.3 We add the geom_bar function to define a bar plot. This add the two bars to the plot

```
plot <- ggplot(data=df, aes(x=hospitals, y=annual_spending, fill=
    hospitals)) +
            geom_bar(stat="identity") +
    theme(axis.text.x = element_text(size = 12, angle = 45), axis
    .text.y = element_text(size = 12)) +
    xlab("Hospitals") +
    ylab("Annual spending") +
    ggtitle("Annual spending per hospital")

print(plot)
```

Listing 6.4 We can also fill the bars based on the class of the data and add additional styling to the axis text as well as adding a plot title

The ggplot package was build on the "the grammar of graphics" created by Wilkinson [30]. In his book, Wilkinson talks about the concept of using graphical objects rather than chart types, giving the example of a pie chart being an instance of a polar graphic [30]. The aesthetic attributes described can be used to represent different dimensions of data. Examples include position, size, shape, rotation, colour, and labels to name a few [30]. Creating plots by understanding and applying

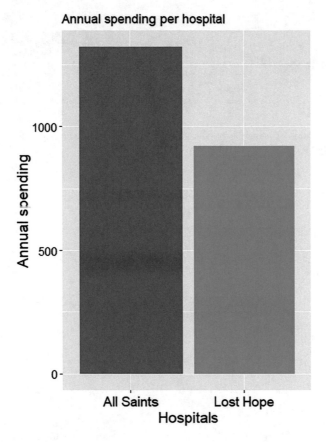

Fig. 6.23 Final bar chart

an underlying grammar can be very expressive and allow for the construction of bespoke plots and charts.

This concept of layered graphics can help to build bespoke plots and visualisations to extend the standard chart and graph types. Rather than having an all-inclusive extensive library of predefined plots, one can use layered components to build up many different types of graphics. These components can include the data and its associated aesthetic mappings, geometric objects, scales and facets as well as co-ordinates and various statistical transformations [28]. An example can be seen in Fig. 6.24 where this techniques was used to recreate Minard's graphic of Napoleon's Russian campaign (introduced in Fig. 6.1).

There is now also a version of ggplot for use in Python. Other options for Python include the *seaborn* and *matplotlib* libraries. Listings 6.5 to 6.7 give an example of producing a simple bar and scatter plot using matplotlib. The outputs can be seen in Fig. 6.25.

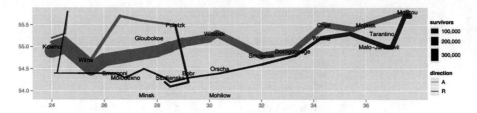

Fig. 6.24 Recreation of Minard's graphic of Napoleon's Russian campaign. (Source: Wickham [28], originally by Taylor & Francis Ltd, www.tandfonline.com)

```
1  import matplotlib.pyplot as plt
2  import pandas as pd
3
4  data = [['Paul Smith', 52, "128/70"], ['Nick Bandera', 18, "
       130/60"], ['Julie Miller', 31, "142/72"]]
5  my_df = pd.DataFrame(data, columns = ["Name", "Age", "BP"])
6  print(my_df)
```

Listing 6.5 Create some basic data using a dataframe

```
1              Name  Age      BP
2  0     Paul Smith   52  128/70
3  1   Nick Bandera   18  130/60
4  2   Julie Miller   31  142/72
```

```
1  plt.rcdefaults()
2  fig, ax = plt.subplots()
3
4  ax.barh(my_df["Name"], my_df["Age"], align='center',color='blue')
5  ax.set_ylabel('Patient name')
6  ax.set_xlabel('Age (years)')
```

Listing 6.6 Example of bar plot

```
1  plt.scatter(my_df["Age"], my_df["HR"], alpha=0.5)
2  plt.title("Scatter plot of age and heart rate")
3  plt.xlabel("Age (years)")
4  plt.ylabel("Heart rate (beats per minute)")
5  plt.show()
```

Listing 6.7 Example of scatter plot

6.10   Using Visualisation in Apps

Charts and graphs can be plotted using frameworks in native apps. For iOS apps this can include frameworks like *Core plot* which can be used for 2D plotting. For native Android development, the *MPAndroidChart* framework provides a range of

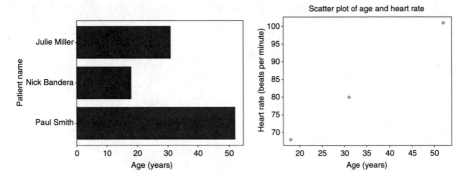

Fig. 6.25 Plots generated with the Python matplotlib library

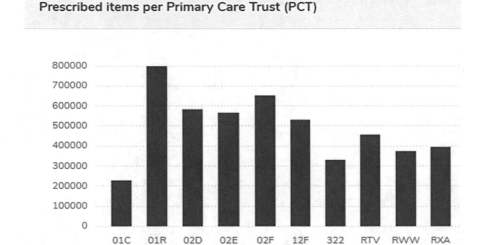

Fig. 6.26 Example of a bar plot created using Chart.js

standard interactive plot types. Another popular alternative is *androidplot*. Data Driven Documents (D3) is a powerful and fully featured JavaScript library for producing a large range of visualisation types. These can be incorporated easily into progressive web apps. Another JavaScript library used to produce interactive web based visualisations is *Chart.js*. An example of a bar chart made using Chart.js can be seen in Fig. 6.26. Table 6.4 provides the sources for the various frameworks and libraries mentioned.

Another option for apps that have server support irrespective of their platform is to produce the plot server side in something like R or Python and then send the plot as a static image to the device. App designers need to consider the available screen size and resolution of the device(s) the app is intended to run on. This relatively smaller space will impact on the layout and presentation of the visualisation you choose to incorporate.

Table 6.4 Some popular tools for generating common visualisation types for different types of app

App type	Visualisation tool	Link
Native iOS	Core-plot	https://github.com/core-plot/core-plot/wiki/Example-Graphs
Native android	Androidplot	http://androidplot.com/
Native android	MPAndroidChart	https://github.com/PhilJay/MPAndroidChart
Progressive web app	D3	https://d3js.org/
Progressive web app	Chart.js	https://www.chartjs.org/docs/latest/

6.10.1   Collecting Data from Users

So far we have considered the layout and composition of outputs presented to the end user. We may also want to consider applying these concepts to the presentation of any input our intervention may require. If we are collecting data from users for an intervention or for research purposes that require active user input (i.e. not collected from passive sensors) then we also want to apply such aesthetic principles to streamline the input process. A standard approach to interface design for data collection is proposed by Vickers et al. who present 10 'golden rules' [27] as summarised here:

The 10 golden rules of interface design for collecting patient data adapted from Vickers et al. [27]

1. Consider that things that are obvious to engineers or informaticians are not necessarily obvious to patients. The perspective of the patient is key to the interface development process and should be stressed continuously.
2. Quick and easy may actually be a burden to the patient. Patients with various impairments and lack of computer experience may struggle to use the interface quickly and efficiently.
3. The types of questionnaires that are developed for research purposes may not be suitable for clinical use. Skipping questions and branching based on logic can be used to improve the experience and relevance for individual patients.
4. Technical medical jargon should be replaced by simpler words and terms.
5. Fields that must be completed in order to submit information and the use of 'open' text field questions can be problematic. It might not be possible or desirable to provide answers to certain required questions. Thus they should only be used when absolutely necessary (e.g. in order

---

(continued)

to use branching logic to ask subsequent related questions). With open text, thought needs to be given to what to do with those responses and why they are being asked. Fields can be limited to a certain number of characters to avoid excessively long responses.

6. Questions about clinical care should only be asked if you intend to act on the information provided.

7. Completing the questions should hold some value for the patients and be in their best interests, for example using responses to initiate discussion in a subsequent clinical consultation.

8. Subgroups of users can dramatically increase workload. Interfaces should be accessible and meet the needs of all users. This can add to the work involved in providing such interfaces (e.g. password management).

9. Observe patients interacting with your tools and question them about this experience. This information can be used to improve the user experience and layout of the tools developed.

10. It is difficult to gain patient trust but easy to lose. Questions that do not make sense to the patients' context or indicate a lack of forethought etc. can erode patients' trust and cause annoyance.

6.10.2   Involving Users in Visualisation Design

The best way to ensure understanding of the visualisations produced is to work with the end users to develop the required visual outputs that deliver the most comprehension for the target user group. An example of this can be seen in Fig. 6.27 where participants were presented with a series of visualisations. Participants' comments were recorded as were the results of questions created to illicit comprehension of the visualisation.

We present two further case studies to illustrate the variation in approaches and lessons learnt from our own previous work.

Case study 1: Feeding symptom and medication information back to users
In our previous work, we aimed to develop an experience sampling app to measure symptom severity and frequency as well as medication adherence. We also wished to feed this back to users in a meaningful manner, along with relevant weather information to help users plan their activities around weather conditions that affected their symptoms.
One of the key aspects to take into account in this context was the target population. We needed to consider how familiar and comfortable our target

(continued)

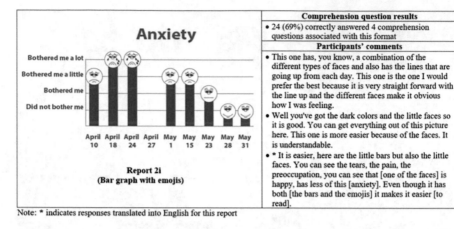

Note: * indicates responses translated into English for this report

Fig. 6.27 Figure reproduced from Stonbraker et al. (2020) highlighting an example participant feedback about a proposed visualisation [24]. (Source: Stonbraker et al., by permission of the American Medical Informatics Association)

users would be with different forms of data visualisations, and how information could be presented to enable users to take action to improve their own health and well being. This is particularly critical in certain illnesses that disproportionately affect those from lower socioeconomic groupings with lower levels of education and health literacy (due to the link with unhealthy behaviours).

Initially, we therefore conducted a user engagement session during which we discussed our ideas with 5–8 people with the relevant disease. As people seemed comfortable with the idea of simple charts like line and bar charts, we then created mock-ups of different charts, which we again discussed with our user engagement group. Visualising the relationship between medication adherence and symptom fluctuation in one graph proved challenging. We presented participants with the two graphs shown in Fig. 6.28. These graphs were mock-ups that served as a starting point for identifying user preferences and generating further discussions. We asked about participants' opinions regarding the visualisations but also assessed their ability to accurately interpret the information.

Notably, participants in the user engagement session were receptive to graphs that were simple, clean and minimal, whereas graphs that were perceived as "busy" were met with reluctance and reticence. Consider the following interaction. The user was able to interpret the graph shown in the bottom half of Fig. 6.28, but immediately shied away from the graph shown in the upper half:

(continued)

Interviewer: *"We've been playing around a bit with, trying to put some sort of information in the graph about your medication as well. So, this is a first idea of what we came up with and we were wondering what you thought of that."* [points to the lower graph]
Participant: *"Yes, I quite agree with that. Like you say, down here and up to there, is where you've took your medication and then when you've stopped taking it, they just go sky-high."*
Interviewer: *"[. . .] What do you think of this version?"* [points to the upper graph]
Participant: *"No. [. . .] There's too much of it."*
Despite feeding these insights back to the wider team, an extremely busy and complicated graph was nevertheless subsequently included in the final app. The graph was the result of an attempt to incorporate all relevant weather data (temperature, humidity, wind speed, night/day times, pressure, lunar phase cycle) in a single graph. While this comprehensiveness may have some appeal, users were unable to interpret this graph without additional explanations.

Similarly, although our user experience work suggested the best approach to visualising symptom data was a simple line graph, the graph subsequently included in the final app was a complicated stacked bar chart that was not suitable for the nature of the data (Fig. 6.29).

Participants highlighted further problems, such as the use of green and red colouring in graphs, which would be problematic for individuals with deuteranomaly and protanomaly (red-green colour blindness). Participants had useful suggestions for improving the graphs:
Participant: *"Well, I was going to suggest, why couldn't you have, rather than two colours, which again is [inaudible 0:19:50] – because I was in education, sorry – two colours, you never know who can see the two colours easily or not. [. . .] Why don't you do an open and a closed one? Closed when they've taken it, and an open one if they don't. Because it's very obvious then there's a difference."*
Importantly, our work highlighted that visualisations need to clearly show how the information displayed is *personally relevant* and how it can be translated into *action* [6]:
Participant: [Examining graph] *"But I don't know whether that would make any difference to me, I don't know whether it's relevant."*
Conclusions:
We learned the following key lessons from this work:

- Visualisations must be kept simple, clean and minimal. This may seem obvious, however, our experiences above show that this simple lesson is worth emphasising.

(continued)

- It is important to consider the target population, especially when apps are developed for people suffering from (chronic) illnesses. Consider the demographic profile of the target group and whether users are likely to be health literate and familiar with the use of technology and with the interpretation of visual data.
- Also consider any health burdens your users are likely to be suffering from. If users are unwell, they will most likely not be receptive to interpreting complex visualisations that require additional cognitive resources.
- It is critical to consult users on their opinion of, and ability to interpret, visualisations. Users can provide useful advice and suggestions on how to make visualisations easier to interpret.
- Importantly, you need to consider that users who take part in such usability sessions are likely to be more motivated and health literate than the average user in the target group.
- Visualisations must always stand on their own. A good way to test this is to ask users to interpret a mock-up graph in a usability evaluation. If users require additional explanations, the graph is unsuitable or needs more work.
- Visualisations need to emphasise personal relevance and it should be easy for users to draw conclusions about suitable actions they can take.

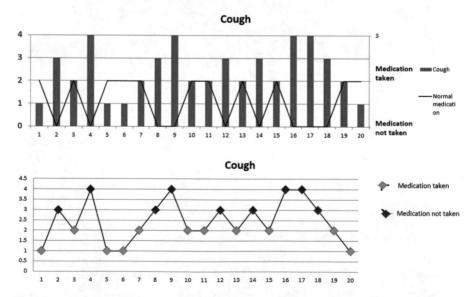

Fig. 6.28 Graphs depicting symptom variation with medication adherence, shown to users during user engagement sessions to generate discussions

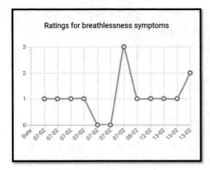 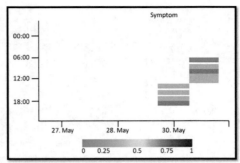

Fig. 6.29 Graph showing the visualisation for symptom data derived from our user engagement work (left) and the graph subsequently included in the app (right)

Case study 2: Feeding activity tracker information back to users with chronic, progressive disease

Chronic obstructive pulmonary disease (COPD) is an inflammatory lung disease that invovles obstruction to airflow from the lungs, resulting in symptoms such as breathlessness, coughing and wheezing. Although the disease cannot be cured, its progression can be slowed down, and symptoms may improve, with appropriate medication and lifestyle changes. Regular physical activity is key to self-management of COPD. In many countries, pulmonary rehabilitation programmes are offered to patients that include exercise training as a key component, however around 90% of patients do not make use of this service, and many of those who begin the programme drop out prior to completion.

Arguably, other means of enabling and motivating patients to pursue physical activity are needed. Off-the-shelf consumer physical activity trackers appear to offer an opportunity to plug this gap: they are relatively cheap and easy to incorporate into daily lives (particularly compared to more involved programmes like pulmonary rehabilitation). Patients could easily monitor their step count per day, set themselves realistic goals, and monitor progress over time using in-built visualisations.

Excited by this opportunity, we pitched this idea to people living with COPD at a Patient and Public Involvement event which we organised in order to bring together relevant researchers and people living with COPD to help generate research ideas and identify priority areas.

The insights of this consultation were somewhat sobering. Participants pointed out a key flaw in our logic. Visualisations in activity trackers are designed to show trends over time, helping users to increase and improve their activity levels. However, COPD is a *progressive* condition with no cure.

(continued)

This means that symptoms – and mobility – will worsen over time. They may worsen less quickly than if no lifestyle changes are made, but the overall trend will nevertheless be downward (Fig. 6.30). Off-the-shelf activity trackers may thus highlight progressive deterioration, resulting in decreased motivation. Motivation is an important determinant of behaviour, and is significantly associated with physical activity levels [17].

Conclusion: The key lesson learned here is that it is critically important to carefully consider your target population and the characteristics of any relevant associated illnesses, symptoms or other health outcomes, to avoid inadvertently visualising aspects of poor health that are de-motivating or anxiety-inducing. As Goodman and Foucault point out, "too much access to information can be de-motivating" ([14], p. 801), especially when coupled with unrealistic expectations. This is not to say that activity trackers and associated visualisations might not prove useful for people with COPD; however visualisation designers need to carefully consider what variables are most likely to constitute useful indicators of progress in a given population.

6.11   Summary of Key Points

We can use visualisations in several ways and for several purposes. One reason is to explore and present our data. This may be done when analysing data produced by an intervention with subsequent visualisations produced for stakeholders in the form of reports, presentations or academic publications. The second main reason is to display information back to users of your intervention. This can

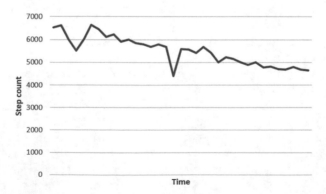

Fig. 6.30 Presenting trends over time may be demotivating, particularly for users with chronic, progressive health conditions

include health and medication tracking apps that summarise a user's activities in these regards. The user may choose to share such data summaries in the form of visualisations with their healthcare team, where it may be factored into decisions made. Producing visualisations for either purpose should aim to present the data clearly and accurately, and should avoid misleading or confusing people and distorting the data in any way. A good visualisation will be clear and easy to read. It will summarise key data for insights and highlight the primary message. A good visualisation can be used to communicate a story about the data to a user in a way that can be much easier to access than in numerical or tabular form, especially for large volumes of data. The choice of visualisation type and how it is presented are key factors in achieving this goal.

- Avoid visual clutter (chart junk)
- Avoid distorting the data and misleading people
- Use appropriate and consistent scales
- Break up complex plots by using multiple plots and/or interactive dynamic plots to allow filtering of data
- Apply the principles of good visualisation to reduce cognitive load and increase comprehension
- Consider the need to support visualisations for multiple devices and for different presentations for a variety of user groups
- Developing visualisations with the intended target group can lead to better comprehension
- The numerical and graph literacy levels of the end user should be considered when designing visualisations

6.12 Quiz

1. Which of the following is **not** a preattentive attribute?

   (a) Colour
   (b) Shape
   (c) Fixation duration

2. The most suitable visualisation type to compare two categories of information is...

   (a) A bar chart
   (b) A pie chart

3. Which of the following are good reasons to use visualisations

   (a) To explore the structure and relationships in our data
   (b) To communicate results to different users
   (c) To obfuscate the underlying data so we can present data to back up a specific agenda

4. People reason better when given information in the form of

    (a) Probabilities
    (b) Frequencies

5. Which of the following should **not** be routinely applied to visualisations

    (a) Axis titles should be present, clearly labelled and show the units of measure
    (b) Error bars should be included when comparing groups
    (c) Multiple statistical and textual annotation to provide context

Answers to the quiz can be found in "Solutions to Quizzes".

6.13 Exercises

1. With regard to the research poster in Fig. 6.8.

    (a) Write a list of the Gestalt laws that it applies
    (b) Write a list of the pre-attentive attributes it uses
    (c) Which kind of layout does it use?
    (d) Is the message the poster is trying to convey clear?
    (e) Reflect on how the poster could be improved

2. What is the best type of plot to visualise the data in the Table 6.5 and why?
3. Using a tool of your choice, produce your suggested visualisation for the data in Table 6.5.

Recommended Reading

1. Card S, Mackinlay J, Shneiderman B. Readings in information visualization: using vision to think. San Diego: Academic; 1999.
2. Wilkinson L. Statistics and computing: the grammar of graphics. 2nd ed. Chicago: Springer; 2005.
3. Tufte E. The visual display of quantitative information. 2nd ed. Cheshire: Graphic Press.

Table 6.5 Average scores (0 lowest to 5 highest) for impact of various respiratory symptoms over 4 months in the year 2019

	Pain	Breathing	Mucus	Cough	Tiredness
Jan	3	5	4	4	3
Feb	4	4	3	4	2
Mar	3	3	2	3	3
April	2	3	2	2	1

References

1. Abela A. Advanced presentations by design: creating communication that drives action. New York: Wiley; 2013.
2. Alahmadi A, Davies A, Royle J, Vigo M, Jay C. Evaluating the impact of pseudo-colour and coordinate system on the detection of medication-induced ECG changes. In: CHI 2019, 4–9 May 2019, Glasgow. 2019. p. 1–3. https://doi.org/10.1145/3290605.3300353
3. Alahmadi A, Davies A, Vigo M, Jay C. Can lay people identify a drug-induced QT-interval prolongation? A psychophysical and eye-tracking experiment examining the ability of non-experts to interpret an ECG. J Am Med Inform Assoc. 2019;26(5):1–8. https://doi.org/10.1093/jamia/ocy183
4. Anscombe F. Graphs in statistical analysis. Am Stat. 1973;27(1):17–21. https://doi.org/10.1007/978-3-540-71915-1_35
5. Davies A, Cunha M, Kamilla Kopec-Harding, Metcalfe P, James Weatherall, Jay C. Biomarker data visualisation for decision making in clinical trials. Int J Med Inform. 2019;132:1–19. https://doi.org/10.1016/j.ijmedinf.2019.104008
6. Davies A, Mueller J, Hennings J, Caress A, Jay C. Recommendations for developing support tools with people suffering from Chronic Obstructive Pulmonary Disease: co-design and pilot testing of a mHealth prototype. JMIR Hum Factors. 2020;7(2):1–17.
7. Davies A, Scott A. Starting to read ECGs: the basics. London: Springer, 2014. https://doi.org/10.1007/978-1-4471-4962-0
8. Desolneux A, Moisan L, Morel J-M. From gestalt theory to image analysis: a probabilistic approach. New York: Springer; 2008.
9. Dill J, Earnshaw R, Kasik D, Vince J, Wong PC. Expanding the frontiers of visual analytics and visualization. London: Springer; 2012.
10. Dowding D, Merrill JA, Onorato N, Barron Y, Rosati RJ, Russell D. The impact of home care nurses' numeracy and graph literacy on comprehension of visual display information: implications for dashboard design. J Am Med Inf Assoc. 2018;25(2):175–82. https://doi.org/10.1093/jamia/ocx042
11. Eddy DM. Probabilistic reasoning in clinical medicine: problems and opportunities. In: Kahneman D, Slovic P, Tversky A, editors. Judgment under uncertainty. New York: Cambridge University Press; 1982. p. 249–67. https://doi.org/10.1017/CBO9780511809477.019
12. Galesic M, Garcia-Retamero R. Graph literacy: a cross-cultural comparison. Med Decis Making. 2011;31(3):444–57. https://doi.org/10.1177/0272989X10373805
13. Gapminder. Gapminder: gapminder foundation is fighting devastating ignorance with a fact-based worldview that everyone can understand; 2020. https://www.gapminder.org/
14. Goodman E, Foucault BE. Seeing fit: visualizing physical activity in context. In: CHI '06 extended abstracts on Human factors in computing systems – CHI EA '06, New York: ACM Press; 2006. https://doi.org/10.1145/1125451.1125609
15. Kannankeril P, Roden DM, Darbar D, Sibley D. Drug-induced long QT syndrome. Pharmacol Rev. 2010;62(4):760–81. https://doi.org/10.1124/pr.110.003723
16. Khan A, Breslav S, Glueck M, Hornbæk K. Benefits of visualization in the Mammography Problem. Int J Hum Comput Stud. 2015;83:94–113. https://doi.org/10.1016/j.ijhcs.2015.07.001
17. Knittle K, Nurmi J, Crutzen R, Hankonen N, Beattie M, Dombrowski SU. How can interventions increase motivation for physical activity? A systematic review and meta-analysis. Health Psychol Rev. 2018;12(3):211–30. https://doi.org/10.1080/17437199.2018.1435299
18. Kopanitsa G, Veseli H, Yampolsky V. Development, implementation and evaluation of an information model for archetype based user responsive medical data visualization. J Biomed Inf. 2015;55:196–205. https://doi.org/10.1016/j.jbi.2015.04.009
19. Krause A, O'Connell M. A picture is worth a thousand tables. New York: Springer; 2012. https://doi.org/10.1007/978-1-4614-5329-1

20. Merz M. (Interactive) graphics for biomarker assessment, chapter 7. In: Krause A, O'Connell M, editors. A picture is worth a thousand tables: graphics in life sciences. London: Springer; 2012, p. 429.
21. Reani M, Davies A, Peek N, Jay C. How do people use information presentation to make decisions in Bayesian reasoning tasks? Int J. Hum Comput Stud. 2018;111:62–77. https://doi.org/10.1016/j.ijhcs.2017.11.004
22. Reani M, Davies A, Peek N, Jay C. Evidencing how experience and problem format affect probabilistic reasoning through interaction analysis. Front Psychol. 2019;10:1–16. https://doi.org/10.3389/fpsyg.2019.01548
23. Sarikaya A, Correll M, Bartram L, Tory M, Fisher D. What do we talk about when we talk about dashboards? IEEE Trans Vis Comput Graph. 2019;25(1):682–92. https://doi.org/10.1109/TVCG.2018.2864903
24. Stonbraker S, Porras T, Schnall R. Patient preferences for visualization of longitudinal patient-reported outcomes data. J Am Med Inform Assoc. 2020;27(2):212–24. https://doi.org/10.1093/jamia/ocz189
25. The University of Manchester. BRIT analytics; 2020. https://www.britanalytics.uk/
26. Tufte ER. The visual display of quantitative information. 2nd ed. Cheshire: Connecticut Graphics Press LLC; 2001. p. 197.
27. Vickers AJ, Chen LY, Stetson PD. Interfaces for collecting data from patients: 10 golden rules. J Am Med Inform Assoc. 2020;27:498–500. https://doi.org/10.1093/jamia/ocz215
28. Wickham H. A layered grammar of graphics. J Comput Graph Stat. 2010;19(1):3–28. https://doi.org/10.1198/jcgs.2009.07098
29. Wickham H. ggplot2: elegant graphics for data analysis. New York: Springer; 2016. https://ggplot2.tidyverse.org
30. Wilkinson L. Statistics and computing: the grammar of graphics. 2nd ed. Chicago: Springer; 2005.

Chapter 7
Usability Testing and Deployment

7.1 Introduction

Those unfamiliar with the field of User Experience (UX) may mistakenly believe that it is about making attractive user interfaces and is essentially concerned with aesthetics. UX is in fact much more widely concerned with the entire experience a user has when interacting with a product or service. UX is not a consideration that should take place some time after the engineering of a product or system. It should instead ideally be considered throughout all stages of the product life-cycle and is often an essential component of the success (or failure) of products and services. If the product is not designed in such a way as to facilitate its use easily, correctly and in some cases even enjoyably, users will cease using the product or alternatively the product is misused and does not achieve its full potential. Most well designed systems apply UX methods throughout the project life-cycle to inform the design of the product itself, rather than being 'bolted' on at the end of the project, or worse, ignored entirely.

UX as a discipline has gained momentum over the years since its emergence from the field of Human Computer Interaction in the late 1970s and early 1980s to coincide with the personal computing revolution, where access to computing became more widely available. There is some overlap between the fields of Human Computer Interaction (HCI) and User Experience (UX), with UX emerging as a discipline from HCI. The main difference is that HCI tends to be more academically inclined and focuses on theories, such as understanding the human behaviour behind interactions with software and computers. UX tends to be more focused on applying techniques, usually in a business/industry setting. There is considerable overlap between the two areas. The domain is interdisciplinary, with people tending to stem from different backgrounds, including (but not limited to), computer science, psychology, sociology, anthropology and business. UX is a powerful tool when applied to the design and evaluation of products and can bring a lot of added value.

© Springer Nature Switzerland AG 2020   229
A. Davies, J. Mueller, *Developing Medical Apps and mHealth Interventions*, Health
Informatics, https://doi.org/10.1007/978-3-030-47499-7_7

Fig. 7.1 An infusion pump.
(Photo by Allie Smith on
Unsplash)

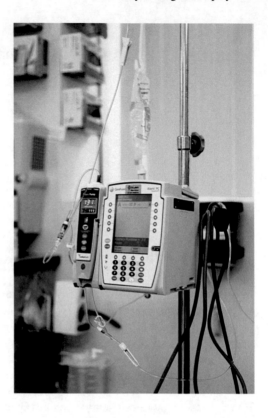

Literature concerning the evaluation of medical devices usually focuses on the evaluation of prototypes rather than on the earlier user research that helps to specify the context of use and the requirements of both the end user and the organisations involved in the development of such devices [28]. Consider a hospital infusion pump like that seen in Fig. 7.1.

Devices like these are used to infuse medication and other substances directly into the bloodstream of patients, usually in a hospital setting. Prescribed doses of drugs are delivered over a time period. A doctor or nurse would need to calculate the drop rate or flow rate of an intravenous infusion. Some of these devices can perform these calculations themselves, whereas other do not. Given that medical complications can arise if the patient gets too much or too little of a drug, setting the rate of the pump correctly is very important. If the device is badly designed and not intuitive, it can increase the chances of an error occurring even if the engineering of the device is good. This example serves to highlight that good engineering practices can be undermined by poor usability design, including bad interface design. Even if there are no functional errors (e.g. software errors), poor design could make 'human error' more likely. Apps are frequently created by people with little or no knowledge of UX principles [15] making them prone to such issues.

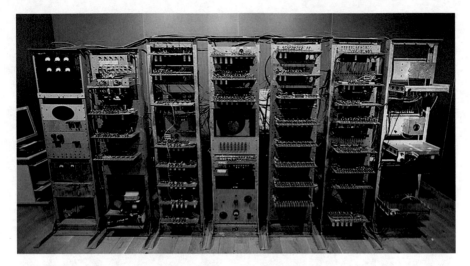

Fig. 7.2 Replica of the Manchester 'Baby' from: https://commons.wikimedia.org/wiki/File:Manchester_baby_head_on.JPG. (Author: Geni. Reproduced under the Creative Commons Attribution-Share Alike 4.0 International, 3.0 Unported, 2.5 Generic, 2.0 Generic and 1.0 Generic license https://creativecommons.org/licenses/by-sa/4.0/)

7.2   Human Computer Interaction

Human Computer Interaction (HCI) as a discipline came into being in the 1980s following the personal computing revolution. Prior to this, computers were large and expensive items such as the Manchester 'Baby' (Small-Scale Experimental Machine) seen in Fig. 7.2. Machines like this were used exclusively by specialists until the personal computer revolution made computers smaller and more accessible.

This saw computers being used in schools, offices and homes. With this development the field of HCI, which was concerned with the way humans interact with such technology, came into being. This includes the factors that determine use of such technology and tools, as well as methods and theories that can be applied to building usable systems.

7.3   User Centered Design

User-Centered Design (UCD) refers to a design process whereby the users of an intended system or product are involved throughout the development processes and the design process is centered around the needs and requirements of the end user. One of the early examples of the application of UCD is the Xerox Star 8010 from the year 1981. This was a commercially-available workstation which was the first to include many technologies that are common to personal computing now. The Star had a Graphical User Interface (GUI) not too dissimilar to modern Windows or Mac operating systems today. It modeled the office paradigm visually with icons representing files and folders, and even had a pointing-device (mouse) [23]. These sorts of features although common-place today were at the time revolutionary. The team used user testing to experimentally determine different design options.

Case study: The 8010 "Star"
Produced by Xerox in 1981, the 8010 Star workstation was ahead of its time in many ways and boasts many features of modern computers that were not widely available at the time. This included using an office metaphor to make the computer 'invisible' to users. It had icons and folders, a pointing device (mouse) and WYSIWYG (what you see is what you get) editing among other things. Importantly the development process included extensive user testing and prototyping making it an early example of user centered design (Fig. 7.3).

A further and more modern example of placing the user experience at the center of the design process is that of the Apple iPhone.

Case study: The Apple iPhone
The development of the iPhone is often touted as a prime example of good UX design. The iPhone is frequently praised for its simple, elegant, minimalist and intuitive design, and Apple is renowned for its dedication to UX research.

It has been argued that Apple has a stronger focus on developing innovative user experiences than developing innovative technology [36]. For example, when Apple launched the iPod, it was not the first portable music player on the market. Arguably, Apple did not come up with revolutionary technology when it developed the iPod, but it did radically change how users experienced this product, e.g. how they loaded music onto their players, and how they were able to browse through their music library [36]. Similarly, although Apple was not the first business to launch a smartphone, iPhones did stand out from among other smartphones on the market due to user-oriented features such as high-resolution screens that made reading on small devices easier.

Steve Jobs, the co-founder and CEO of Apple Inc., is believed to have been one of the main driving forces behind this focus on user experience, as is evidenced in Walter Isaacson's authorised biography [21]. Apple is widely known for emphasising design and interactivity and prioritising user experience over other, more technical aspects [20].

In particular, Apple is known for focusing not only on use of their product, but the entire user experience from initially ordering the product, to unpacking

(continued)

it, setting it up and finally using it [7]. This manifests for example in a focus on user-centred web design on Apple's website where customers can order and purchase the product [38]. This includes detailed and informative descriptions of the product as well as simple, intuitive navigation through the web pages until checkout is reached. Many Apple users describe the user experience of Apple products not only as "good" or "user-friendly" but as actually "fun".

Key conclusions:

- User experience describes a whole process, extending beyond use of the actual product (e.g. consider how people will find your app, how easy it will be to download and set up).
- User experience research and development needs to consider the emotional aspects; where possible users should feel pleasure in using the products rather than simply being able to use them without problems.
- Investing in user experience research tends to pay off in terms of enhanced user engagement. Apple users are often described as "fans" instead of mere "customers".

7.4 Design and User Testing

User centered design principles should be applied throughout the development cycle for the best results. As mentioned elsewhere in this book, the first stage after determining a need for an intervention would be to gather user requirements. This can be done in a number of different ways as described in other Chaps. 2 and 3 and is summarised briefly here:

Requirements gathering methods:

- Interviews (structured, semi-structured, unstructured)
- Focus groups
- User stories
- Surveys
- Scenarios
- Personas
- Stakeholder analysis
- Task mapping

Figure 1.

Set 1 (Cox)

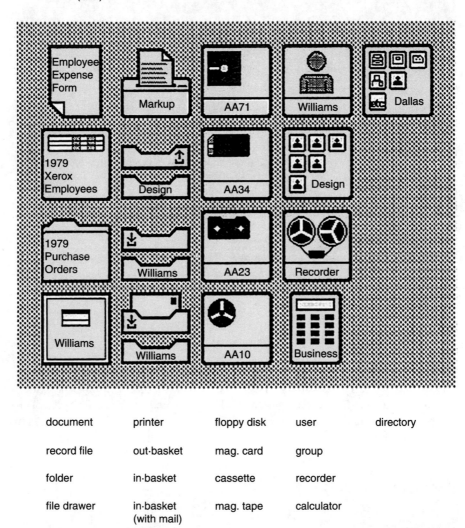

document	printer	floppy disk	user	directory
record file	out·basket	mag. card	group	
folder	in·basket	cassette	recorder	
file drawer	in·basket (with mail)	mag. tape	calculator	

Fig. 7.3 Icons on the Star from: https://commons.wikimedia.org/wiki/File:Icons_on_the_Star.jpg. (Author: Interactiontechniques. Reproduced under the Creative Commons Attribution-Share Alike 4.0 International license. https://creativecommons.org/licenses/by-sa/4.0/deed.en)

7.5 Usability Studies

A usability study is a way of evaluating a product by formally testing it with users. Various metrics are used to quantify this interaction including validated surveys, observation, and recording of physiological changes related to various emotional states. Experimental designs that measure task performance are also used. UX studies are often carried out in specially designed UX labs that may have specialised equipment, such as eye-trackers, cameras and other sensors. They are also sometimes designed to mimic a natural environment or work setting. UX studies can also be carried out on products that have been released into the 'wild' to see how real users interact with them outside of more formal lab-based settings.

7.5.1 Sample Size

In medicine the randomized controlled trial (RCT) is often used to demonstrate the effectiveness of an intervention. Before data are collected a *power analysis* is typically carried out. This is done to inform the researchers of the required minimum sample size needed to detect an effect at a certain level of statistical significance for a given predetermined statistical test. Usability studies in contrast often use far fewer participants and do not use techniques like power analysis to determine sample size.

Using a similar method to that of software engineering regarding determining when to stop testing for bugs, Nielsen and Landauer produced a well known paper where they introduced a mathematical model for finding UX problems [33]. The headline of this work is that 5 participants in a user study can reveal up to 80% of usability problems. This was determined by looking at the number of problems detected across 11 studies with a variable number of participants with the assumption that the issues were independent of one another. They modeled this using the formula below.

$$found(i) = N(1 - (1 - \lambda)^i)$$

Where the number of problems found at least once (i) is determined by the total number of interface problems (N) and λ is the probability of detecting an issue given the number of participants i [33]. Through repeated evaluations the accuracy improves for N and λ. This assertion of 5 being the magic number for UX testing has been challenged by more recent studies [3].

Taking a pragmatic perspective focused on getting a product to market as fast and cost-effectively as possible has led some practitioners to use the Rapid Iterative Testing and Evaluation (RITE) method instead (Fig. 7.4).

Access to participants and the type of tests that may be required is a much more complex issue in the field of healthcare. Patients may be vulnerable, access to clinical environments for 'in-the-wild' testing may be problematic and interfere with routine clinical care and the devices being tested may also carry a higher level of risk. Health apps are a little easier to manage unless they themselves are considered medical interventions. It may also work better with chronic patients that have an investment in managing or tracking their condition. They often have established support groups and charities that may help to facilitate recruitment for focus groups etc.

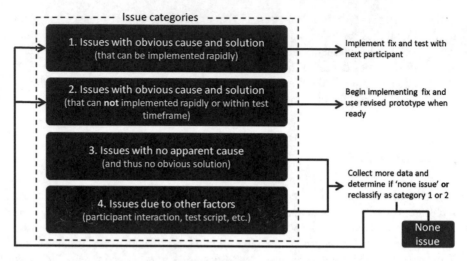

Fig. 7.4 General rules for the RITE method, based on [31]

7.6 Accessibility

Accessibility in this context refers to accessible computing. This is the ability of people to access computer systems despite various impairments or disabilities. It is preferable to design your intervention to be as accessible to as many people as possible and not to exclude people by design. It has also been postulated that many acute and chronic health conditions manifest with impairments related to their health conditions that may affect them in a similar way to a disability or other impairment even if they would not be considered to be a classically defined primary disability [18]. Impairments can also be transitory and can affect people who are otherwise healthy, for example temporarily being unable to type because one has cold hands after being outside in cold winter temperatures. The W3C's Web Accessibility Initiative (WAI) has developed a set of accessibility guidelines for the Web called WCAG (Web Content Accessibility Guidelines) [37]. These guidelines are also applicable to mobile apps with or without web content. The specific mapping of guidelines to mobile can be found here https://www.w3.org/TR/mobile-accessibility-mapping/. WCAG is a technical standard for developers and researchers which is in turn built on a set of accessibility principles. Making a website or web app accessible doesn't usually require a large amount of additional effort or development resource, especially if it is done bit by bit during development as part of the process. Many of the guidelines relate to using a standard structure, for example headings and sub-headings, and providing text alternatives for items like images, icons and buttons. Such information can be used by screen readers. An example can be seen in Listing 7.1 where a HTML image tag also has some alternative text that can be read with screen reader software.

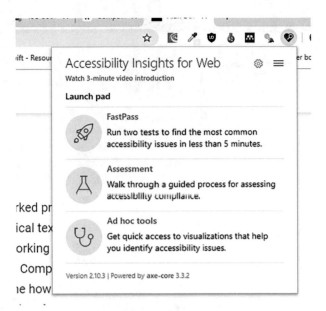

Fig. 7.5 Accessibility Insights for Web Google Chrome browser extension menu options. (From https://chrome.google.com/webstore/detail/accessibility-insights-fo/ pbjjkligggfmakdaogkfomddhfmpjeni?hl=en Used with permission from Microsoft)

```
1 <img src="pyramid.png" alt="Hierarchy of evidence pyramid." />
```
Listing 7.1 Example of alt text for an image

When applying these guidelines retrospectively, it can be helpful to use a tool to identify any areas that might not meet the guidelines. One such useful tool that was created by Microsoft is *Accessibility insights* (https://accessibilityinsights.io/). This offers Google Chrome and Edge extensions (Fig. 7.5), as well as a downloadable version for Windows applications. This can also be very useful when developing and testing hybrid web apps through a browser. The tool provides a report detailing any elements that do not comply to the guidelines (Fig. 7.6). This can also be highlighted directly on the web page with overlays on the identified elements.

> **Screen reader:** Software that speaks aloud the different UI components and other media on a screen for the benefit of people with visual impairments. This can give information on images, icons, menus and other elements, as well as reading aloud any plain text on the screen using Text-To-Speech (TTS). On some systems this information can also be provided in Braille.

The UK's National Health Service (NHS) has also provided an evidence based resource for user interface (UI) styles, components and patterns (https://beta.nhs.

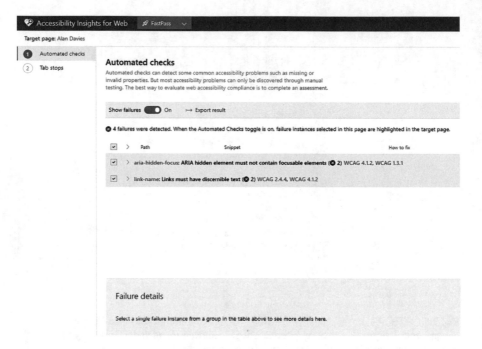

Fig. 7.6 Accessibility Insights for Web website report showing WCAG guideline links. (From https://chrome.google.com/webstore/detail/accessibility-insights-fo/pbjjkligggfmakdaogkfomddhfmpjeni?hl=en Used with permission from Microsoft)

uk/service-manual/styles-components-patterns). This can help developers to style their pages like those of the NHS website in terms of look and feel. For UK health based applications this can provide a familiar look and experience. The various UI components have also been researched and guidance for their use is also given along with the HTML code and Nunjucks template code (a template engine based on jinja2).

7.7   Affective Computing

The term affective computing has been attributed to Rosalind Picard presented in her MIT technical report in 1997 [34]. Affective computing refers to the ability of computers to recognise, express, model, communicate and respond to human emotional states [1]. The term *affect* comes from psychology and is related to experience, emotion and feelings. The *valence* of an emotion relates to the positive or negative categorisation of the emotion. Affective computing is a challenging area given the idiosyncratic nature of human emotion, and the fact that some emotional states are inaccessible and cannot be captured. Furthermore, some emotions are difficult to differentiate. Many of the existing methods used as proxies to detect emotional states are only able to identify arousal (physiological alertness/attentiveness). There is also a large degree of variation, even for the same emotion for the same person over the course of short time periods [1]. There is also an ethical perspective to this given that the ability to detect emotional states could be potentially used for manipulation.

Despite all of these challenges, the ability to detect a user's emotional state and adapt the interaction with a product/service remains an opportunity to provide tailored experiences that would increase positive interactions with the system in question. Consider the possibility of changing recommendations for a user based on their mood, or even the layout or options presented in a given system or presenting additional help if frustration is detected. Emotion is also connected to many background processes including perception, decision making, memory, empathy and social interaction [1].

7.8 Physiological Methods

It is challenging to quantify someone's experience as this tends to be individual and subjective. We can ask people what they think using methods mentioned previously, such as interviews and focus groups and the 'Think Aloud' protocol. These methods are often used in UX testing. They are subject to certain limitations, such as recall bias and selective reporting.

We can instead (or as well as) use psychophysiological methods to examine participants' arousal and valence to try and gain some understanding of their emotional responses during an interaction [17]. This can be useful if participants become frustrated or bored with a system, as we can detect this with such methods and report on it. We can also detect if certain tasks are especially cognitively demanding. In practice these physiological methods are often used in conjunction with other methods like interviews, observations and task performance to enhance our understanding of how users interact with a system. Measuring these emotions and behaviours offers us valuable insights that can be used to evaluate a user's mental and emotional state as they interact with a product or system [35]. One such physiological method that was pioneered in the late 1800s with the observation of eyes was later developed into eye-tracking methodology, with the first eye-tracker created in around 1908.

7.8.1 Eye-Tracking

The tracking of participants' eye-movements has been frequently applied to usability studies and HCI research as well as medical research itself (i.e. [10, 24, 26]). The various eye-tracking metrics can inform us of different aspects of how a system

Table 7.1 Some common eye-tracking metrics

Metric	Description
Fixation duration	A period of time when the eye is relatively still
Dwell time	Total time form entry to exit of an AOI
Fixation count	Number of fixations in an area
Number of transitions	The count of transitions between areas
Time to first fixation	Time taken until an area is first fixated upon

Note: *AOI* area of interest

is working. This ranges from obvious examples, such as being able to tell if a participant noticed something by looking directly at it, to more complex proxies of human behaviours such as determining cognitive load and thus task complexity.

Researchers can add *Areas of Interest* (AOIs) to a stimulus (an image, a website, app, etc.). This allows the researcher or UX practitioner to draw a shape (or complex polygon) over a particular region of the stimulus space that they are interested in retrieving data from. These AOIs can be added to static images, web page elements or videos. Some of the common metrics used in eye-tracking can be seen in Table 7.1.

With AOIs we can ask questions like: how long did users spend looking at a particular feature? Did they notice a particular feature at all? How long did it take the participant to notice a particular feature? Some metrics are task dependent, such as fixation duration. Increased fixation duration can be both a sign of increased cognitive load when carrying out a complex task, or a sign of boredom in an information-poor setting [19].

7.8.1.1   Mobile Eye-Tracking

Eye-tracking can be applied to mobile devices to test apps in a similar way to desktop applications and websites. Figure 7.7 shows a mobile device stand that can be used to capture gaze data of participants using a mobile device. Eye-tracking glasses also exist to allow for more natural interaction with a mobile device and to avoid the need for such stands.

7.8.1.2   Eye-Tracking Visualisations

Eye-tracking visualisations are an intuitive way of communicating findings from eye-tracking evaluations. There are several common types of visualisation that are often applied to eye-tracking data. One is the *heatmap*, which can be used to show aggregate information, such as fixation count or duration as seen in Fig. 7.8 which shows an electrocardiogram (ECG) viewed by multiple participants (experts in ECG interpretation). The 'hotter' red areas show the longest duration of gaze or the highest number of fixations.

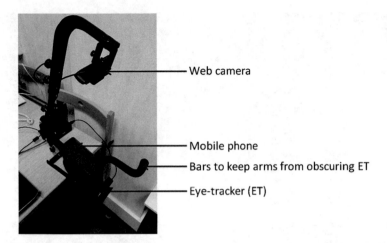

Fig. 7.7 Tobii Pro mobile device stand with an X2-60 eye-tracker set up to record a mobile device in a HCI lab

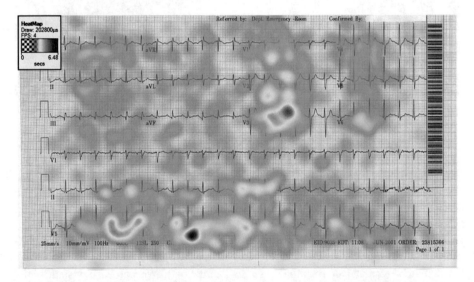

Fig. 7.8 Heatmap superimposed onto a 12-lead ECG showing the aggregated gaze of participants from a research study

These sorts of plots, and the associated *opacity/focus map* which shows transparency through a black overlay to the image below can be used to intuitively show the level of the reported measure [8]. Another commonly used visualisation is a *gazeplot*, which can show one or more participants' scanpaths (Fig. 7.9). A scanpath is the ordered sequence of fixations a participant makes as they transition their gaze around a stimulus.

The figure shows several participants' (denoted by the different colours) visual movements over a stimulus, in this case a chest x-ray image. Each circle represents

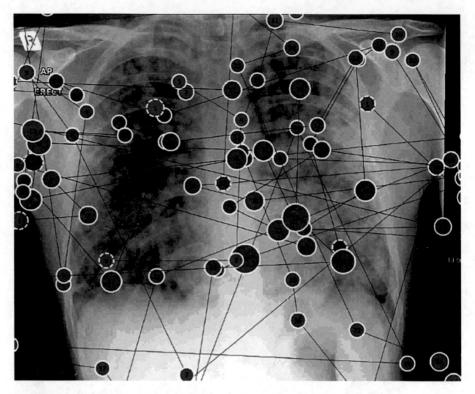

Fig. 7.9 Gazeplot showing several participants' scanpaths superimposed onto a chest x-ray

a fixation and the size of the circle indicates the duration of fixations with larger circles indicating a greater fixation duration. The numbers inside the circles represent the sequence in which the participants transitioned their gaze around the image from 1 to n. These types of visualisation can be used to explore common visual strategies that may be used by participants. These visualisations are limited by number of participants. Too many participants and the visualisation becomes unreadable. In such cases scan paths are better compared with different metrics in a matrix format (for examples [13, 25] and [14]). We can also visualise the transitions made between areas to see if there is some connection between these areas. Figure 7.10 shows the aggregated frequency of visual transitions between leads of an electrocardiogram (ECG) with darker cells representing more transitions. Cells along the diagonal show repeated fixations in the same region (lead). Such visualisations help to deal with larger numbers of participants while still remaining readable. We can also represent scanpaths as a string of letters, with each letter representing an AOI that was fixated on in sequence.

Figure 7.11 shows an example of adding AOIs (A, B and C) to an application (Brazil Breathing). We can then see what two participants' scanpaths might look like.

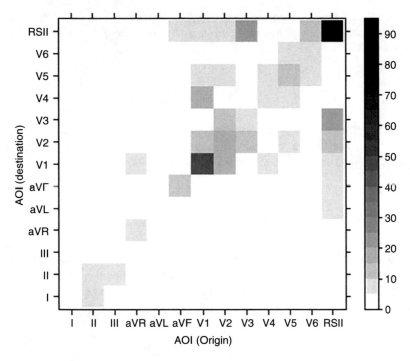

Fig. 7.10 Aggregated visual transitions between ECG leads (as AOIs)

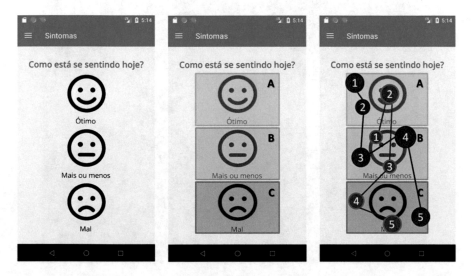

Fig. 7.11 Fictitious example of AOIs added to the 'Brazil Breathing' app with 2 participants scanpaths

These scanpaths can then be represented as a string of characters representing the order in which they transitioned their gaze between the different AOIs e.g.

$$p_1 = \{A, A, B, B, C\}$$

$$p_2 = \{B, A, B, C, C\}$$

We can then use string similarity measures such as the *Levenshtein string edit distance* to compute the similarity of such scanpaths. Again the results can be displayed in matrix form to account for multiple participants.

7.8.2   *Electroencephalography (EEG)*

The EEG can be used to extract correlates of emotional states. Electrical activity from the brain can be detected as it is generated by cumulative electrical fields as electrical impulses travel along neurons [9]. Potential differences in these fields can be amplified to analyse brain activity [9]. Electrodes are used do detect these fields (Fig. 7.12).

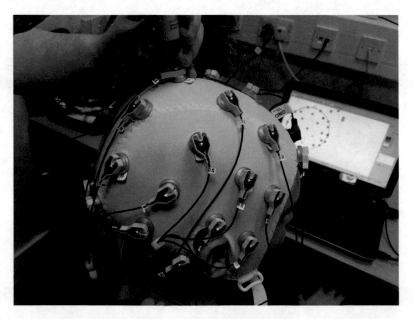

Fig. 7.12 EEG sensors being applied during a lab based experiment

7.8.3 Electromyogram (EMG)

Electromyogram (EMG) is used to detect electrical activity in skeletal muscles. This is often performed medically with another test for nerve conduction studies to determine the function of nerves. In UX studies we often use EMG to detect facial expressions associated with frowning and smiling. This is done by detecting electrical activity in the related facial muscles, the Corrugator muscle for frowning and the Zygomatic muscle for smiling.

7.8.4 Electrocardiogram (ECG)

The ECG detects electrical activity in cardiac (heart) muscle via electrodes attached to the body. This activity is outputted as a waveform (Fig. 7.13). The horizontal axis represents time with the vertical axis representing electrical amplitude [12]. The waveform consists of various waves, intervals and segments and represents a single heart beat. Changes in the morphology (shape and appearance) of these different components can indicate an underling pathology.

In terms of usability studies, the ECG is usually used to examine *heart rate variability*. This is done by looking at the period between beats (the R-R interval). Heart rate variability has been linked to increased mental effort and stress.

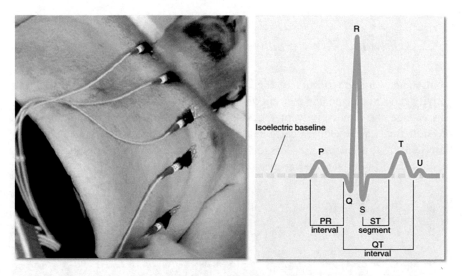

Fig. 7.13 (Left) electrodes attached to body, (Right) the ECG waveform. (Adapted from [12]. Reprinted/adapted by permission from Springer Nature Customer Service Centre GmbH: Springer Nature, Starting to Read ECGs: The Basics by Alan Davies and Alwyn Scott, © Springer-Verlag London (2014))

Example: Using EEG, ECG and EMG to evaluate individuals' emotional reactions to different web interface designs
Lee and Seo [27] used various physiological measures, including EEG, ECG and EMG alongside typical usability metrics to assess users' emotional reactions to different web interface designs.

Ten male college students participated in their study. The participants were asked to navigate four different car companies' websites and complete various tasks (e.g. identify the model of a car), while brain waves and heart activity were measured using EEGs, ECGs and EMGs. After the participants had viewed and interacted with the websites, they were asked to select their preferred website. The authors then compared participants' brain and heart activity for the four different websites.

The traditional usability metrics used included user performance measurements, keystroke analyses, satisfaction questionnaires, and interviews.
Conclusion: The authors observe that, overall, the traditional usability metrics led to similar conclusions as the physiological measurements. Both methods were able to predict users' website preferences with satisfactory accuracy, although ECG signals provided less accurate predictions than the other methods. It is important to note that these methods are particularly useful in detecting usability issues that the users would not (for whatever reason) express verbally.

7.8.5 Galvanic Skin Response (GSR)

Continuous variation occurs in the skin's electrical nature. This electrodermal activity can be detected and measured using Galvanic Skin Response (GSR). Sweat can change the conductivity of the skin which in turn can be used to indicate physiological and psychological states of arousal. This is usually carried out in lab based settings by attaching sensors to the fingers which people wear whilst engaging in some usability-related task or evaluation.

Example: Using Galvanic Skin Response (GSR) to supplement traditional usability metrics in the evaluation of an e-government website
Foglia et al. [16] undertook an evaluation of an e-government website which included an animated face (AF) to guide users' navigation. They used GSR alongside traditional usability metrics to show how these different measures are related, and to test whether effects observed using traditional metrics can be detected using physiological measures.

(continued)

Forty-three participants were recruited into their study. Participants were asked to complete two tasks using the government website. The first task was to fill in a registration form, and the second was to pay for a parking fine ticket. To assess the effects of the AF, participants were divided into two groups. One group completed the first task with the AF and the second task without the AF, while the other group completed the first task without the AF and the second task with the AF. This allowed both within-group and between-group comparisons.

Using traditional metrics, the authors note that, when viewing the website with the AF, participants rated the website more positively, visited less pages in order to complete the task, and rated it as requiring less mental effort (using the Subjective Mental Effort Questionnaire).

Using GSR measurements, the authors note that participants showed higher GSR values and steeper skin conductivity peaks when the AF was present, indicating higher physiological arousal. The authors conclude that, overall, participants were more emotionally involved when the AF was present, and that GSR can be used as a technique to quantify emotional responses in usability studies.

Limitations of using GSR for usability evaluations
Importantly, the authors note several limitations of using GSR in usability evaluations:

- GSR can identify increases and decreases in physiological arousal which may be related to differen emotional states; however in order to specify the emotion or the reason for the emotional change, traditional usability metrics are needed
- GSR measurements cannot distinguish between arousal and stress
- Individual users may vary substantially in their GSR signal patterns; some users have relatively flat traces without steep peaks and smooth decreases, which renders the analysis difficult
- Due to this individual variation, making comparisons between different users is difficult; within-individual comparisons may therefore be more useful

7.8.6 Facial Recognition

People's facial expressions can also be an indicator of their emotional state. Traditionally this was manually coded by an observer during a usability study. With improvements in technology this can also now be automated to some degree with computer vision and machine learning techniques. There may however be some cultural differences in expression as well as certain conditions (e.g. stroke, muscular dystrophy) which may make it difficult for some to produce the common facial expressions.

Example: EmotionKit, a framework for deriving user emotions and relating them to user interface events
Johanssen et al. [22] developed EmotionKit, which is a framework that uses facial recognition to detect user emotions which can be used in usability evaluations. It uses the in-built camera found in consumer smartphone devices and is thus well suited to assess the usability of smartphone applications.

The authors tested their framework by presenting 12 users with interactive mobile applications involving various usability problems. The content of their mobile application was about the history of the Munich subway system; this topic was chosen as it is unlikely to elicit any particular emotions in itself and thus confound the results.

While the users navigated through the application, EmotionKit was used to detect their facial expressions. Concurrently, two observers noted down any relevant observations such as changes in facial expressions (e.g. "smiling" or "wondering face" [22], p. 3). Additionally, participants were interviewed regarding their experiences after using the web application.

Subsequently, the authors compared observation notes, participants' responses and the outputs of EmotionKit. For example, a usability problem one user encountered was a five-second delay between two screens of the application. The participant described being confused by the long loading time. The emotions detected by EmotionKit were initially *fear*, followed by *contempt* and *sadness* after the second screen finally appeared.

Conclusions: Overall, the authors conclude that the emotions detected by EmotionKit were broadly congruent with the observers' notes, and that it was possible to detect usability problems using this method. They suggest using their EmotionKit framework in conjunction with interaction event data (e.g. logging which fields users clicked on) in order to explore usability problems.

It should be noted that many of the physiological methods discussed here are prone to being affected by various external factors such as environmental temperature, light levels, pre-existing physical/medical conditions and certain medications (and/or illicit drugs). Many usability studies also use combinations of the methods above to examine experience from several different perspectives. For example using interviewing and physiological methods in tandem. This can help address unconscious aspects that the participant themselves may not be aware of. This is also the case for HCI research that can combine and leverage different approaches to gain more understanding of a phenomena. One such example of an approach that combined elements of Affective computing with eye-tracking visualisations was applied to identify accessibility and usability issues with different user groups using the web. The method combined an algorithm for detecting a 'trending' visual scanpath with an algorithm to detect changes in arousal level determined by pupil size [29]. This can relate to stress or attraction etc and is dependent on the context to which it is applied. This was applied to 38 participants (19 neurotypical and 19 with Autistic spectrum disorder) as they viewed 8 different web pages. Data from the groups was aggregated and visualised to show where attention was focused as well as their level of arousal. Participants with Autistic spectrum disorder exhibited lower levels of arousal to effective web content which was consistent with existing literature on Autistic spectrum disorder [29]. This example highlights the potential of combining methods to gain deeper insights into how humans interact with computers.

7.9   Guidelines for the Inclusion of Human Factors in Approval Checking

More recently, guidelines concerning the inclusion of Human Factors in medical device products have been produced. These include:

- IEC 62366
- AAMI HE75, 2018
- MHRA (Human Factors and Usability Engineering – Guidance for Medical Devices Including Drug-device Combination Products), 2017
- FDA (Applying Human Factors and Usability Engineering to Medical Devices), 2016

The sources provide useful guidelines on the application of human factors to medical devices and the standards to be reached. The Medicines and Healthcare Products Regulatory Agency (MHRA) highlight some human factors considerations and how they fit into the overall product lifecycle (Fig. 7.14) [30].

7.10   In the Wild Evaluation

After an intervention has been developed and tested and has undergone a more formal lab based usability study with a number of representative end users, the next step can involve continuing to gather usability data once the application has been released. The term "in the wild" is often used to denote the fact that it is now outside of this more controlled development and testing environment. This stage could involve deploying the application to a larger group of users prior to wide-scale deployment or can be the full-scale deployment of the intervention. Continual

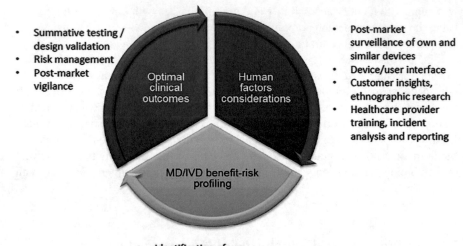

- Summative testing / design validation
- Risk management
- Post-market vigilance

Optimal clinical outcomes

Human factors considerations

- Post-market surveillance of own and similar devices
- Device/user interface
- Customer insights, ethnographic research
- Healthcare provider training, incident analysis and reporting

MD/IVD benefit-risk profiling

- Identification of use
- Use environment
- Risk assessment of use and use error
- Prioritise tasks and user interface related to safety
- Formative testing and design iteration

Fig. 7.14 How human factors form part of benefit-risk management throughout the product life-cycle. (Source: Medicines and Healthcare products Regulatory Agency (MHRA). Human Factors and Usability Engineering – Guidance for Medical Devices Including Drug-device Combination Products. Technical Report September, Medicines and Healthcare Products Regulatory Agency, London, 2017. Licensed under the Open Government Licence v3.0. http://www.nationalarchives. gov.uk/doc/open-government-licence/version/3/ from [30])

usability monitoring is advisable as the group of end users may use the app in very different ways to a smaller subset of people used for usability testing.

Attrition is a known problem facing digital health interventions [4] and apps are no exception to this. Trying to get people to continue using your intervention over a sustained time period is challenging. App stores provide information on the number of downloads and in which countries the downloads take place. This information is helpful but it doesn't show you how many people continue to use the intervention after download and whether or not they are using the app as you intended them to.

Figure 7.15 shows a visualisation of usage of a prototype app post release on the app store. The app is for symptom tracking for COPD patients using ecological momentary assessment. The aim was for patients and carers to fill this in ideally once a day. You can see in the figure that 37 people used the app to report their symptoms over a four month period. Each of the small rectangles represents one or more episode of self-reporting. The red superimposed rectangles show that out of the 37 participants only 3 were using the app as we intended them to. The rest of the participants submitted data on a few occasions or even just once. One participant, highlighted with the red circle (P18), submitted the data rapidly 10 times on a single day and then never again [11].

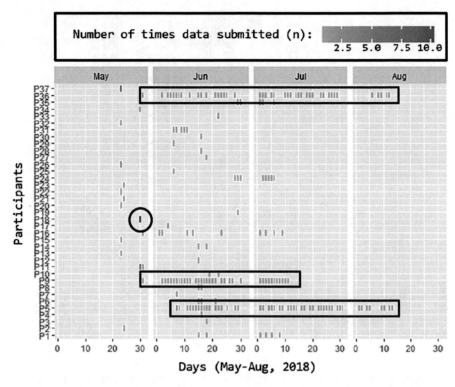

Fig. 7.15 Participant self-reporting of symptom impact gathered over a 4 month window from May to August 2018. (Source: Alan Davies, Julia Mueller, Jean Hennings, Ann Caress, and Caroline Jay. Recommendations for developing support tools with people suffering from Chronic Obstructive Pulmonary Disease: co-design and pilot testing of a mHealth prototype. JMIR Human Factors, 2020 [11]. Distributed under the terms of the Creative Commons Attribution License https://creativecommons.org/licenses/by/4.0/)

Being able to gain insights like this into how people are using your intervention is very useful as it allows you to start to understand user behaviours and target strategies to improve areas that are not working as expected.

One way to obtain such insights is to collect *event* data. This can include very detailed interaction data such as the number of times a button is pressed, scrolling pages, number of times people view help information and transitions between screens in the app. Figure 7.16 displays a heatmap showing the number of transitions between different pages on the app. For example we can see that transitioning between the *home* and *symptoms* pages happened the most frequently. We can also see which pages/screens are viewed the most and least. Event data in this study were collected using an event capturing system developed by Apaolaza et al. [2].

Event data usually consists of the *event* or action itself and a *timestamp* to show when the event took place. Listing 7.2 shows an example of a single event extracted from the event data. The data are stored in JavaScript Object Notations (JSON) form

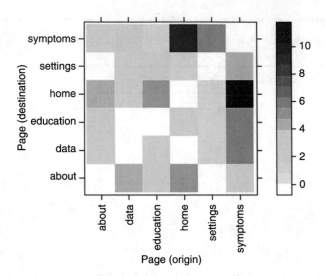

Fig. 7.16 Transitions between different screens/pages of the app. (Source: Alan Davies, Julia Mueller, Jean Hennings, Ann Caress, and Caroline Jay. Recommendations for developing support tools with people suffering from Chronic Obstructive Pulmonary Disease: co-design and pilot testing of a mHealth prototype. JMIR Human Factors, 2020 [11]. Distributed under the terms of the Creative Commons Attribution License https://creativecommons.org/licenses/by/4.0/)

(for more about this format see Chap. 5). As the app was a progressive web app and used web technologies. We can see that when a user lifts their finger from the screen it is captured as a *mouseup* event. We can see the finger co-ordinates represented by *mouse*, we can also see the document object model (DOM) element that was tapped on, in this case a *span* HTML element. We can also see the page that it was on (file:///android_asset/www/index.html) and associated timestamps.

```
1   ...
2   {"_id":
3     {"$oid":"5b0ed4380c53e11a28866cb7"},
4     "event":"mouseup",
5     "mouse":{
6       "coordX":99,
7       "coordY":314,
8       "offsetX":77,
9       "offsetY":38,
10      "but":"1"
11    },
12    "node":{
13      "dom":"id(\"rb-17-0\")/SPAN[1]",
14      "id":"rb-17-0",
15      "inheritedId":true,
16      "class":["button-inner"],
17      "type":"SPAN",
18      "textContent":" "
19    },
```

```
20    "episodeCount":1,
21    "timestampms":1.527698513988e+12,
22    "sessionstartms":1.527697243577e+12,
23    "timezoneOffset":−60,
24    "sd":"COPD_APP",
25    "sid":"<removed for anonymity>",
26    "url":"file:///android_asset/www/index.html",
27    "urlFull":"file:///android_asset/www/index.html"
28 }
29 ...
```

Listing 7.2 Example event extracted from event data

We can use such data to identify behaviours and strategies applied as well as common usage patterns. This can be examined for single users or aggregated to view overarching behavioural and usage patterns.

7.11 Applying HCI to Healthcare

There is a contention between the type of user centred design that we have discussed and that of medical device development. In the former case working with participants to generate health apps and interventions is more straightforward than if the product is a medical intervention. In this latter case more regulations and requirements need to be adhered to. This adds to complexity especially for small companies and individuals. In the case of the highest risk, medical devices (class 3 according to the NICE evidence standards framework, [32]), carrying out the iterative design with end users cannot take place prior to marketing and deployment [5]. This makes it more challenging to apply HCI/UX methods to the design of such interventions. Figure 7.17 highlights some questions that can be asked at various stages of the development of health interventions.

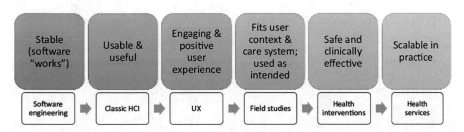

Fig. 7.17 Evaluation questions. (Reprinted from International Journal of Human Computer Studies, 131:41–51, Ann Blandford, *HCI for health and wellbeing: Challenges and opportunities*, page 48, © Elsevier Ltd. All rights reserved (2019), with permission from Elsevier [5]. Original image adapted from [6], distributed under the Attribution 4.0 International (CC BY 4.0) license https://creativecommons.org/licenses/by/4.0/)

7.12 Summary of Key Points

To ensure that the use of your intervention is a pleasant and intuitive experience for your intended users, you need to consider the usability and accessibility aspects of your intervention. If using the product causes frustration or confusion for your users, or worse, if it is unsafe, they are likely to discontinue using your intervention regardless of its other advantages. What might seem obvious and intuitive to the developer or designer may not be so for the intended user group. The best way to find out if the intervention is delivering value is to build it with users and test the usability of the product at all stages to ensure it meets users' needs and works as intended. Ultimately if your intervention is easy to use (or even enjoyable), people will continue to use it and your brand and reputation will increase in value.

- HCI and UX are similar and overlap but have different foci
- UX emerged from HCI and is grounded in user-centred design (UCD) principles
- Methods used in both HCI and UX are mixed and taken from multiple disciplines
- The aim of UCD is to build systems with the user at the centre of the design process
- It can be difficult to apply UCD techniques and UX evaluation in healthcare settings
- More successful products tend to focus on the usability of the product or system
- Event data analysis can be helpful to identify how the product/intervention is being used in a real world setting by real end users
- Physiological analysis methods can be used in usability studies to gain information about people's behaviour and emotional states as they interact with a product or service

7.13 Quiz

1. Which of the following is **not** a commonly used requirements gathering method?

   (a) Focus groups
   (b) User stories
   (c) Data flow diagrams
   (d) Interviews

2. Sample sizes for usability studies use a power analysis to determine the correct sample size?

   (a) True
   (b) False

3. Which of the following image tags are considering accessibility?

```
1    <img src="fido001.png" />
2    <img src="dog.png" alt="Image of a dog" />
3    <img src="dog.png" onclick="data.loadDataScape()" />
4
```

    (a) Line 1
    (b) Line 2
    (c) Line 3

4. Physiological methods to detect human emotional states include:

    (a) Eye-tracking
    (b) Electroencephalography
    (c) Electrocardiogram
    (d) Electromyogram
    (e) Electrononogram

5. Capturing event data from how users interact with an app provides useful insights into behaviour and usage patterns

    (a) True
    (b) False

Answers to the quiz can be found in "Solutions to Quizzes".

7.14 Exercises

1. Read Picard's report on Affective Computing: R. W. Picard *Affective Computing*. M.I.T Media Laboratory Perceptual Computing Section Technical Report No. 321. Cambridge: MIT 1997
You can find a copy here: https://affect.media.mit.edu/pdfs/95.picard.pdf
Reflect on the following points:

    (a) Is it likely that in the near future we will be able to accurately detect human emotion?
    (b) What are the moral and ethical considerations of this (e.g. emotional manipulation)
    (c) Would there be situations where machines displaying and responding human emotions is desirable?
    (d) Is the Turing test (section 1.3.2 of the report) a suitable test for determining if a machine can really think?

2. Install the 'Accessibility insights' plugin https://accessibilityinsights.io/ and carry out a *FastPass*. Use this to check a web app or PWA if you have one. Alternatively a web site of your choosing.

(a) How many accessibility issues did you detect?

(b) Did you expect to find more or less issues?

(c) Reflect on how you can design your intervention to improve accessibility for your users

Recommended Reading

1. Bojko A. Eye tracking the user experience: a practical guide to research. New York: Rosenfeld; 2013.
2. Davies A, Mueller J, Hennings J, Caress A, Jay C. Recommendations for developing support tools with people suffering from Chronic Obstructive Pulmonary Disease: co-design and pilot testing of a mHealth prototype. JMIR Human Factors. 2020;7(2):1–17.
3. Blandford A. HCI for health and wellbeing: challenges and opportunities. Int J Hum Comput Stud. 2019;131:41–51.
4. Tullis T, Albert B. Measuring the user experience: collecting, analyzing, and presenting usability metrics. 2nd ed. Amsterdam: Morgan Kaufmann; 2013.
5. Shariat J, Saucier CS. Tragic design: the impact of bad design and how to fix it. Sebastopol: O'Reilly; 2017.

References

1. Picard R. Affective computing: challenges. Int J Hum Comput Stud. 2003;59(1–2):55–64. https://doi.org/10.1016/S1071-5819(03)00052-1
2. Apaolaza A, Harper S, Jay C. Understanding users in the wild. In: Proceedings of the 10th international cross-disciplinary conference on web accessibility – W4A'13. New York. ACM Press; 2013. p 1. https://doi.org/10.1145/2461121.2461133
3. Barnum C, Bevan N, Cockton G, Nielsen J, Spool J, Wixon D. The "magic number 5": is it enough for web testing? In: ACM CHI 2003, Florida, 5–10 Apr. vol. 5. p. 698–9; 2003. https://doi.org/10.1145/765891.765936
4. Bauer AM, Iles-Shih M, Ghomi RH, Rue T, Grover T, Kincler N, Miller M, Katon WJ. Acceptability of mHealth augmentation of collaborative care: a mixed methods pilot study. Gen Hosp Psychiatry. 2018;51:22–29. https://doi.org/10.1016/j.genhosppsych.2017.11.010
5. Blandford A. HCI for health and wellbeing: challenges and opportunities. Int J Hum Comput Stud. 2019;131:41–51. https://doi.org/10.1016/j.ijhcs.2019.06.007
6. Blandford A, Gibbs J, Newhouse N, Perski O, Singh A, Murray E. Seven lessons for interdisciplinary research on interactive digital health interventions. Dig Health. 2018;4:205520761877032. https://doi.org/10.1177/2055207618770325
7. Boag P. The iPhone X user experience: from purchase to daily use; 2017. https://boagworld.com/news/iphone-x-user-experience-purchase-daily-use/
8. Bojko A. Eye tracking the user experience: a practicle guide to research. New York: Rosenfeld Media; 2013.
9. Casson AJ, Abdulaal M, Dulabh M, Kohli S, Krachunov S, Trimble E. Electroencephalogram. In: Tamura T, Chen W, editors. Seamless healthcare monitoring: advancements in wearable, attachable, and invisible devices. chapter 2. Gewerbestrasse 11, 6330 Cham, Switzerland: Springer International Publishing AG; 2018. p. 45–82.
10. Davies A, Harper S, Vigo M, Jay C. Investigating the effect of clinical history before electro-cardiogram interpretation on the visual behavior and interpretation accuracy of clinicians. Sci Rep. 2019;9(1):0–10. https://doi.org/10.1038/s41598-019-47830-0

11. Davies A, Mueller J, Hennings J, Caress A, Jay C. Recommendations for developing support tools with people suffering from Chronic Obstructive Pulmonary Disease: co-design and pilot testing of a mHealth prototype. JMIR Human Factors. 2020;7(2):1–17.

12. Davies A, Scott A. Starting to read ECGs: the basics. London: Springer; 2014. https://doi.org/10.1007/978-1-4471-4962-0

13. Davies A, Vigo M, Harper S, Jay C. The Visualisation of eye-tracking scanpaths: what can they tell us about how clinicians view electrocardiograms? In: Proceedings of the 2nd workshop on eye tracking and visualization, ETVIS 2016; 2016. p. 79–83. https://doi.org/10.1109/ETVIS.2016.7851172

14. Davies A, Vigo M, Harper S, Jay C. Using simultaneous scanpath visualization to investigate the relationship between accuracy and eye movement during medical image interpretation. J Eye Mov Res. 2018;10(5):1–11. https://doi.org/10.16910/jemr.10.5.11

15. Firth KH. User experience design: the critical first step for app development. Nurs Educ Perspect. 2019;40(1):65–6. https://doi.org/10.1016/j.jbi.2016.02.002

16. Foglia P, Prete CA, Zanda M. Relating GSR signals to traditional usability metrics: case study with an anthropomorphic web assistant. In: 2008 IEEE instrumentation and measurement technology conference. IEEE; May 2008. p. 1814–8. https://doi.org/10.1109/IMTC.2008.4547339

17. Ganglbauer E, Schrammel J, Deutsch S, Tscheligi M. Applying psychophysiological methods for measuring user experience: possibilities, challenges and feasibility. Hum-Comput Interact. INTERACT 2011 (Lect Notes Comput Sci). 2011;6949:714–715. https://doi.org/10.1007/978-3-642-23768-3

18. Harper S, Mueller J, Davies A, Nicolau H, Eraslan S, Yesilada Y. The case for "health-induced impairments and disabilities". In: W4A'20, Taipei; 20–21 Apr 2020. p. 8.

19. Holmqvist K, Nyström M, Anderson R, Dewhurst R, Jarodzka H, Van de Weijer J. Eye tracking: a comprehensive guide to methods and measures. New York: Oxford University Press; 2011.

20. IMore. Apple and the user experience business model | iMore. https://www.imore.com/apple-and-user-experience-business-model

21. Isaacson W. Steve jobs: the exclusive biography. New York: Simon & Schuster; 2011.

22. Johanssen JO, Bernius JP, Bruegge B. Toward usability problem identification based on user emotions derived from facial expressions. In: 2019 IEEE/ACM 4th international workshop on emotion awareness in software engineering (SEmotion). IEEE; May 2019. p. 1–7. https://doi.org/10.1109/SEmotion.2019.00008

23. Johnson J, Roberts TL, Verplank W, Smith DC, Irby CH, Beard M, Mackey K. The Xerox Star: a retrospective. Computer. 1989;22(9):11–26. https://doi.org/10.1109/2.35211

24. Krupinski EA, Calvin NF, Harold Kundel L. Enhancing recognition of lesions in radiographic images using perceptual feedback. Opt Eng. 2013;37(3):813–8.

25. Kumar A, Netzel R, Burch M, Weiskopf D, Mueller K. Multi-similarity matrices of eye movement data. In: Proceedings of the 2nd workshop on eye tracking and visualization, ETVIS 2016; Oct 2016. p. 26–30. https://doi.org/10.1109/ETVIS.2016.7851161

26. Law B, Stella Atkins M, Lomax AJ, Mackenzie CL. Eye gaze patterns differentiate novice and experts in a virtual laparoscopic surgery training environment. In: Proceedings of the 2004 symposium on eye tracking research & applications. New York: ACM; 2004. p. 41–8.

27. Lee H, Seo S. A comparison and analysis of usability methods for web evaluation: the relationship between typical usability test and bio-signals characteristics (EEG, ECG); 2010. https://www.semanticscholar.org/paper/A-Comparison-and-Analysis-of-Usability-Methods-for-Lee/7a0c07018860ba9432d0607492422bc5c452bd59

28. Martin JL, Clark DJ, Morgan SP, Crowe JA, Murphy E. A user-centred approach to requirements elicitation in medical device development: a case study from an industry perspective. Appl Ergon. 2012;43(1):184–190. https://doi.org/10.1016/j.apergo.2011.05.002

29. Matthews O, Eraslan S, Yaneva V, Davies A, Yesilada Y, Vigo M, Harper S. Combining trending scan paths with arousal to model visual behaviour on the Web: a case study of neurotypical people vs people with autism. In: ACM UMAP 2019 – proceedings of the 27th

ACM conference on user modeling, adaptation and personalization, Larnaca; 2019. p. 86–94. https://doi.org/10.1145/3320435.3320446

30. Medicines and Healthcare products Regulatory Agency (MHRA). Human factors and usability engineering – guidance for medical devices including drug-device combination products. Technical Report September, Medicines and Healthcare Products Regulatory Agency, London; 2017. https://doi.org/10.1016/j.molliq.2015.09.041

31. Medlock MC, Wixon D, Terrano M, Romero RL, Fulton B. Using the RITE method to improve products; a definition and a case study; 2002. see https://pdfs.semanticscholar.org/5340/ef8a91900840263a4036b0433a389b7097b2.pdf

32. National Institute for Health and Care Excellence. Evidence standards framework for digital health technologies; 2019. https://www.nice.org.uk/Media/Default/About/what-we-do/our-programmes/evidence-standards-framework/digital-evidence-standards-framework.pdf

33. Nielsen J, Landauer TK. A mathematical model of the finding of usability problems. In: ACM proceedings, Interchi 93, Amsterdam; 1993. p. 206–213. https://doi.org/10.1145/169059.169166

34. Picard RW. Affective computing. Technical Report 321. Cambridge, MA: MIT; 1997. https://doi.org/10.1109/IISA.2017.8316379

35. Tullis T, Albert B. Measuring the user experience: collecting, analyzing and presenting usability metrics. 2 ed. Amsterdam: Morgan Kaufmann; 2013.

36. UXTeam. User Experience (Not Technology) Is The Secret To Apple's Success; 2020. https://www.uxteam.com/blog/user-experience-innovation-not-technology-is-the-secret-to-apples-success/

37. W3C. Web Content Accessibility Guidelines (WCAG) Overview; 2019. https://www.w3.org/WAI/standards-guidelines/wcag/

38. Wulff B. The Apple Effect – Proof that UX is worth every penny; 2015. https://www.userzoom.com/blog/the-apple-effect-proof-that-ux-is-worth-every-penny/

Chapter 8
Designing an mHealth Evaluation

8.1   Introduction

An understanding of research methodologies and the principles of experimental design are advantageous when applied to the evaluation of an intervention, and/or to carry out research activities with collected data. This chapter introduces some of the principle methodologies that can be applied, including different types of study design that use quantitative or qualitative methods. For the best results evaluation and data analysis methods should be planned and agreed prior to the designing and development of an intervention or data collection application.

This chapter examines some of the primary study designs used to evaluate health interventions, and uses examples and case studies to show how these designs can be applied to evaluate, test and improve mHealth interventions. We also look at some qualitative approaches, such as interviews, focus groups and observation studies that can provide rich information about the success (or otherwise) of an intervention.

8.2   Designing an Evaluation: Initial Considerations

As noted in previous sections of this book (e.g. Chap. 3), the process of developing health apps should be iterative, involving several cycles of development, testing and evaluation. We can therefore distinguish between testing of apps for the purpose of further development, and definitive evaluations to test the clinical and/or cost effectiveness of the final product.

Testing for development purposes is likely to include qualitative and mixed-methods approaches such as Think Aloud testing. Studies to assess clinical effectiveness will focus on quantitative methods with some form of meaningful comparator, though qualitative elements can be embedded within or appended to these methods to provide context and enable more in-depth understanding.

© Springer Nature Switzerland AG 2020   259
A. Davies, J. Mueller, *Developing Medical Apps and mHealth Interventions*, Health Informatics, https://doi.org/10.1007/978-3-030-47499-7_8

A definitive evaluation of clinical effectiveness should only be embarked on when the total treatment package has been tested and adapted to a point where it is unlikely to change substantially and the intervention can be implemented reliably [21]. The total treatment package includes the app, the context of use and the delivery method (e.g. dissemination via clinicians or online platforms). When this treatment package is deemed relatively stable, it may be appropriate to undertake a definitive study to establish the effectiveness of the app.

8.2.1 Asking the Right Questions

While designing a study to evaluate a health app, it is important to consider a few key questions that will drive future decisions. Murray et al. [21] define thirteen key questions and decisions that are relevant when evaluating a digital health intervention (DHI). The authors recommend that all or most of these questions should be addressed in the course of an evaluation. This highlights that app evaluations should not be viewed as one-dimensional assessments of a single outcome, but rather as a series of evaluations that are ultimately brought together to assess the overall utility of the app.

While these questions should be answered through the evaluation itself, we highlight here how consideration of these questions early on will help inform decisions regarding the design of the evaluation.

Defining the problem

(1) Is there a clear health need that this DHI is intended to address?
(2) Is there a defined population that could benefit from this DHI?

Critically, the app will need to address a clear health need and target a defined population to allow a sensible approach to evaluation. If the aim of the app is unclear, it will be difficult to establish the primary outcome measure. For example, an app aiming to "target obesity" is too ambiguous to allow meaningful evaluation, as various primary outcomes could fall within this category (e.g. improvements in dietary behaviours, reduction of sedentary behaviour, increase of physical activity, weight loss. . .). Similarly, an ill-defined target population will impede establishment of a clear recruitment strategy. Clear inclusion and exclusion criteria are key to good study design as they help reduce the risk of bias. These two questions are also designed to encourage investigators to begin with "a detailed and often theory-based characterisation of the nature of the problem and the context in which the intervention will be used" [21], p. 4.

Defining the likely benefit of the DHI

(3) Is the DHI likely to reach this population, and if so, is the population likely to use it?
(4) Is there a credible causal explanation for the DHI to achieve the desired impact?

Considering the likely benefit of the app is key to determining suitable outcome measures, analysis methods, and for determining the magnitude of the expected effect of the intervention. If we cannot reasonably expect a clinically meaningful effect of the app on the target population, an evaluation will be inconsequential and will potentially waste valuable resources. This may seem obvious, but the point does require careful consideration and the complete treatment package needs to be critically examined. For example, an app designed to help older adults reduce their risk of falls is unlikely to reach the target population and thus be effectual if the app is simply placed on an app store without further advertising or signposting. Referral via clinicians or other groups/organisation that are able to contact elderly, frail people may need to be added to the treatment package. Thus, methods of advertisement and recruitment need to be thought through in detail, particularly when the target population is difficult to reach or engage, as is often the case for health-related apps. This question also highlights the importance of assessing the recruited sample against the target population. For example, when evaluating an app designed to facilitate weight loss in overweight individuals at risk of diabetes, we will need to appraise whether our app users (and the comparison group if relevant) actually were overweight and at risk of diabetes. If not, and we have instead brought about weight loss in an already healthy-weight sample, the app should not be considered effective.

(5) **What key components are needed for the DHI, which components impact on the predicted outcome, and how do they interact with each other?**
(6) **What strategies should be used to support tailoring the DHI to participants over time?**

When thinking about different potential outcomes of the app, it also worth considering whether they may interact and how they may be interrelated. For example, an app for parents of under 5-year-old children may enhance parents' medical domain knowledge around child health, which might increase their parenting self-efficacy (their belief in their own parenting abilities), which in turn may reduce help-seeking for minor health issues. Such considerations are important during study design as they help decide which outcomes need to be measured, and it will also inform the analysis.

(7) **What is the likely direction and magnitude of the effect of the DHI or its components compared to a comparator that is meaningful for the stage of the research process?**
(8) **How confident are we about the magnitude of the effect of the DHI or its components compared to a comparator that is meaningful for the stage of the research process?**

The relationship between the app and its hypothesised outcomes needs to be critically examined. A credible causal explanation should be apparent from the outset, ideally informed by theory and/or existing evidence. For example, in a previous project, we sought to design a study to evaluate the effectiveness of a child health app for parents in reducing unnecessary emergency attendance. When we consulted parents, many expressed doubts about whether the app would bring about the desired effect, because, while it provided information about common childhood health problems, it was less clear on when (not) to seek help and did not include specific components (aside from education) to target help-seeking behaviour.

Another important consideration is the direction and magnitude of the expected effect of the intervention, as this will impact on calculations for the desired sample size of the study. This is discussed further in Sect. 8.7.

(9) **Has the possibility of harms been adequately considered? And the likelihood of risks or adverse outcomes assessed?**

(10) **Has DHI cost and its cost impact on users and health systems been adequately considered and measured?**

(11) **What is the overall assessment of the utility of this intervention? How confident are we in this overall assessment?**

When considering the likely benefit of the app, risks and potential harm also need to be appraised. These will need to be assessed alongside outcome measures measuring the desired impact of the app. This is discussed further in Sect. 8.12. Costs and health economic evaluations are covered in Sect. 8.10. Once all questions raised above have been addressed and answered by the evaluation, an overall assessment of the utility of the app can be made.

Decisions to be made based on our current knowledge

(12) **Should we change research priorities?**
(13) **Should we change clinical practice?**

The final two questions in Murray et al.'s [21] list should be answered at the end of the evaluation. Based on the overall evaluation, we may need to change research priorities and/or clinical practice.

8.2.2 Specific Aspects of Apps That Affect Evaluation Design Choices

In general, the principles of designing and conducting evaluations of complex interventions are applicable to app evaluations. However, there are specific features of apps which need to be taken into account if an evaluation is to provide meaningful evidence that supports sensible decision-making. These include:

The context in which the evaluation is undertaken: Consideration of the context is necessary to appraise the generalisability of the results outside of the evaluation environment. For example, in lab-based setting, participants may be motivated to engage with and use an app. However, when deploying an app "in the wild" where users use the app in their everyday lives or usual work practice, there may be a high drop out rate.

The trade-off between external and internal validity: Enhancing *external validity* means the results are more likely to be applicable in "real world" settings, while enhancing *internal validity* means reducing bias and increasing our confidence in the results. For example, our previous research involved testing a digital intervention designed to help people appraise their own symptoms [18, 19]. The intervention was a website, and designed to be used by people in their own homes. To enhance internal validity, one could conduct the study with healthy participants in a lab-based setting, and instruct them to imagine they are experiencing certain symptoms from a specified symptom vignette. This way you can better control how people use the intervention and for which symptoms. However, this may not accurately reflect how people would use the intervention in reality. To enhance external validity, one could conduct the study with people who actually have symptoms, in their own homes. This more accurately reflects reality, but this makes it very difficult to control participants' situations, and therefore it is less clear whether changes detected in the evaluation are due to the intervention, or other factors which were not controlled.

How people use the app: When evaluating an app, it is important to assess not only whether people use it and whether this leads to desired outcomes, but also *how* people use it. This is particularly important for apps because they are often used remotely. You may have developed an effective intervention, but it cannot achieve its full potential if people, for whatever reason, do not use it or do not use it as intended. Therefore you should ensure to measure process outcome such as frequency of use and which features are used by collecting event data within the app (and possibly supplementing this with self-reported data).

Specification of the intervention and delivery platform: This involves specifying which components form part of the intervention and how they are delivered (e.g. completely online or with some face-to-face interaction). Results will only be reproducible if all intervention components are clearly specified [21]. However, this may be hard to achieve, particularly when apps are tailored to individual user characteristics, preference and choices.

Choice and specification of the comparator: Choosing an appropriate comparator may be difficult because people accustomed to using digital interventions are often also accustomed to seeking out resources online [21]. Therefore it will be difficult to control whether comparators do indeed receive no intervention. Also, if the trial takes place online, people may drop out if they dislike the study group they have been assigned to, leading to differential dropout, and therefore biasing findings. Dropout and attrition in online evaluation are discussed further in Sect. 8.11. Comparison groups are discussed in Sect. 8.8.

8.3 Choosing a Study Design

There is a wide range of different study designs that can be applied to explore effects as well as acceptability and feasibility of mHealth interventions. The choice of study design will depend on a number of factors, including ethical and practical factors as well as your aims and objectives and the nature of the topic.

Figure 8.1 provides an overview of commonly used study designs.

8.3.1 Quantitative or Qualitative

The first key consideration is whether a quantitative or qualitative approach is most suited to your aims, though combinations of these are also possible for maximum insights. *Quantitative* research seeks to generalise from a sample to the wider population by using numerical comparisons and inferential statistics. *Qualitative* research on the other hand seeks to explore and gain a deep understanding of a phenomenon or event. Qualitative research is preferred over quantitative research when the research seeks to explore questions of *how* and *why*, and when the research aims to gain an understanding of participants' subjective experiences.

Quantitative research is more suitable when you wish to numerically establish relationships between different variables and when you aim to draw inferences about other people based on your study findings. Qualitative research is typically carried out with smaller samples and involves unstructured data (e.g. responses to open-ended questions, field notes) and as such is not suitable for making generalisations about the wider population.

Another important difference lies in the measurement of outcomes. Quantitative research can only assess pre-defined outcomes (e.g. participants in a survey can only respond to pre-defined questions with pre-defined answer options), whereas qualitative research allows exploration of unexpected or unintended outcomes due to its flexible, open-ended nature.

For example, prior to the development of a physical activity app for people with diabetes you may wish to understand, in-depth, how people with diabetes feel about physical activity, and why they exercise (or why not). A qualitative study would be useful here because it would allow you to identify facilitators and barriers to physical activity and how they play into people's decision-making and behaviour. By asking participants about their physical activity behaviour in an open-ended manner, you will be able to explore factors you may not have foreseen. A quantitative survey would be less useful because, in this case, you would have to establish a list of facilitators and barriers first, and participants would only be able to select from the pre-defined list. The survey would be more useful as a second step, after having established a list of potential barriers and facilitators, to determine how prevalent they are in the population. Based on this, you could select the most common barriers as targets for your intervention.

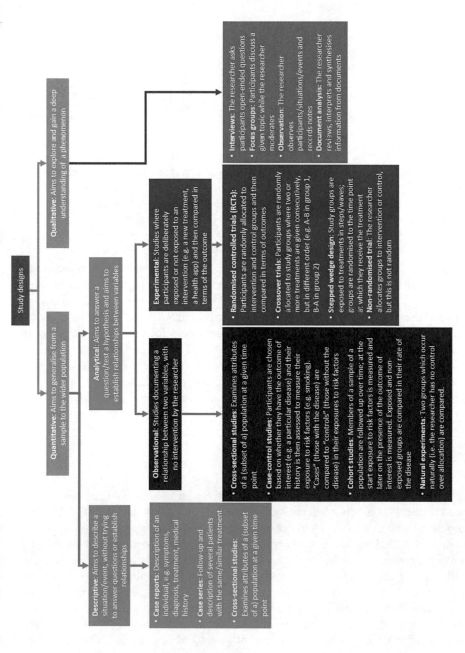

Fig. 8.1 An overview of study designs. (Modified from Ranganathan et al., 2018 [30])

Table 8.1 A comparison of qualitative and quantitative research methods

	Qualitative	Quantitative
Research questions	Why? How?	How often?
Data collection	Interviews, focus groups, observation	Measurements
Data analysis	Finding themes in participants' descriptions	Numerical comparisons and inferential statistics
Outcomes	Allows identification of unintended outcomes	Allows only measurement of predefined outcomes

Qualitative approaches are often useful when testing the usability and acceptability of an app. Once you have a first draft of your app, for example, it is helpful to ask a small group of potential users to use the app while vocalising their thoughts ("Think Aloud"). You can use field notes or video/audio recording to explore whether users experienced any difficulties or issues while using the app. Again, a qualitative approach is necessary here to explore unexpected and unintended outcomes.

Quantitative designs are needed when assessing the effectiveness of interventions. Qualitative studies are not suitable for determining effectiveness because they can only elucidate individual users' subjective experiences. For example, consider an app designed to provide information to parents about child health in order to reduce unnecessary attendance at emergency services. To assess whether the app has an effect on emergency attendance you would need to measure emergency attendance and compare numbers from before and after implementation of the app and/or between those who used the app and those who did not use it. Table 8.1 summarises the key differences between qualitative and quantitative methods.

8.3.2   Descriptive or Analytical

If you have decided that a quantitative approach is best suited to your aims, you will need to decide between a descriptive and an analytical study design [30]. This will depend on your aims. *Descriptive* designs are used when the researcher only wishes to give a detailed account of a situation, phenomenon or event, without wanting to answer a particular research question. This type of design is often appropriate for early-stage, preliminary work. For example, if you are developing an app for patients with a rare disease, it may be helpful to first write up a descriptive *case report* about a patient with the disease (or a *case series* about several patients) which you can then refer to during development of early ideas. Alternatively, you may wish to conduct a *cross-sectional survey* among the patient group and describe key characteristics about the patient group and the disease (e.g. age, symptoms).

If the researcher aims to address some form of research question or establish relationships between different variables, an *analytical* study design will need to be chosen.

Note that some study designs such as cross-sectional studies can be either descriptive or analytical. This depends on the aims and objectives of the individual study. For example, an app development company may collect app event data from their users simply to obtain an overview of the current usage of different features of their app in order to decide whether to expand or curtail certain app features. This would be classed as descriptive. However, the app company could make the same data available to researchers who wish to explore the usage of app features in relation to geolocation, e.g. to answer the question whether users from more socioeconomically deprived areas are more or less likely to access certain features than users from wealthier areas. This would serve to answer a specific question and would therefore be classed as analytical.

Similarly, case studies may be purely descriptive or analytical. We may look at app usage of a specific user over time simply in order to describe the user's interaction with the app and identify any usability issues to inform further app development, which would be largely descriptive. However, we could also follow up individual users in order to explore their experiences in-depth, gain a deeper understand of different users' interactions with technology and answer wider questions (e.g. how does a user with visual impairments interact with a health app over time).

8.3.3 Observational or Experimental

The next key consideration will be whether an observational or experimental study design is most appropriate and feasible.

In *observational* studies, the researcher collects and analyses information from a sample of the population without intervening. In other words, the researcher measures different variables as they occur naturally. In *experimental* studies, on the other hand, the researcher actively allocates study participants to different groups (usually a group receiving some form of intervention and a control group that does not receive the intervention) which are then compared.

Experimental studies are generally considered to constitute a higher form of evidence than observational studies because they have a lower risk of error and bias. For example, imagine you wish to assess the effectiveness of an educational app for cancer patients. If you simply compare people who downloaded and used the app to a group of people who did not use it, it will not be clear whether any measured associations are due to use of the app, or due to pre-existing differences between the two groups. Cancer patients who download and use an educational health app are likely to have higher (health) literacy and educational levels, and may be generally healthier than other cancer patients, as those who do not use the app may be too unwell to do so. However, if you *randomly* allocate people to either use the app or to receive usual care, the two groups are less likely to differ prior to the study. Any differences between the two groups measured at the end of the study are then more likely to be attributable to use of the app.

As such, experimental studies with random allocation to study groups ("randomised controlled trials") allow *causal inferences*, whereas observational studies only allow us to assess *correlations* between variables.

Although randomised controlled trials are considered the gold standard for determining causal relationships, they are not always possible or feasible. Randomised controlled trials tend to be expensive and time-intensive. The overall cost can range from USD 43 to USD 103,254 per patient, and USD 0.2–611.5 million per RCT [35]. RCTs often take several years to plan, implement and execute.

Another important consideration is whether random allocation to experimental groups is ethical. For example, consider a study that aims to determine the relationship between breastfeeding and development of infant illnesses. It would be highly unethical to randomly assign women to either breastfeed or not breastfeed their babies, and therefore an observational design – where the decision of whether or not to breastfeed remains with the individual mothers – would be more suited for this research question.

If limited time or resources are available for the evaluation of your app, or if randomisation is not possible or ethical, you may wish to consider observational study designs that are quicker and cheaper to conduct. One compromise is to undertake a *natural experiment*, which means that you compare people who used your app with those who did not, but participants choose their group naturally, based on their own preferences. As discussed above, there is a risk of bias in such studies. You will need to meticulously consider and assess variables that could potentially confound the relationship between app usage and your outcome of interest. Confounders are variables that are related to *both* the exposure (in this case usage of the app) and the outcome (e.g. quality of life, or symptom severity/frequency). Because they are related to exposure and outcome, they can create the appearance of a relationship. For example, higher levels of socioeconomic status are often related to higher usage of health apps, and also with improved health outcomes. As such people who use health apps may appear to be healthier because of their app usage, when in reality this is due to their socioeconomic status enabling them better access to healthcare and healthy lifestyles. Common confounders in mHealth studies include (health) literacy levels, educational levels, socioeconomic status, and gender. Therefore it is important to consider potential confounders prior to conducting the study, so that these variables can be measured and controlled for in analyses.

8.3.4 Pragmatic or Explanatory

A key consideration in designing an evaluation study relates to the question of whether you intend to conduct a *pragmatic* or an *explanatory* study. This will depend on your aims. Explanatory studies aim to determine which specific components of an intervention are effective and how they relate to specific outcomes and behaviours in order to inform theory. A pragmatic study, on the other hand, seeks to assess whether an intervention is effective in a given context. As such, pragmatic studies evaluate "real-world" implementations of interventions and aim to establish whether the intervention will be effective when contextual limitations and constraints are factored in [28].

Both approaches have advantages and disadvantages. Pragmatic studies are conducted in naturalistic settings and therefore have high *external validity*, meaning their findings are more likely to be generalisable to the wider population. However, they tend to be limited in their theoretical, explanatory power [31]. For example, a study comparing a complex clinical decision app against usual care in one mid-sized hospital can show whether this app is effective in this particular setting. It will not illuminate, however, which specific components are (in)effective. It will also be difficult to ascertain whether the app is more or less effective in particular circumstances, e.g. for particular patient groups.

Explanatory studies, on the other hand, have high *internal validity* because they are typically conducted in controlled settings where extraneous variables can be controlled. The flipside of the coin, however, is that its findings will be less generalisable to the "real world" where many extraneous variables are at play [32]. For example, the study described above could also be conducted in a more controlled setting than directly in clinical practice. It could involve providing doctors with a set of fictional patient scenarios, and assessing how the decision-making app works when specific parameters within these scenarios are varied. It could also involve several comparison groups with different versions of the app, varying specific features and functions. This would make it easier to establish causal links between specific patient characteristics, app components and outcomes. However the findings would be less applicable to clinical practice, where patient presentations are less clear-cut and various other variables will affect decision-making.

In an ideal world, studies would initially be explanatory, followed by a pragmatic study in the setting of implementation. However, due to limited time and financial resources, this approach is not always feasible. A thorough consideration of the aims and the best approach to address them is therefore advisable.

8.4 Experimental Studies

Ideally, evaluations of any form of interventions should involve deliberate exposure to the intervention to enable comparisons between those who have been exposed to those who have not been exposed. This provides a better indication of causality than simply allowing people to choose whether they wish to use the intervention themselves because, as previously noted, such choices can inherently entail bias which can lead to misleading findings. If deliberate exposure is possible, an experimental design should be considered for app evaluation. We will now explore some common forms of experimental design. Note that this list is not exhaustive; other forms of experimental evaluation exist and combinations of different designs are also possible.

8.4.1 Randomised Controlled Trials (RCTs)

Perhaps the best known and most common form of experimental design, the randomised controlled trial (RCT) is often considered to provide the highest form of empirical evidence (surpassed only by meta-analyses which combine data from several randomised controlled trials). An overview of the study design is provided in Fig. 8.2. Briefly, RCTs involve *randomly* allocating study participants to different study groups, and then comparing participants in terms of specific outcomes.

In RCTs, a sample is first drawn from the wider population that we are interested in. For example, if we have designed a child health app for parents of under five year old children, our population of interest would be "all parents of under five year old children (in a given geographic area)". As we cannot recruit and test *all* parents, we would then draw a sample from this population. Ideally, this should be a representative sample. For example, if our study participants are more educated and wealthy than the average parent of under five year olds, any conclusions drawn from our study will not apply to the wider population; it will be limited to our specific sample.

The key feature of this type of study is that it involves *randomisation*. This refers to the random allocation of participants to study groups, which usually consist of an intervention group which is exposed to the intervention and a control group which is not exposed to the intervention. By allocating individuals randomly, it is assumed that any individual differences between study participants are equally distributed across the groups, thus meaning that the two groups should not differ systematically prior to exposure (or non-exposure) to the intervention.

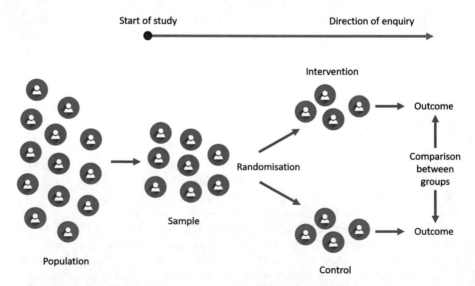

Fig. 8.2 Overview of the study design used in randomised controlled trials

For example, in evaluating an app we may be concerned that younger users will be more receptive to and therefore respond more positively to the app than older users. If we allow study participants to choose their group allocation, we may find that younger users predominantly choose the intervention group and older users choose the control group. This would mean that we cannot determine whether any differences measured between intervention and control relate to the app, or simply to differences between different age groups. By randomly allocating users, we would assume that participants of different ages should be evenly distributed across the two groups. Therefore, random allocation is key for determining causal relationships between interventions and outcomes, because it eliminates selection bias and reduces confounding. Any observed differences between intervention and control groups can be attributed directly to the intervention rather than external factors.

RCTs often employ further methods to enhance rigour and thus increase confidence in the study findings. Clinical drug treatment trials are often *double blinded*, meaning neither the investigator nor the participants know which groups receives treatment and which receives a placebo. This eliminates measurement and reporting bias. In single-blinded trials, either only the investigators or the participants are blinded to allocation.

In studies evaluating digital health interventions, blinding and use of placebos is more difficult and may be impossible in some scenarios, though there are some options that may be applicable, such as the use of active control groups (see Sect. 8.8).

At times, it may be advantageous or more feasible to randomise groups of participants rather than individual participants. This study design is known as a *cluster-randomised trial*. Clusters can be any groupings of individuals such as schools or clinics. For example, Ning et al. [23] conducted a study to evaluate the effectiveness of an app for caregivers of preschoolers. The app was designed to prevent unintentional injuries among children. Schools were randomly allocated to either intervention (caregivers received an educational app about pediatric diseases and parenting skills with additional components focused on unintentional injury prevention) or control (caregivers received only the educational app without the additional component).

A clustered design is beneficial in this case because there is otherwise a high risk of *contamination* between study groups. This means participants allocated to the intervention might interact with participants allocated to the control and inform them about elements of the intervention. For example, in Ning et al.'s study caregivers might talk amongst themselves about the app, and intervention caregivers might show other caregivers the additional component about injury prevention. Alternatively, they might simply tell them about strategies learned from this additional component. Or – less intentionally – they might put strategies learned via the app into practice and control caregivers may observe and take up these practices via social learning. Either way, this would mean that intervention effects might occur in the control group, thus "contaminating" the control group. Such effects are particularly important to consider for app evaluation studies, because app content is often easy to share with others.

Another advantage of clustered designs is that they can facilitate linking up with existing databases such as national registries and publicly available health data, which often hold data in aggregated form. Take, for example, a study aiming to evaluate the effects of an educational app on emergency attendance in England. The researchers could use publicly available data from Public Health England's "Fingertips", a web platform that provides easy access to a wide range of health and health related data [29]. However, data on Fingertips are aggregated at general practice level. It would therefore not be possible to link data from individual patients with data on emergency attendance. By randomising by practice instead of individual level, we would know exactly which practices were intervention practices and which were controls, and could therefore compare emergency attendance in intervention and control practices using Fingertips data.

8.4.2 Crossover Trials

In crossover trials, participants are randomly allocated to study groups where two or more treatments are given consecutively, but in different order [34]. The most common form is a simple AB/BA study. In this design, participants in the AB study group first receive treatment A followed by treatment B while participants in the BA group receive the two treatments in reverse order. This means that the effects of the two treatments can be observed in the same participant, and comparisons can also be made between the two groups. This means we can assess *within-subjects* effects as well as *between-subjects* effects. This way it is possible to obtain a greater number of data points with a small sample, i.e. it increases the statistical power of the study to detect intervention effects without increasing the required sample size.

The main limitation of this type of trial is that it is limited to interventions with short term effects, as outcomes need to be measurable in the time period before switching to the other treatment form, and effects of the first treatment should not interfere with effects of the second treatment. Interventions that take years to show effects or that bring about long-term effects are not suitable.

> **Example: Using a randomized crossover design to compare different communication systems in a hospital**
> Patel et al. [26] used a randomized crossover design to compare the effects of using either a pager system or an app-based communication system for communication among doctors and nurses in a hospital. One group first used the conventional pager system followed by a two-week "washout period", followed by use of the app-based communication system. The other group

(continued)

used the two systems in reverse order. This way, the authors were able to compare quality of information transfer, time taken to respond to messages, and users' satisfaction with each device between the two different systems. Due to the crossover design, each participant served as their own control, reducing effects of selection bias.

8.4.3 Stepped Wedge Design

In a stepped wedge design, study groups are exposed to treatments in "steps" or "waves". Groups are randomised to the time point at which they receive the treatment. Thus, by the end of the study, all participants will have received the intervention, but the time at which they are exposed to it is randomly allocated. Typically, there are several data collection points. At the start, none of the participants have been exposed to the intervention, i.e. this data collection point serves as a baseline. At the next data collection point, the first participant (or group of participants) have received the intervention but the others have not. At each data collection point, an additional participant (or group of participants) is added.

Due to the stepped design, we are able to measure effects of the intervention on the different participants at each data collection point as they are added. Similarly to the crossover trial, comparisons can be between and within participants, enhancing the statistical power of the study. Instead of individual participants we can also expose clusters to the intervention in a stepped wedge cluster randomised trial.

A main advantage of this design is that eventually all study sites/participants are exposed to the intervention, thus addressing any ethical concerns around withholding potentially effective interventions. Moreover, phased introduction of interventions can yield information that can inform future scale up considerations.

Example: Using a stepped-wedge, cluster randomised controlled trial design to evaluate the effects of a community health worker managed mobile health intervention
Peiris et al. [27] used a stepped-wedge, cluster randomised controlled trial design to evaluate the effects of a community health worker managed mobile health intervention for people assessed at high cardiovascular disease risk in rural India. The intervention consisted of several elements, including a tablet-based clinical decision support system to support doctors in assessing cardiovascular disease risk. Eighteen primary health centres (PHCs) were randomised to receive the intervention at different time points. Figure 8.3

(continued)

shows a schematic representation of the design. In the first 6 months, non of the PHCs were exposed to the intervention. In months 7–12, six PHCs commenced the intervention while the remaining 12 remained in the control phase. In months 13–18, a further 6 PHCs commenced the intervention, until finally all 18 PHCs were exposed to the intervention in months 19–24. Importantly, random allocation was undertaken prior to commencement of the intervention at any PHC.

8.5 Observational Studies

We will now examine three types of observational study designs in more depth. Case-control studies, cohort studies and cross-sectional studies are commonly used in epidemiological research to study the relationships between diseases and different factors on a population level. They can also lend themselves well to evaluation of interventions when randomised trials are not appropriate or infeasible.

8.5.1 Cross-Sectional Studies

Cross-sectional studies are observational studies that measure attributes of a population at a single point in time, usually in form of a survey. Cross-sectional

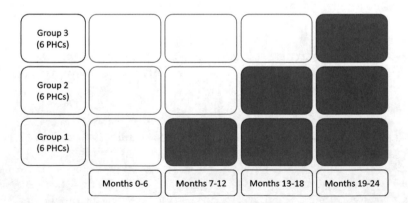

Fig. 8.3 Overview of the stepped wedge cluster-randomised design used by Peiris et al. [27]. All cells represent data collection phases. Shaded cells represent intervention periods and blank cells represent control periods

studies generally provide limited information for evaluations because they cannot establish a temporal link between different variables, as all variables are measured at a single point in time. Moreover, they do not involve the introduction of any form of intervention. Therefore, they cannot be used to infer causality (only correlations).

The main advantage of cross-sectional studies is that they are relatively quick and cost-effective to conduct. A cross-sectional design may be useful to obtain a descriptive overview of your user group and their perceptions of the app. For example, you could send a questionnaire out to all users of your app and enquire about their opinions regarding the app and their perceptions of whether this has influenced their behaviour or their health outcomes. This may provide useful insights but it is important to note that the results derive from participants' subjective views and retrospective recall of events and should therefore not be interpreted as an objective evaluation. For example, users may report that their usage of a fitness app has increased their physical activity levels despite this not being the case, e.g. because this outcome would be considered socially desirable, or because they overestimate their own current activity levels.

While the same can be said for RCTs that rely on self-reports, findings from RCTs are nevertheless stronger. Due to randomisation, we would expect any errors in measurement (e.g. recall inaccuracies) to occur to the same degree in all study groups, and therefore any differences measured are considered relevant.

An important limitation of the design described above (i.e., a survey among users of your app) is the lack of a comparison group. The design could be improved by also including people who did not use your app in the survey. Comparisons can then be made, but it is important to bear in mind that results may be biased and/or confounded, and no conclusions can be drawn about the causal link between use of the app and user attributes or behaviours. For example, if you find that users of your fitness app report higher physical activity levels than people not currently using the app, this may simply be because app users are generally more motivated to increase their fitness levels than the average population.

8.5.2   Cohort Studies

In cohort studies a sample of the population is followed over time to explore whether certain exposures are linked to specific diseases. At the start of the study, the sample should be disease-free so that a clear temporal link can be established between exposures (e.g. smoking) and subsequently occurring disease (e.g. cancer). This temporal link gives a stronger indication of causality than data derived from cross-sectional or retrospective studies. Figure 8.4 visually depicts the cohort design.

A drawback of cohort studies is that they may take a long time to complete (in many cases decades) and are consequently more expensive to conduct. They are also not suitable for rare diseases as a large sample size would be needed to identify a large enough number of people with the disease. Cohort studies are usually *prospective* i.e. participants are enrolled before disease onset. They can

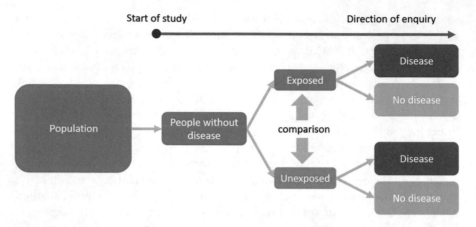

Fig. 8.4 Schematic representation of cohort studies. As the figure shows, studies begin with a disease-free sample of the population and follow up participants over time to determine which exposures they have been exposed to and who develops the disease

also be *retrospective*, meaning that an existing dataset is used, e.g. data from a previously conducted cohort study or routinely collected data (such as primary care data provided by Public Health England Fingertips [29]).

Cohort studies in the classic epidemiological sense are not usually suitable for the evaluation of specific interventions. As noted above, they often take a long time to complete as they begin with a disease-free population and participants need to be followed up until disease can realistically occur. In most cases it will be more time-efficient to conduct a randomised trial. However, a cohort study may be a useful approach if an intervention has already been rolled out and when it is not possible to control who receives the intervention. This would be the case, for example, if an app has already been uploaded to app stores and it is not possible to take it down (e.g. if the app company has a contract with clinical commissioning groups in place). In this case, it may be useful to recruit a large sample and measure whether people have been exposed to the app or not, and then follow participants up over time to measure whether they develop certain outcomes.

> **Example: Using a cohort design to follow up long-term app usage**
> A cohort approach can also be useful in terms of evaluating feasibility and other process outcomes due to the longitudinal collection of data. For example, Wheaton et al. [37] followed up a cohort of women in rural Australia who were provided with an app designed to promote breastfeeding. Data were collected via online questionnaires at baseline as well as 3 and 6 months postpartum. The questionnaire included questions regarding participants' use of the app and infant feeding. As such, the researchers were able to assess

(continued)

usage of their app "in the wild" and over time, providing useful insights into usability, acceptability and implementation. Note that this is not a true cohort design as it included only *exposed* individuals (i.e. those exposed to the app).

8.5.3   Case-Control Studies

In case-control studies, study participants are first selected based on their disease status, and categorised into cases (those with the disease) and controls (those without the disease). They are then compared regarding factors that they have been exposed to, to determine whether cases and controls differ in their exposure. For example, case-control studies have been used to test for differences between people with and without cancer in their exposures to e.g. smoking, alcohol, and red meat consumption. In fact, it was a case-control study that first identified the link between smoking and lung cancer in 1950 [6]. Figure 8.5 shows a schematic representation of case-control studies.

The main advantage of case-control studies is that they are relatively quick and cheap to conduct. Compared to cohort studies, in which data need to be collected over long time frames (usually years, often decades), case-control studies can be completed within much shorter timescales. Moreover, case-control studies lend themselves well to diseases that are relatively rare. Cohort studies begin data collection prior to development of the disease, and would therefore require large sample sizes to identify a sufficiently large number of people with the disease if it is

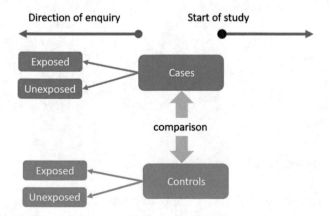

Fig. 8.5 Schematic representation of case-control studies. As the figure shows, studies begin with the identification of cases (people with the disease) and controls (people without the disease) and try to establish what happened before disease occurred, i.e. what exposures are linked with the disease

rare. In contrast, case-control studies begin data collection after disease onset and it is therefore possible to specifically identify those with a relevant diagnosis without inflating the sample size.

A drawback of case-control studies is that they cannot provide a clear temporal link between disease and exposure, because exposure is measured retrospectively. Thus causality is less clear. Another drawback is that they cannot be used to calculate disease incidence because participants are specifically selected based on their diagnosis and are thus not representative of the population.

Example: Using a case-control design to evaluate a mobile diagnostic tool
Fujita et al. [8] used a case-control design to evaluate a mobile diagnostic tool for Carpal Tunnel Syndrome (CTS) screening. The intervention consisted of an iPad-based app that recorded the speed and timing of finger movements while playing a short game. The app then analysed these finger movements in order to differentiate between those with and without CTS. To evaluate the app, Fujita et al. recruited 22 participants with CTS (cases) and 11 participants without CTS (controls). They then compared diagnoses via the app with diagnoses made by hand surgeons based on electrophysiological testing. This allowed them to determine the app's sensitivity (percentage of participants correctly classed as having CTS) and specificity (percentage of participants correctly classed as non-CTS).

As this example shows, RCTs are not always the best method for app evaluation. In an RCT, we would randomise participants to either receive the intervention or not receive the intervention. Comparing people who used the diagnostic app with those who did not use the app would not have been useful in this case. A case-control study was appropriate here because a comparison of people with and without the disease using the same app was needed. A limitation, however, is that due to the lack of randomisation, confounding could influence the results. Cases and controls may differ on other parameters aside from CTS which influence hand movements (e.g. age) and it is therefore difficult to determine whether the app responded to CTS or other pre-existing differences.

8.5.4   Quasi-experimental Studies

Quasi-experimental studies (or "natural experiments") are studies where the researcher has no control over group allocation, i.e. the groups occur "naturally". Examples include studies comparing men and women or older and younger people. Another classic example is the study by Hodges and Tizard published in 1989 [10], which compared children who had been in foster care with those who had grown up with their biological families.

Quasi-experimental approaches can be used for app evaluation when group allocation is either not feasible or ethical, for example when an app has already been implemented, or when the region of implementation is fixed. For example, a clinical commissioning group in a certain part of England might commission a company to develop an educational app to promote vaccination uptake in parents. Thus the intervention site is fixed as the local area for which the commissioning group is responsible. For evaluation purposes, a suitable comparison site could be chosen from a different area (e.g. an area of similar size and socioeconomic profile). However as this constitutes a natural experiment without allocation, there is a risk of confounding and any differences between the sites cannot be clearly linked to the app.

8.6   Feasibility and Pilot Studies

Regardless of the chosen study design, it is often advisable to conduct a feasibility and/or pilot study prior to the definitive study.

A *feasibility study* seeks to assess whether a planned study will be viable given clinical, cultural, logistic, economic and ethical influences [28]. A feasibility study aims to test whether planned study procedures or intervention components will be workable and practicable.

A *pilot study* will usually employ the same methods as those planned for the larger evaluation study, but on a smaller scale [28]. The aim is to test whether all planned procedures and components can work together smoothly, and to provide statistical parameter estimates for sample size calculations. In order to ensure a study has a sufficiently large sample, investigators typically require an estimate of the magnitude of the effect that can be expected of the intervention (the *effect size*) and an estimate of the variability of the outcome measure (e.g. the *standard deviation*). Such parameters can be difficult to estimate without prior empirical data. Data from pilot studies can be used to make these estimates and thus inform the sample size calculation. Recommendations for the required sample size for pilot studies vary, but some sources suggest recruiting at least 30 participants per study group [3].

> **Example: Testing the feasibility of taking a digital approach to understanding rheumatoid arthritis**
> Crouthamel et al. [5] were interested in whether an entirely digital approach using social media and a mobile app could be used to understand health outcomes in people with rheumatoid arthritis. They conducted a feasibility

(continued)

study to test whether the app would be acceptable to users, whether it would be possible to recruit participants online via ResearchKit, and whether the recruited sample would be representative of the general rheumatoid arthritis population. They also used the feasibility approach to evaluate algorithms developed to support the objective measurement of symptoms via the app. As this example shows, feasibility studies can provide valuable information that will help plan the larger study, enhancing efficiency and reducing the risk of wasting time and resources on infeasible procedures. The information regarding recruitment rates can, for example, be used to plan timelines for the main study and to put together realistic cost estimates. Feasibility studies do not necessarily need to replicate the design of the subsequent definitive study. The study conducted by Crouthamel et al. could, for example, be used to inform planning for a randomised trial despite its observational design.

8.7 Sample Size

Sample size calculations for app evaluation studies are critical because effect sizes for health apps are often small, meaning that a large sample size is required to provide the study with sufficient statistical power to detect existing effects. In a meta-analysis evaluating the effectiveness of app-based mobile interventions on nutrition behaviours and nutrition-related health outcomes, for example, effect sizes ranged from 0.19–0.30 (using Hedge's g), which is considered a small effect [4]. A study aiming to measure an effect size of 0.2 (comparing two independent means) with 80% power and an error probability level of 0.05, for example, would require a total sample size of approximately 788 participants.

To ensure a sensible power analysis and sample size calculation can be carried out, it is advisable to thoroughly research the literature on effect sizes found in previous, similar interventions, and to ideally conduct a pilot study prior to the larger study to obtain the required estimates.

8.8 Control Groups

If you have decided to undertake a quantitative evaluation of your app, you will need to decide on some form of meaningful comparison. The choice of an appropriate means of comparison will depend on various factors. Often, it is not sufficient or appropriate to simply include a control group that does not receive any form of treatment. Below are some common forms of control/comparison that can be used in app evaluation studies.

Usual care: In many cases, it would be unethical not to provide any form of treatment to the control group. This is particularly true for studies in health-related settings. Participants often have health problems for which there are already some established forms of care. Aside from the obvious ethical implications of not providing treatment, it is also more practically relevant to test interventions against existing forms of care, as commissioners will want to know whether implementation of a new intervention results in incremental benefits compared to existing ones.

Active control groups: Instead of exposing control groups to no intervention or "usual care", researchers will sometimes use *active control groups*. In active control groups participants receive some form of treatment that is similar to the intervention but lacks the key "active ingredient(s)" that are hypothesised to lead to improvements in the health outcome under study. For example, if you have developed an app that uses cognitive behavioural therapy to treat anxiety, you could develop a second app which merely provides educational information or meditation exercises. You can then design a study to test whether your app brings about significantly better improvements than this simple control app. This enhances rigour in two ways. Firstly, it provides a stronger test for your app; if a much simpler app leads to the same improvements as your more complex app, it is not worth spending resources on implementation and dissemination of the more complex – and likely more costly – app. Secondly, it addresses *placebo effects*. Placebo effects occur when a beneficial effect is brought about by an intervention that does not relate to the properties of the intervention itself but is due to participants' mere *belief* in the effectiveness of the intervention. In study designs using active control groups, it may be possible to blind participants to their group allocation to reduce bias.

Within-subjects comparisons: Although many study designs will involve a separate group against which the intervention group can be compared, this is not always possible or required. Study participants' outcomes may also be compared to their own previous outcomes in a pre/post evaluation. An advantage is that we can collect more datapoints with a smaller sample. The main issue with this form of comparison is that it is difficult to control for other factors which may affect outcomes in the study period. Therefore, this type of design is often used for feasibility and pilot testing rather than definitive evaluation assessment. For example, Short et al. [33] used a pre post design with 12 participants to pilot-test an mHealth app referral service aimed at assisting cancer survivors to increase their physical activity. Participants were assessed at baseline and immediately post-intervention. Using this design, the authors were able to obtain preliminary estimates for statistical parameters needed to determine the appropriate sample size for a larger definitive trial.

To design a study that provides meaningful and robust results, you will need to consider the study aims and the potential impact of a study. For example, if the study aims to help commissioners decide whether to implement a new intervention, a comparison against existing forms of treatment (i.e. usual care) is likely to be most useful.

		Factor 1: tailoring	
		Tailored	*Untailored*
Factor 2: Inclusion of	*Yes*	Intervention	Comparison group 1
components to address beliefs	*No*	Comparison group 2	Comparison group 3

Fig. 8.6 Schematic presentation of the factorial design used by Mueller et al. [19] to evaluate a digital health intervention. The study included two factors (*tailoring* and *inclusion of components to address beliefs*) with two levels each

However, if the aim is to identify why particular components of an intervention are effective in order to develop theory, a more complex set of comparison groups may be needed. In such cases researchers will often employ a *factorial* design with several levels in each factors. For example, Mueller et al. [19] developed a digital health intervention that used information tailoring and inclusion of components to address peoples' beliefs to change behaviour. The evaluation study involved a factorial design with the two factors *tailoring* and *inclusion of components to address beliefs*. Each study group received a different combination of the two factors, shown in Fig. 8.6. This meant that the study was able to compare the impact of each factor alone, the impact of both factors together, and the impact of neither of the two factors, and thus assess differential effects.

8.9   Choosing a Study Design: Minimum and Best Practice Standards

The UK National Institute for Health and Care Excellence (NICE) has developed a framework for digital health technologies (DHTs) to ensure they meet evidence standards for clinical and cost effectiveness [22]. This framework can help us understand what good levels of evidence for DHTs should look like. The framework can be used by those developing DHTs to inform their evidence development plans. It can also be used by commissioners to decide whether the appropriate level of evidence is present for a given DHT to warrant its implementation within the UK health and care system. It covers both clinical effectiveness (Section A) and the economic impact (Section B) of DHTs.

Importantly, this framework highlights that evaluation of DHTs does not always have to involve randomised controlled trials (RCTs). While RCTs provide the strongest evidence for causal relationships, it may not be appropriate or feasible to conduct randomised trials in some contexts. The framework demonstrates that other forms of evidence may be acceptable.

To identify the appropriate level of evidence for a given DHT, the Framework first requires you to categorise the DHT according to its primary function. There are four evidence tiers which are based on their primary aim and the level of risk they pose for the users, from low risk (tier 1) to high risk (tier 3b):

1. **Tier 1**: *System services* "with no measurable patient outcomes but which provide services to the health and social care system", e.g. electronic prescribing systems
2. **Tier 2**: DHTs whose primary aim is to *inform*, provide *simple monitoring* or *communication* (includes communication between members of the public, patients and healthcare professionals), e.g. fitness wearables and simple symptom diaries
3. **Tier 3a**: DHTs with the primary aim of *preventative behaviour change* (for public health issues such as smoking, diet, exercise etc.) or *self-management* of specific conditions, e.g. smoking cessation or weight management apps; apps that allow users to record information about their condition
4. **Tier 3b**: DHTs with the primary aim of providing *treatment*, *active monitoring* (i.e. any tracking of patient location and/or of data relating to a specified condition), *calculating* (any form of calculator impacting on treatment/diagnosis/care) or *diagnosis*

For example, a DHT designed to promote behaviour change to prevent a health problem (e.g. an app promoting healthy diets and physical activity to prevent Type 2 diabetes) would be classed as evidence tier 3a, whereas a DHT which provides or guides treatment (e.g. an app functioning as a decision tool used by healthcare professionals to decide whether antibiotics should be prescribed or not) would be classed as evidence tier 3b.

Once the appropriate evidence tier has been selected, the framework can be used to find the relevant study design for this evidence tier. The framework highlights minimum and best practice standards. For example, according to the framework, the relevant designs for demonstrating effectiveness for an app in evidence tier 3a are:

- Minimum evidence standard: High quality observational or quasi-experimental studies demonstrating relevant outcomes. These studies should present comparative data.
- Best practice standard: High quality intervention study (quasi-experimental or experimental design) which incorporates a comparison group, showing improvements in relevant outcomes.

Note that DHTs in evidence tiers 3a and 3b also need to meet the standards in tiers 1 and 2. The framework also provides different evidence standards for different evidence categories. For example, for a DHT in tier 2, the categories are *reliable information content*, *ongoing data collection to show usage of the DHT*, *ongoing data collection to show value of the DHT*, and *quality and safeguarding*. Not all evidence categories require empirical evaluations. To show reliable information content, for example, the best practice standard includes "evidence of endorsement, accreditation or recommendation by NICE, NHS England, a relevant professional body or recognised UK patient organisation" ([22], p. 16). Note that DHTs in tier 2 do not need to demonstrate effectiveness.

Economic evaluations recommended in the NICE Framework are presented in Sect. 8.10.

8.10   Costs and Economic Evaluations

The purpose of economic evaluations of health apps is to inform decision makers such as clinical commissioners about the economic value, sustainability and cost-effectiveness of the interventions. Economic evaluations of health apps are critically important because, despite often-cited claims of their ability to reduce costs, evidence for their cost-effectiveness is limited [11].

Assessing cost effectiveness involves measuring costs by combining resource use (e.g. amount of money and staff time spent) with unit costs for health and social care and weighing that against the value of health improvements brought about by the intervention [17]. This should include not only the immediate costs of development but also the long term costs of maintaining, updating and disseminating the app [21]. Economic evaluations should also consider how these costs could be met and who will take responsibility for them [17].

Economic evaluations of health interventions can take different forms, depending on the perspective taken. Common approaches include [11, 17]:

- **Cost-utility analysis**. This compares costs and benefits, and measures benefits in terms of *quality-adjusted life-years*. This is a measure of length of life weighted by quality of life to reflect not only if life has been prolonged but also the quality of the gained life years (scaled from 0 to 1, where 0 = dead and 1 = perfect health).
- **Cost-effectiveness analysis**. This measures benefits in terms of natural or clinical units, such as the number of avoided disease cases
- **Cost-consequence analysis**. This is an extended form of cost-effectiveness analysis, where multiple benefits are measured. The different benefits are reported separately rather than in a single cost-outcome ratio.
- **Cost-benefit analysis**. This is the most common type of evaluation within other (non-health) public policy fields, such as environment and transport appraisals. The benefits of programs are measured in monetary terms (i.e. a monetary value is placed on health outcomes).
- **Cost-minimisation analysis**. This method is often used in the health sector to compare different medical interventions in terms of their cost so that the option with the lowest cost can be selected [7]. It can only be used to measure and compare costs of interventions that have the same benefits (i.e. the same outcomes would be used to measure their effectiveness).

The type of conducted evaluation will depend on the research question as well as the extent to which the intervention interacts with the context it is implemented in, and the resulting diversity in costs and benefits [17]. It will also depend on the funder/payer of the intervention because different funders will take different perspectives. Cost-utility analysis and cost effectiveness analysis are often used when the health sector is the payer of the intervention. Cost-consequence analysis and cost-benefit analysis are often used when taking a public sector/societal perspective (e.g. when a local authority is the payer of the intervention), because it usually allows the inclusion of non-health benefits. Cost-minimisation analysis is used when taking a societal perspective (when you are interested in costs to wider society, including health care services, social services, and individual patients) or a third-party payer perspective [7].

How "benefit" is measured will depend on the purpose of the individual app and what it aims to achieve.

Benefits that should be considered (dependent on the relevant perspective) [17]:

- health effects (e.g., number of days spent symptom-free)
- measures of time spent in a healthy state
- monetary valuation of healthy time (or other health outcomes). For example, the UK National Institute for Health and Clinical Excellence (NICE) uses a cost-effectiveness threshold ranging between £20,000 and £30,000 per quality-adjusted life year to establish whether the technology represents an efficient use of limited NHS resources [15]. This means that they would consider a new technology as worthy of being funded if it can enhance the quality of life of patients by 1 (this is a standardised score) for every £20–30,000 of funding that is put in.
- measurement of life satisfaction
- measurement of patients' own perception of whether they are able to live a meaningful life
- non-health outcomes such as improvements in self-management capacities, increased health literacy, reductions in stress and anxiety, improvements in social interactions, self-confidence, better work productivity etc. [2]

Costs that should be considered [17]:

- **Development:** For health apps, development costs constitute the largest proportion of the costs. These costs can be substantial, usually amounting to tens of thousands or even hundreds of thousands of pounds sterling. Development costs include costs for software engineering but also wider costs such as costs for requirements gathering from users and stakeholders, costs for other preparatory work such as literature reviews to identify existing evidence, costs for developing the intervention, and costs for user testing.
- **Maintenance and running costs:** Depending on the individual app, these costs may be as low as simply the cost of hosting the app on a server or they may be more costly, for example if the app needs to be signposted by clinicians.
- **Updating the content, features and software:** This is important to ensure compatibility with updates by other software manufacturers in order to uphold functionality.

8.10.1 Economic Evaluation According to the NICE Evidence Standards Framework for Digital Health Technologies

The NICE Framework [22], introduced in Sect. 8.9, also provides guidance to help developers and others understand what information is needed for an effective economic analysis. The Framework depicts how the economic impact standard components come together to produce economic analysis outputs. The Framework distinguishes between different commissioning decisions and their associated level of economic risk to the payer. Pilot studies and local commissioning decisions are considered a "low" risk. Local, regional or national commissioning for cost-saving DHTs (e.g. if the DHT is expected to involve considerable implementation costs but is expected to be cost-saving overall) would be assigned a "medium" risk. Commissioning decisions on the national level for cost-incurring DHTs (e.g. service redesign costs) would be considered a "high" risk.

Based on this, the Framework assigns an economic analysis level of either *basic*, *low financial commitment* or *high financial commitment*, respectively. Based on the economic analysis level, it recommends different economic analysis methods and specifies the outputs this would produce.

For example, for pilot studies and local commissioning decisions the Framework assigns a "low" level of economic risk to the payer, and a "basic" level of economic analysis. For the basic level, the Framework suggests *budget impact analysis*, which will provide estimated yearly budget impact for years 1 to 2.

At the national level, the level of economic risk depends on whether the DHT under evaluation is expected to be *cost-saving* (medium risk) or *cost-incurring* (high risk). For economic analyses with low financial commitment, the Framework recommends cost-consequence analysis. For DHTs "with health outcomes funded by the NHS and Personal Social Services" or DHTs "funded by the public sector with health and non-health outcomes" or for DHTs that "focus on social care", the Framework recommends cost-utility analysis ([22], p. 30).

8.11 Non-response and Dropout in Online Evaluations

Due to the nature of apps and how they are accessed and disseminated, evaluations of apps are often conducted online. Non-response and attrition are common issues in online studies [36]. Dropout is particularly problematic when participants drop out for systematic reasons [1], e.g. when study arms differ in acceptability rather than randomly. Findings will be biased if this leads to group differences on potentially confounding variables.

For example, in a previous research study, we assigned participants to one of four study groups, each receiving different forms of health information. Some participants received tailored information, while others received generic information, and some viewed information supplemented with certain components while others viewed information without these components. As such, the information viewed by the four study groups differed considerably in length. The study took place online, which meant that there was a low threshold for dropout. As a result, more participants dropped out from some groups than others [18].

This not only led to unequal group sizes, but also to age differences between the groups. Thus we could not discern if any differences measured between the groups were due to the different forms of information or due to age differences.

In general, issues related to attrition can be addressed by undertaking an intention-treat-analysis, where all participants are included according to the group they were randomised to, regardless of whether they were exposed to the intervention or whether they dropped out before they were exposed [16].

Aside from bias issues through differential dropout or non-response, these issues can also lead to reduced generalisability of the findings. For example, if an evaluation retains more women or more highly educated participants than the general population targeted by the app, it will mean that the sample is not representative of its target populations and findings cannot be easily generalised.

This has important implications for the database design of health apps. Databases should ideally collect and – if possible – retain (anonymised) data from all app users, including those who discontinue use or drop out of the evaluation. This enables comparison of those who drop out with those who continue in order to explore any systematic differences which could cause bias. It also enables an intention-to-treat analysis in randomised trials (although it should be noted that, under the General Data Protection Regulation, users can request for their personal data to be removed unless it has been fully anonymised).

8.12 Considering Harm and Risk

Aside from assessing effectiveness, evaluations of apps need to give serious consideration to the possibility of harm. Evaluations need to actively address this by including specific elements that look for potential risks. Risks and harms will depend on the individual app, but some common sources include [25]:

- breaches of privacy and information governance
- inadequate security arrangements, e.g. lack of encryption of personal data
- unintended consequences such as negative emotional effects on patients e.g. anxiety or frustration
- inaccurate (medical) information
- inappropriate decision support leading to incorrect decisions and behaviours, e.g. a clinical decision aid app which recommends the wrong medication
- unintended costs to individual consumers or healthcare systems (e.g. a symptom appraisal app which recommends presenting to emergency services for trivial symptoms)

- lack of compliance with professional standards, e.g. accountability, truthfulness and transparency
- unnecessary medicalisation/pathologisation of natural fluctuations in health outcomes
- deceptive or misleading promotion of apps
- opaque financial transactions (leading to e.g. unintentional subscriptions or in-app purchases)
- ineffective apps may be used to replace existing effective medical interventions, leading to aggravation of symptoms or delayed diagnosis

Expected harms should be systematically identified and quantified. This can be undertaken as part of an evaluation. For example, an app aiming to increase physical activity among older adults with chronic health conditions may inadvertently cause stress and anxiety, by making those who are less active feel guilty. Thus, stress and anxiety should be measured alongside physical activity levels.

However, there may also be *unexpected harms*. These will require alternative strategies for identification. For example, qualitative interviews and focus groups with users may help to highlight unforeseen harm. Following any evaluation, one should ideally additionally conduct a long-term observational study during widespread implementation to assess any potential harm occurring when the intervention is deployed "in the wild" (as opposed to the more controlled environment typical to most evaluation studies).

The Organisation for the Review of Care and Health Applications (ORCHA) [24] has developed tools for reviewing apps that include criteria on data privacy; such tools may be a helpful resource when evaluating the risk potential of your app.

8.13   Qualitative Studies

Where quantitative methods are good for quantification and measuring pre-defined outcomes, qualitative methods are good for exploring a phenomenon or research question in more depth. As such, they are well suited for evaluating *acceptability* and *usability*. If possible, it is usually advisable to conduct some form of qualitative evaluation alongside studies assessing the effectiveness of an intervention in order to explore unintended and unexpected outcomes and to gain a more complete picture of how app usage has been incorporated into users' lives or workflows. This is important in order to explore *reasons* underlying users' behaviours and decisions.

If, for example, an RCT evaluating a mobile communication app for clinicians finds no effect of the app on the length of existing workflows, this could be due to various reasons. It could be because the app simply has no effect on these workflows, or because the app is creating new issues, thus masking any effects on other workflows. With a quantitative evaluation alone we will struggle to identify these finer nuances because it is difficult – or impossible – to apprehend all possible consequences and outcomes. In a qualitative study, a sub-sample of clinicians can be questioned regarding their experiences using the app and their perceptions of its usefulness, thus allowing opportunities for in-depth exploration.

Example: Using a qualitative realist evaluation to supplement the quantitative evaluation of an app for type 2 diabetes management

Hensel et al. [9] used a qualitative *realist evaluation* as part of a larger randomised trial to evaluate a web-based solution for improving self-management in type 2 diabetes. Realist evaluations aim to explore how interventions lead to outcomes taking contexts and mechanisms of action into account. In other words, they aim to explore not only whether an intervention works but under what circumstances it works (or not). The embedded realist evaluation consisted of telephone interviews conducted at baseline and again towards the end of the intervention. Interviews explored participants' experiences of using the web-based intervention, facilitators and barriers to effective use and facilitators and barriers to diabetes self-management. Analyses revealed that interviewees who reported a range of psychosocial issues and competing priorities as well as low confidence in their ability to self-manage their diabetes also experienced no improvements in blood glucose levels. Conversely, those who reported high or moderate confidence and no competing priorities experienced improvements in blood glucose.

As the example above demonstrates, qualitative elements embedded within quantitative evaluations can provide important insights. While quantitative studies can address the question "Does it work?", qualitative studies can additionally explore "why, for whom, and under what circumstances does it (not) work?".

The following sections explore some common qualitative study designs.

8.13.1 Interviews

Many qualitative methods rely on data collected from interviews and these data are used to provide insights into what people think about a particular subject and why. They are also used to inform design, and to provide retrospective information on why people behaved in a certain way or made particular choices. We can also use interview data to help us study or understand a particular phenomenon and provide rich data. We may use interview findings as part of the design process to ensure that potential users' and other stakeholders' views are listened to and reflected in the design process. We may also use interviews to evaluate a product/intervention once it has been released to determine how well received it was along with identifying usability issues. There are 4 main types of interview consisting of:

1. Structured
2. Unstructured (open-ended)
3. Semi-structured
4. Group (i.e. focus groups)

Interviews can be carried out in person, face-to-face or remotely (via phone, messaging/email or video conferencing).

The type of interview and delivery method are dependent on the task and other practicalities, such as distance or convenience. The types of interview are named according to how much control the interviewer (person carrying out the interview) has over the interviewee (person being interviewed). If for example you wanted to understand users' first impressions/reaction to a new design idea, you would probably choose an informal open-ended type of interview allowing for the exploration of ideas. In contrast to this, if you wanted to gain feedback about a specific design feature then a structured or semi-structured interview or questionnaire would be more appropriate because the goals are more specific.

Structured interviews use predetermined questions and are therefore appropriate when the goals of the interview are well defined and understood. In some cases interviewees choose from a set of written or spoken options. Questions are usually closed and the same questions are used with every participant. *Unstructured interviews* do not have any predetermined content and are more like a conversations that is focused around a specific topic of interest. They also have the potential to delve into great depth or into whole new and unexpected areas. *Semi-structured interviews* combine some of the features of both structured and unstructured interviews, using both open-ended and closed questions. A basic script can be used by the interviewer as a guide and for consistency, but the questions may then go off in new directions depending on the responses.

There are of course some limitations to interviews and these include issues related to many types of self-reported data such as recall issues as people cannot always remember events accurately, and missing detail as they might not know which details are important, or they may not want to share all the details for other reasons. Finally they suffer from issues of replicability. You could potentially generate completely different results with different interview participants.

8.13.1.1 Carrying Out an Interview

If you decide to carry out an interview for design or evaluation then there are certain considerations to be aware of. There is a certain amount of skill required in carrying out a successful interview. Firstly one should set a clear goal for the interview (what are you trying to find out) and be sure it is the most appropriate method for the stated goal. Secondly one should prepare and ideally test out (through piloting) an interview protocol in the case of a structured or semi-structured interview. The questions on the protocol should be related to the goal and ideally one should try and elicit feedback from others to check the content is relevant and the language clear.

The protocol can also help the interviewer by acting as a memory aid to ensure all the key questions are asked.

Many interviews are audio recorded and analysed later, although this is sometimes done by an interviewer asking questions and another person taking notes. If you do decide to audio record the interview then it is important to be familiar with the recording device and test that it works (and is charged etc.) prior to the interview. Usually, one would contact the interviewee prior to the interview and arrange a suitable time and place to carry it out. If you are using face-to-face interviews then the location is important. You ideally need a quiet environment that is free of disturbances (interruptions, noise or other distracting stimuli). You want the interviewee to feel safe and relaxed but the location should not bias the interview in any way. Again the way you interact with the interviewee is important. Ideally one should be aware of cultural issues. For example, in some cultures eye-contact can be viewed as a form of aggression, whereas in other cultures not looking people in the eye can be seen as rude, disrespectful or a sign of untrustworthiness. This also relates to your dress code and nonverbal communication. The clothes you wear may be dictated by cultural norms. Generally smart but causal clothing is preferred as uniforms or other professional dress may affect the power dynamic and alter communication. The *SOLER* acronym can be useful when interviewing people (accounting for cultural variation). It stands for:

- Square (sit squarely facing the interviewee)
- Open (have an open posture, do not cross arms or place barriers between you)
- Lean (lean forwards slightly as this indicates interest)
- Eye-contact (give eye-contact to show interest)
- Relax (if you look relaxed it will help the interviewee also feel relaxed)

Finally when asking the questions, do not use leading questions and avoid the use of jargon. Make sure the questions are clear and specific, for example *"How does the current system work?"* or *"what do you like/dislike about it?"* and *"If you could improve one thing what would it be?"*.

It is important to use open-ended questions wherever possible to invite elaboration and detail by the participant, and to avoid leading the participant. Closed-ended questions are questions that can be answered with a simple Yes/No answer. Open-ended questions require more elaborate responses. Words which typically indicate open-ended questions include:

- What
- How
- Why
- When
- Tell me about...

For example, consider the following exchange derived from an interview study that assessed how participants used a health app for symptom monitoring:

Interviewer: *"Do you think this might be useful; this graph?"*
Participant: *"Yes, I do"*

As you can see, the interviewer used a closed-ended question, and received only a very short answer. Now consider the following exchange, from the same study:

Interviewer: *"So, if you could just describe what you think it [the graph] might show?"*

Participant: *"Just showed the ratings for breathlessness symptoms, its giving me a graph of how my ratings would be over a day. Or maybe a few days. But yeah, it just shows how variable breathlessness can be."*

In the second example, the interviewer phrased the question in a more open-ended manner, inviting the participant to describe the graph rather than simply state whether they think it is useful. Consequently the interviewee provided a more elaborate response, which allowed the interviewer to assess whether the interviewee had been able to interpret the graph correctly.

8.13.2   Focus Groups

Focus groups are a form of group interview, where research participants discuss an issue amongst themselves (rather than with the researcher). The researcher may facilitate and moderate the discussion and ask questions, but interactions among the group are central to the methodology [12]. Participants are encouraged to discuss and comment on each others' contributions and thus expand on and explore different points of view.

Focus groups are often viewed simply as an easy means to interview a larger number of people at lower cost, however, careful consideration should accompany the choice of the method. Focus groups can be useful when participants may be reluctant to be interviewed on their own. One-to-one interview settings can often seem overly intense or formal, and the presence of a larger group (possibly even a group who know each other) may help create a more comfortable atmosphere. Focus groups are also a useful means for exploring a variety of perspectives on a topic, because group interactions can lead to forms of communication that would simply not be accessible in one-to-one settings, such as joking or arguing [12]. Focus groups can also allow the researcher to tap into dynamics such as group norms and cultural values which may not become apparent during direct questioning in an interview.

Despite these benefits, there are situations in which focus groups are less helpful. One risk is that particularly vocal individuals can monopolise the group discussion, making it more difficult for others to share their insights. Another concern is that group dynamics may mean that opinions at variance with those of the majority of the group are less likely to be shared. Focus groups may also be less useful for pursuing specific research questions and aims, as group discussions tend to digress from the original subject as participants share different experiences and opinions. Finally, one should bear in mind that focus groups are not likely to be suited to the discussion of sensitive topics that may be attached to stigma, embarrassment or blame.

Because focus groups constitute a useful means for idea generation and brain-storming, they are often used to gather initial ideas for health app development and for designing plans for evaluation. In a recent project, for example, we sought to design a study to evaluate an app for parents of under 5 year old children. To help design this study in a feasible and acceptable manner, we undertook a focus group with parents and briefly presented the app and our initial ideas. The parents then discussed the ideas among themselves. This generated several ideas for additions to our study as well as highlighting problems. For example, parents in the focus group highlighted that we would need to budget for some form of child care to enable parents to take part in certain parts of the evaluation, an aspect we had not considered before.

We also used focus groups to help generate ideas for the development of an app for self-management of chronic obstructive pulmonary disease. Through group discussions, participants came up with novel and intriguing ideas, such as the creation of novel in-app features that could help those with chronic lung problems navigate everyday activities better.

For the testing phase of our app, however, we found individual interviews to be more helpful than focus groups. For the testing phase participants needed to be able to fully engage with the app which would be difficult in a group session. Moreover, participants had very differing levels of familiarity with technology. In a group setting, those struggling with usage of the app might feel less confident in showing their difficulties.

Example: Using focus groups as part of the evaluation of an app for premenopausal women
In some situations, however, focus groups may be useful for app evaluations as well. Mann et al. [14] aimed to evaluate the content, usability and acceptability of an app designed to improve intake of bioavailable dietary iron in premenopausal women. The authors provided women aged 18–50 with the app on their smartphones and asked them to use the app over a 2-week period. Subsequently, the women took part in one-hour focus group sessions with 6–7 participants per group, where they discussed which sections and features of the app they liked or disliked and why. This helped the authors identify suggestions for improvement to inform ongoing development. It should be noted, however, that there is a risk that the desire for harmony or conformity within the group may have led to less popular opinions being subdued.

8.13.3   Observation

Qualitative research often entails observation, either exclusively or in conjunction with interview methods. Typically, participants are observed while they perform some form of task or are involved in some form of activity. Observation may occur in real-time and/or subsequently using video recordings. The researcher records observations either in a structured or unstructured format. In the structured format, observations are coded according to specific criteria and are thus brought into a format which can be analysed quantitatively. For example, the presence of a specific behaviour can be coded as *present* or *not present*, or it can be rated on a Likert scale. In an unstructured format, the researcher records free-text notes of what they are observing. Unstructured observations can be analysed qualitatively to identify recurring and important themes and concepts.

Observational methods are often helpful because participants' reports of their behaviour may not always be congruous with their actual behaviour. Observation may allow insights into actual behaviour (though this may be influenced by the presence of an observer) and also allows the researcher to take the context into account during interpretation [20].

An important consideration in observation studies is whether informed consent needs to be obtained. In some research paradigms, the researcher maintains a distance from the observees and the role of the researcher remains concealed. In other paradigms the observer becomes a participant in the situation they are observing, interacting with the observees. The role of the observer can be either concealed or known. The advantage of concealed observation is that it mitigates the risk of biased findings as participants adapt their behaviour due to observation. The drawback is that this has obvious ethical implications. Observation can also be combined with interview methods, e.g. by interviewing participants while also taking notes regarding the wider context and physical environment.

Another limitation to consider is that observation is always filtered through the perception and interpretation of the observer. The observer is unable to perceive and record all details of a given situation. This would simply exceed the limitations of human processing of information. Some form of editing and filtering will occur invariably. Moreover, analysis of the data requires interpretation, which will be influenced by preconceptions, beliefs and assumptions of the researcher (though the same can be said of any form of analysis, including quantitative analysis).

Observational methods can be very useful during testing of smartphone apps. For example, to test an initial prototype version of a smartphone app for people with chronic obstructive pulmonary disease, we asked participants to navigate through the app while vocalising their thoughts about it. Participants' verbalisations were audio-recorded. Additionally, we took notes as we observed how they navigated the app, recording whenever participants' interactions signalled some form of difficulty using the app. As such, we were able to tap into participants' accounts as well as our observation of their actual interactions with the app. This was critical because participants' vocalisations did not always concur with their interactions. For example, when asked about their opinion regarding certain features, participants tended to reply that they liked them. However observation at times clearly showed that participants struggled with these features, needing multiple attempts to perform actions and often undertaking accidental actions. This highlights that simply asking users to report their opinions regarding apps is not a sufficient form of evaluation. Users may edit their responses to avoid conflict, criticism or to avoid appearing incapable.

8.14   Review by External Organisations

Once you have a completed treatment package, you may wish to have your app reviewed externally to enhance credibility. The Organisation for the Review of Care and Health Applications (ORCHA) is the world-leading organisation for reviewing health apps [24]. ORCHA has produced several tools and services that can be used by:

- app developers, to help them create better apps
- health professionals, to help them identify suitable apps which they can recommend (or even prescribe) to their patients
- governments and health & social care organisations, to help them identify apps which are likely to have beneficial impacts

For a fee, ORCHA will conduct an independent review of health apps. The outcomes of the review can be used for further product development, and/or they can be shared with potential customers to help market the app. If an app receives a sufficiently high score, ORCHA will award it with a quality badge and will feature it in one of their app libraries [24]. ORCHA has also developed tools such as the ORCHA-24, which includes 24 app assessment criteria to evaluate data privacy, clinical efficacy and user experience [13].

8.15   Summary of Key Points

Evaluating mHealth interventions is critically important. Health apps have the potential to play an important role in dealing with the challenges entailed in the rising pressures on healthcare services. However, without rigorous evaluations, the true potential of mHealth cannot be unlocked. Commissioners, policy-makers and other decision-makers need sound evidence to inform their decisions of whether to invest in the implementation of health apps. App developers and researchers also require this evidence to inform the successful development of future interventions and to help further our knowledge. This chapter provides an overview of commonly used study designs, from descriptive, observational studies to rigorous randomised controlled trials and in-depth qualitative explorations, along with their benefits and limitations. Thinking critically about different study designs and their respective advantages and disadvantages is a crucial step in designing a successful evaluation of an mHealth intervention. It is important to remember that only experimental studies with random allocation to study groups allow causal relationships to be established, but experimental studies are not always the most appropriate design. Observational studies may provide valuable and useful insights when applied correctly.

- Ideally, evaluation and data analysis methods should be planned and agreed prior to the designing and development of an intervention
- A definitive evaluation of clinical effectiveness should only be embarked on when the total treatment package has been sufficiently tested and adapted
- Quantitative research is suitable when you wish to numerically establish relationships between different variables and when you aim to draw inferences about other people based on your study findings
- Causal relationships between variables (i.e. whether X causes Y) can only be established using experimental studies with random allocation of study participants to different groups
- Common observational study designs include cross-sectional studies, cohort studies, case-control studies, and quasi-experimental studies
- Qualitative research seeks to explore and gain a deep understanding of a phenomenon or event based on people's subjective experience; as such it is often useful for initial intervention development and testing stages
- Experimental studies with random allocation are not always feasible or ethical, or they may be considered too resource-intensive for a given evaluation; in such cases observational study designs should be considered
- Pilot and feasibility studies should usually precede larger definitive evaluation studies to test and optimise study procedures
- The UK National Institute for Health and Care Excellence (NICE) Evidence standards framework for digital health technologies can be used to ensure evaluations meet evidence standards for clinical and cost effectiveness
- Evaluations should also consider and assess potential sources of harm and risk

8.16   Quiz

1. Which of the following designs could you use to evaluate the clinical effectiveness of an mHealth intervention? (several may apply)

   (a) A randomised controlled trial
   (b) A cluster-randomised controlled trials
   (c) An observational, pre post comparison study
   (d) A qualitative study

2. What type of study is a natural experiment?

   (a) A sub-type of randomised controlled trials
   (b) An observational study

(c) A mixed-methods study design that combines experimental and qualitative methods

3. A researcher wished to compare the effect on activity levels of an app with daily reminders versus weekly email reminders. Participants were randomised to one of two groups. One group first used the app for 1 month, then received the email reminders for 1 month. The other group first received the emails and then the app. Physical activity was tracked in both groups using a wrist-worn activity tracker. This study design is a...

(a) Stepped-wedge design
(b) Randomised controlled trial with reverse-order groups
(c) Cross-over trial
(d) Case-control study

4. What type of health economic evaluation would be most suitable to evaluate the cost-effectiveness of a health app funded by a country's national health service? (several may apply)

(a) Cost-utility analysis
(b) Cost-effectiveness analysis
(c) Cost-benefit analysis
(d) Cost-consequence analysis

Answers to the quiz can be found in "Solutions to Quizzes".

8.17   Exercises

1. According to the NICE Evidence Standards Framework for Digital Health Technologies, what would be the minimum evidence standard for "Demonstrating effectiveness" for an app which connects to a fitness wearable device that allows people to monitor their general health?
2. Read the following open-access publication:
   Iribarren, S. J., Cato, K., Falzon, L., & Stone, P. W. (2017). *What is the economic evidence for mHealth? A systematic review of economic evaluations of mHealth solutions.* PloS One, 12(2), e0170581. http://doi.org/10.1371/journal.pone.0170581
   Based on the paper, answer the following questions:

   a. What was the predominant economic evaluation method used to economically evaluate mHealth interventions?
   b. What were the main quality issues in the economic evaluations assessed in the paper?
   c. What comparison groups did the studies with the highest quality use?

Recommended Reading

1. National Institute for Health and Care Excellence. Evidence standards framework for digital health technologies; 2019. Retrieved March 15, 2019, from https://www.nice.org.uk/Media/Default/About/what-we-do/our-programmes/evidence-standards-framework/digital-evidence-standards-framework.pdf
2. McNamee P, Murray E, Kelly MP, Bojke L, Chilcott J, Fischer A-T, West R, Yardley L. Designing and undertaking a health economics study of digital health interventions. Am J Prev Med. 2016;51(5):852–60. https://doi.org/10.1016/j.amepre.2016.05.007
3. Murray E, Hekler EB, Andersson G, Collins LM, Do-Herty A, Hollis C, Rivera DE, West R, Wyatt JC. Evaluating digital health interventions. Am J Prev Med. 2016;51(5):843–51. https://doi.org/10.1016/j.amepre.2016.06.008
4. Ranganathan P, Aggarwal R. Study designs: part 1 – an overview and classification. Perspect Clin Res. 2018;9(4):184–86. https://doi.org/10.4103/picr.PICR_124_18
5. Bhopal RS. Concepts of epidemiology: integrating the ideas, theories, principles, and methods of epidemiology. 2nd ed. Oxford: Oxford University Press; 2016.
6. Porta M. Dictionary of epidemiology. Oxford: Oxford University Press; 2008.
7. Ritchie J, Spencer L. Qualitative data analysis for applied policy research. In: Huberman AM, Miles MB, editors. The qualitative researcher's companion. London: Sage; 2002. p. 305–30.

References

1. Bell ML, Kenward MG, Fairclough DL, Horton NJ. Differential dropout and bias in randomised controlled trials: when it matters and when it may not. BMJ. 2013;346:e8668. https://doi.org/10.1136/bmj.e8668
2. Benning TM, Alayli-Goebbels AFG, Aarts M-J, Stolk E, de Wit GA, Prenger R, Braakman-Jansen LMA, Evers SMAA. Exploring outcomes to consider in economic evaluations of health promotion programs: what broader non-health outcomes matter most? BMC Health Serv Res. 2015;15(1):266. https://doi.org/10.1186/s12913-015-0908-y
3. Browne RH. On the use of a pilot sample for sample size determination. Stat Med. 1995;14(17):1933–40. https://doi.org/10.1002/sim.4780141709
4. Cohen J. Statistical power analysis for the behavioral sciences. 2nd ed. Hillsdale: Lawrence Earlbaum Associates; 1988.
5. Crouthamel M, Quattrocchi E, Watts S, Wang S, Berry P, Garcia-Gancedo L, Hamy V, Williams RE. Using a researchkit smartphone app to collect rheumatoid arthritis symptoms from real-world participants: feasibility study. JMIR mHealth uHealth. 2018;6(9):e177. https://doi.org/10.2196/mhealth.9656
6. Doll R, Hill AB. Smoking and carcinoma of the lung. Br Med J. 1950;2(4682):739. https://doi.org/10.1136/BMJ.2.4682.739
7. Duenas A. Cost-minimization analysis. In: Encyclopedia of behavioral medicine. New York: Springer; 2013. p. 516. https://doi.org/10.1007/978-1-4419-1005-9_1376
8. Fujita K, Watanabe T, Kuroiwa T, Sasaki T, Nimura A, Sugiura Y. A tablet-based app for carpal tunnel syndrome screening: diagnostic case-control study. JMIR mHealth uHealth. 2019;7(9):e14172. https://doi.org/10.2196/14172
9. Hensel JM, Shaw J, Jeffs L, Ivers NM, Desveaux L, Cohen A, Agarwal P, Wodchis WP, Tepper J, Larsen D, McGahan A, Cram P, Mukerji G, Mamdani M, Yang R, Wong I, Onabajo N, Jamieson T, Bhatia RS. A pragmatic randomized control trial and realist evaluation on the implementation and effectiveness of an internet application to support self-management among individuals seeking specialized mental health care: a study protocol. BMC Psychiatry. 2016;16(1):350. https://doi.org/10.1186/s12888-016-1057-5

10. Hodges J, Tizard B. Social and family relationships of ex-institutional adolescents. J Child Psychol Psychiatry. 1989;30(1):77–97. https://doi.org/10.1111/j.1469-7610.1989.tb00770.x

11. Iribarren SJ, Cato K, Falzon L, Stone PW. What is the economic evidence for mHealth? A systematic review of economic evaluations of mHealth solutions. PloS one. 2017;12(2):e0170581. https://doi.org/10.1371/journal.pone.0170581

12. Kitzinger J. Qualitative research. Introducing focus groups. BMJ. (Clinical research ed.) 1995;311(7000):299–302. https://doi.org/10.1136/bmj.311.7000.299

13. Leigh S, Ouyang J, Mimnagh C. Effective? Engaging? Secure? Applying the ORCHA-24 framework to evaluate apps for chronic insomnia disorder. Evid Based Ment Health. 2017;20(4):e20. https://doi.org/10.1136/EB-2017-102751

14. Mann D, Riddell L, Lim K, Byrne LK, Nowson C, Rigo M, Szymlek-Gay EA, Booth AO. Mobile phone app aimed at improving iron intake and bioavailability in premenopausal women: a qualitative evaluation. JMIR mHealth uHealth. 2015;3(3):e92. https://doi.org/10.2196/mhealth.4300

15. McCabe C, Claxton K, Culyer AJ. The NICE cost-effectiveness threshold. PharmacoEconomics. 2008;26(9):733–44. https://doi.org/10.2165/00019053-200826090-00004

16. McCoy CE. Understanding the intention-to-treat principle in randomized controlled trials. West J Emerg Med. 2017;18(6):1075–8. https://doi.org/10.5811/westjem.2017.8.35985

17. McNamee P, Murray E, Kelly MP, Bojke L, Chilcott J, Fischer A, West R, Yardley L. Designing and undertaking a health economics study of digital health interventions. Am J Prev Med. 2016;51(5):852–60. https://doi.org/10.1016/j.amepre.2016.05.007

18. Mueller J, Davies A, Harper S, Jay C, Todd C. Widening access to online health education for lung cancer. In: Proceedings of the 13th web for all conference on – W4A '16. New York: ACM Press; 2016. p. 1–4. https://doi.org/10.1145/2899475.2899495

19. Mueller J, Davies A, Jay C, Harper S, Blackhall F, Summers Y, Harle A, Todd C. Developing and testing a web-based intervention to encourage early help-seeking in people with symptoms associated with lung cancer. Br J Health Psychol. 2018;24(1):31–65. https://doi.org/10.1111/bjhp.12325

20. Mulhall A. In the field: notes on observation in qualitative research. J Adv Nurs. 2003;41(3):306–13. https://doi.org/10.1046/j.1365-2648.2003.02514.x

21. Murray E, Hekler EB, Andersson G, Collins LM, Doherty A, Hollis C, Rivera DE, West R, Wyatt JC. Evaluating digital health interventions. Am J Prev Med. 2016;51(5):843–51. https://doi.org/10.1016/j.amepre.2016.06.008

22. National Institute for Health and Care Excellence. Evidence standards framework for digital health technologies; 2019. https://www.nice.org.uk/Media/Default/About/what-we-do/our-programmes/evidence-standards-framework/digital-evidence-standards-framework.pdf

23. Ning P, Chen B, Cheng P, Yang Y, Schwebel DC, Yu R, Deng J, Li S, Hu G. Effectiveness of an app-based intervention for unintentional injury among caregivers of preschoolers: protocol for a cluster randomized controlled trial. BMC Public Health. 2018;18(1):865. https://doi.org/10.1186/s12889-018-5790-1

24. Organisation for the Review of Care and Health Applications (ORCHA). (n.d.). ORCHA. Retrieved February 29, 2020, from www.orcha.co.uk

25. Parker L, Karliychuk T, Gillies D, Mintzes B, Raven M, Grundy Q. A health app developer's guide to law and policy: a multi-sector policy analysis. BMC Med Inf Decis Mak. 2017;17(1):141. https://doi.org/10.1186/s12911-017-0535-0

26. Patel B, Johnston M, Cookson N, King D, Arora S, Darzi A. Interprofessional communication of clinicians using a mobile phone app: a randomized crossover trial using simulated patients. J Med Internet Res. 2016;18(4):e79. https://doi.org/10.2196/jmir.4854

27. Peiris D, Praveen D, Mogulluru K, Ameer MA, Raghu A, Li Q, Heritier S, MacMahon S, Prabhakaran D, Clifford GD, Joshi R, Maulik PK, Jan S, Tarassenko L, Patel A. SMARThealth India: a stepped-wedge, cluster randomised controlled trial of a community health worker managed mobile health intervention for people assessed at high cardiovascular disease risk in rural India. PLoS ONE. 2019;14(3):e0213708. https://doi.org/10.1371/journal.pone.0213708

28. Porta M. Dictionary of epidemiology. Oxford: Oxford University Press; 2008.

29. Public Health England. (n.d.). National General Practice Profiles. Retrieved March 25, 2019, from https://fingertips.phe.org.uk/profile/general-practice
30. Ranganathan P, Aggarwal R. Study designs: part 1 – an overview and classification. Perspect Clin Res. 2018;9(4):184–6. https://doi.org/10.4103/picr.PICR_124_18
31. Roland M, Torgerson DJ. Understanding controlled trials: what are pragmatic trials? BMJ. 1998;316(7127):285. https://doi.org/10.1136/bmj.316.7127.285
32. Sedgwick P. Explanatory trials versus pragmatic trials. BMJ. (Clinical research ed.) 2014;349:g6694. https://doi.org/10.1136/bmj.g6694
33. Short CE, Finlay A, Sanders I, Maher C. Development and pilot evaluation of a clinic-based mHealth app referral service to support adult cancer survivors increase their participation in physical activity using publicly available mobile apps. BMC Health Serv Res. 2018;18(1):27. https://doi.org/10.1186/s12913-017-2818-7
34. Sibbald B, Roberts C. Understanding controlled trials. Crossover trials. BMJ. (Clinical research ed.) 1998;316(7146):1719. https://doi.org/10.1136/bmj.316.7146.1719
35. Speich B, von Niederhäusern B, Schur N, Hemkens LG, Fürst T, Bhatnagar N, Alturki R, Agarwal A, Kasenda B, Pauli-Magnus C, Schwenkglenks M, Briel M. MAking Randomized Trials Affordable (MARTA) Group. Systematic review on costs and resource use of randomized clinical trials shows a lack of transparent and comprehensive data. J Clin Epidemiol. 2018;96:1–11. https://doi.org/10.1016/j.jclinepi.2017.12.018
36. Webb TL, Joseph J, Yardley L, Michie S. Using the internet to promote health behavior change: a systematic review and meta-analysis of the impact of theoretical basis. Use of behavior change techniques, and mode of delivery on efficacy. J Med Internet Res. 2010;12(1):e4. https://doi.org/10.2196/jmir.1376
37. Wheaton N, Lenehan J, Amir LH. Evaluation of a breastfeeding app in rural Australia: prospective cohort study. J Hum Lact. 2018;34(4):089033441879418. https://doi.org/10.1177/0890334418794181

Chapter 9
Data Analysis Methods

9.1 Introduction

As highlighted in the previous chapter, evaluating health apps in some form or other is important to ensure the app works as intended, to supply decision-makers with required information, and to drive future developments and improvements of the product. Not every app will require a lengthy and costly evaluation in a randomised controlled trial, and not all apps need to demonstrate clinical effectiveness. For some apps, observational studies or qualitative assessments will be best placed to gain insight into critical questions regarding the app's feasibility and acceptability.

Regardless of the method of evaluation you decide to use, all forms of evaluation have one key commonality: they generate data which then need to be synthesised into a form that allows interpretation. Data in its raw form can rarely answer specific questions or allow you to draw conclusions. Some form of *analysis* is required. This chapter covers different methods of analysing and understanding your data.

We aim to provide an overview of common analysis methods, spanning different data types from various evaluation designs. The chapter begins by examining traditional statistical analysis methods, followed by Machine Learning methods that can be used with less structured data and for large volumes of data (such as those produced by electronic health records). This is followed with an overview of software packages and tools commonly used for data analysis. Finally, we present common qualitative analysis methods. Throughout the chapter, we provide applied examples of how the different methods have been used in existing research with smartphone health apps.

It should be noted that it is beyond the scope of this book to provide an exhaustive overview of analysis methods or to train users in the use of these methods. Rather, the aim of this chapter is to provide readers with a solid basis to understand the purpose and limitations of different analysis methods and to become acquainted with some of the commonly used approaches in these areas. Please see this chapter's

© Springer Nature Switzerland AG 2020
A. Davies, J. Mueller, *Developing Medical Apps and mHealth Interventions*, Health Informatics, https://doi.org/10.1007/978-3-030-47499-7_9

recommended reading section for some excellent resources that cover these areas in much more depth.

9.2   Data Sources and Outcomes in App-Based Research

The use of smartphones and connected devices in health research has opened up new avenues not only in terms of developing and disseminating interventions, but also in terms of new data sources and data collection methods. Data sources that can be utilised in research involving mHealth technologies include:

- Self-reported outcomes, e.g. by asking users to record their symptoms daily within the app
- Event data/log data indicating which features users access, which pages they view, frequency of clicks on different links/buttons etc.
- Sensor data, e.g. accelerometer data from fitness trackers

All of these data forms can be collected using standard, off-the-shelf smartphone devices with in-built sensors (e.g. GPS, accelerometres), though they can also be augmented. For example, sensors can be added to standard devices to measure air quality [35], and research-grade activity trackers (such as ActiGraph, Polar and Omron) can be used which are generally more accurate than consumer-level devices [37]. Biosensors are also becoming increasingly available to consumers, in the form of medical diagnostic devices that consumers can purchase for use at home.

One of the key advantages of using smartphones for data collection is that data can be collected frequently and "in the moment", as opposed to surveys which are often completed retrospectively. Repeated sampling of participants' behaviours and experiences in real time, in their natural environments, is known as *ecological momentary assessment* (EMA). EMA helps to build a more detailed understanding of health and enhances ecological validity, because it involves collecting data in natural environments rather than controlled laboratory settings.

Consider the following example. Shiffman [33] sought to measure how many cigarettes participants smoked per day. The author compared responses from traditional paper diaries to responses derived from electronic diaries for ecological momentary assessment. The results are shown in Fig. 9.1. Using a traditional paper diary, people filled in the diary retrospectively at specific times, meaning they needed to try and remember how many cigarettes they had smoked. As a result of not being able to remember the exact numbers, most participants rounded their estimates to units of 5 (e.g. 15, 20, 25). Using EMA, on the other hand, participants were asked to record this information in a relatively brief, unobtrusive way, several times per day, resulting in more accurate numbers and a much smoother distribution of values.

Event data and log data are crucial for understanding the feasibility, acceptability and usability of smartphone apps. For example, they can show which features and pages users access most frequently, and which ones are never used or viewed at all.

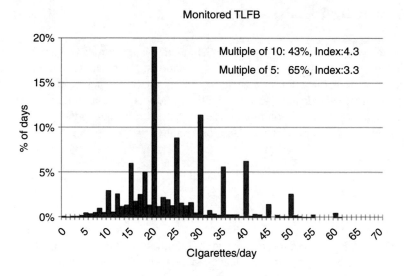

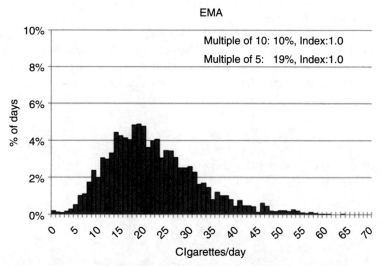

Fig. 9.1 The graphs show reported cigarette consumption using self-report (top graph) and ecological momentary assessment (bottom graph). (Reproduced with permission. Source: Saul Shiffman [33])

Event data and log data are discussed further in Chap. 7. The use of sensor data is discussed in Chap. 4, Sect. 4.4.

9.3   Statistical Analysis Methods

In the following sections, we present statistical analysis methods that are commonly applied in research studies to evaluate interventions. We begin by examining some preparatory steps that should precede the actual analysis, such as the formulation of hypotheses, data cleaning and preparation, and testing of assumptions. We then present some of the most commonly used statistical tests and show how these have been implemented in previous research on health apps.

9.3.1   Hypotheses

The first step to a successful evaluation is the formulation of clear, answerable research questions and/or testable research hypotheses. At the end of the evaluation, it should be possible to state a clear answer to the research question, and, if a hypothesis has been stated, it should be possible to state whether this hypothesis is supported by the evidence or not.

To start, the evaluation needs a clear aim and objectives. The *research aim* is what you intend to achieve, while the *objectives* state the actions you will need to undertake to meet the aim. The aim should clearly state what you are evaluating (the intervention), the target population, the primary outcome(s), and the comparison group.

Example of aims and objectives for the evaluation of a weight loss app targeted towards obese individuals

AIM: To assess the safety, acceptability and effectiveness of an educational smartphone app designed to promote adherence to the Mediterranean diet in reducing body mass index (BMI) at 6-months follow-up in obese individuals (BMI$\geq$30), compared with usual care.

OBJECTIVES

1. Pilot-test procedures for evaluating the smartphone app
2. Evaluate the effect of distributing the app in primary care on change in BMI compared with the control group who receive usual care at 6-month follow-up
3. Examine unintended/adverse outcomes of the app
4. Examine acceptability of the app
5. Examine cost-effectiveness of the app

Once a clear set of aims and objectives have been established, it is useful to formulate testable hypotheses. Whether hypotheses can be established will depend on the topic and the state of existing literature. If insufficient evidence is available to make predictions, a research question may be stated instead. If relevant evidence and/or theory is available, a specific hypothesis should be phrased in form of a statement that predicts outcomes and relationships. Hypotheses should meet the following criteria [1]:

- The hypothesis should state an expected relationship between variables (e.g. "X is associated with Y"; "X influences/has an impact on Y" (causal); "Z is a mediator between X and Y")
- The hypothesis should be testable and falsifiable (it should be clear what outcome is expected if it is true or false)
- The hypothesis should be consistent with existing literature and knowledge
- The hypothesis should be formulated as simply and concisely as possible, ideally in form of a sentence or a formula (e.g. Mean of group 1>Mean of group 2)

Generally, research hypotheses are formulated in form of an *alternative hypothesis* and a *null hypothesis*. The null hypothesis states that there is no relationship between the variables, whereas the alternative hypothesis posits the expected relationship. Even if a relationship is expected, it is important to formulate a null hypothesis because this is the hypothesis tested by statistical tests. Essentially, statistical tests test the probability of the assumption that there is no relationship. As such, it is the null hypothesis that is accepted or rejected in statistical testing, *not* the alternative hypothesis.

Example research question and hypotheses for the evaluation of a weight loss app targeted towards obese individuals

Research question: What is the impact of using an educational smartphone app designed to promote adherence to the Mediterranean diet for six months on BMI among obese individuals?

Null hypothesis: There will be no difference in mean BMI in the intervention group and the control group at 6-month follow-up.

$$Mean BMI_{intervention} = Mean BMI_{control}$$

Alternative hypothesis: Mean BMI in the intervention group will be significantly smaller than in the control group at 6-month follow-up.

$$Mean BMI_{intervention} < Mean BMI_{control}$$

9.3.2   Data Preparation and Cleaning

Quantitative data analysis involves bringing data into a numerical form allowing analysis using traditional statistical methods or data science methods such as Machine Learning. Some data may already be in a suitable format for quantitative analysis, e.g. measurements of participants' heights. Other data may need to be transformed into a numerical format. For example, in order to compare two groups (e.g. men and women) on a given variable, the two groups would usually be assigned a number (e.g. men = 1 and women = 2), thus allowing statistical software programmes to work with the data.

Aside from such coding procedures, data often require substantial cleaning and preparation before meaningful analyses can be conducted, particularly when data have not been collected for the purpose of the evaluation, e.g. when using data from electronic health records or other routinely collected data, or when using unstructured data mined from the Web. It has been estimated that data cleaning and preparation takes up approximately 80% of the total data engineering process [44]. Data cleaning and preparation is critical in order to address the following issues which can mask important patterns in the data:

- **Missing and incomplete data:** This issue affects all forms of data collection including self-reported surveys (participants may forget or choose not to complete sections in surveys), routine clinical data (clinicians may forget or choose not to record information, or may not have the information available), and passively collected sensor data (sensors may be inadequately calibrated or batteries may run out).
- **Inconsistencies:** Data of the same type may be recorded in different ways. For example, in clinical records, complex diseases (e.g. asthma) are coded in various formats, including written notes, symptoms, or combinations of diagnoses [29].
- **Noise:** Datasets often contain large amounts of extraneous information that need to be filtered before a focus on a specific research question is possible. For example, White & Horvitz aimed to explore how people search the Web to appraise their symptoms. They mined search queries from search engine logs and then needed to undertake various procedures to identify search terms focusing on symptoms and filter out irrelevant queries [41].

9.3.3   Data Types

The type of data available for analysis will dictate the types of analyses that are possible. Figure 9.2 shows different types of data based on their *measurement scales*.

The first critical distinction lies between discrete and continuous data. *Discrete data* represent units that are separate and discrete. The units can be counted but not measured, and values between units are not meaningful. An example is "number of

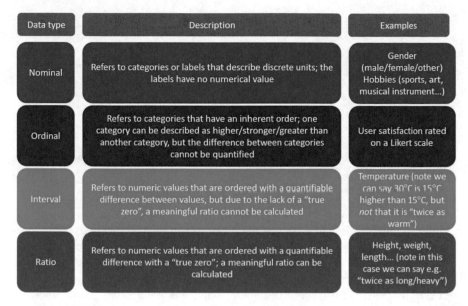

Data type	Description	Examples
Nominal	Refers to categories or labels that describe discrete units; the labels have no numerical value	Gender (male/female/other) Hobbies (sports, art, musical instrument…)
Ordinal	Refers to categories that have an inherent order; one category can be described as higher/stronger/greater than another category, but the difference between categories cannot be quantified	User satisfaction rated on a Likert scale
Interval	Refers to numeric values that are ordered with a quantifiable difference between values, but due to the lack of a "true zero", a meaningful ratio cannot be calculated	Temperature (note we can say 30°C is 15°C higher than 15°C, but *not* that it is "twice as warm")
Ratio	Refers to numeric values that are ordered with a quantifiable difference with a "true zero"; a meaningful ratio can be calculated	Height, weight, length… (note in this case we can say e.g. "twice as long/heavy")

Fig. 9.2 Data types

users using an Android operating system". You can count the number of users, and the value can only take on whole numbers; values between whole numbers (e.g. "2.5 users") are not meaningful. *Continuous data* can be measured and values between the units are meaningful, e.g. length of time a user spent on a given page.

As Fig. 9.2 shows, data types can be further broken down into nominal, ordinal, interval and ratio data. These distinctions are important because they determine the kinds of analyses you can undertake. For example, consider a basic descriptive statistical parameter like the *arithmetic mean*. You can sensibly calculate a mean for something like height, weight or temperature, or user satisfaction rated on a Likert scale (ratio, interval and ordinal data). However, it does not make sense to calculate a mean for a variable like "language" (nominal data).

9.3.4 Descriptive Statistics

Descriptive statistics aim to describe and summarise the sample but do not seek to draw conclusions about the wider population. Common descriptive statistics include measures of central tendency (e.g. arithmetic mean, median, mode) and measures of spread (e.g. standard deviation, standard error, variance). It is important to consider these types of measures in conjunction. A mean alone does not sufficiently describe a sample; we need some form of measure of the variability of the data to understand how well the mean represents individual values in the sample. Consider for example the graphs shown in Fig. 9.3. Both datasets have the same mean ($M = 5$), but, as can

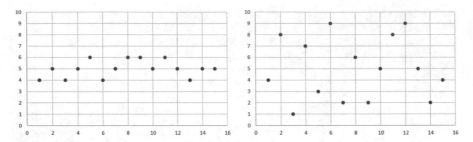

Fig. 9.3 Scatterplots of two different data sets with the same mean but differing standard deviations

be seen from the scatterplots, data points in the left plot are clustered much more closely around the mean than data points in the right plot. The standard deviation in the left plot is 0.76, whereas it is 2.73 in the right plot.

Another useful descriptive statistic is the *correlation*. It describes the extent to which two variables co-vary. It thus gives an indication of the strength of the relationship between two variables. Note that it does *not* give an indication of causation. Causation can only be determined in conjunction with the appropriate study design (i.e. an experimental design with random allocation).

Descriptive statistics are very useful when describing the sample to give the reader an idea of how representative this sample is of the wider population, or of another population the reader may wish to gain insight into. This often includes providing the average age (along with the standard deviation) as well as the age range, the number of male and female participants, the distribution of different education levels, the distribution of different ethnic groups, and other relevant health data such as the number and distribution of different comorbidities.

Such descriptions are particularly important for the evaluation of digital technology such as smartphone apps, because access to digital technology tends to follow the same gradient as health inequalities. This means that there is a risk that samples will consist mainly of those who have access to digital technology, i.e. those who are relatively wealthy and educated. As such, findings are unlikely to be representative of those in disadvantaged or marginalised population groups, who also have the poorest health outcomes.

9.3.5   Assumptions

Before delving into specific analysis methods, it is important to note that *inferential statistical analysis methods* (i.e. methods used to draw conclusions about the population based on the sample) are usually tied to certain *assumptions* about the data. The outputs of the statistical tests are only meaningful when these assumptions hold true. Therefore, the first stage in any data analysis project should always involve an exploration of the data and testing of assumptions.

Fig. 9.4 Normal distribution (bell curve/Gaussian distribution)

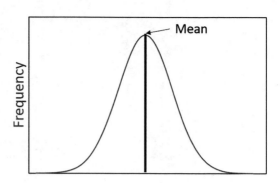

One assumption common to many inferential statistical tests (e.g. t-test, ANOVA and linear regression) is that the sampling distribution of the mean of the outcome under study is *normal*. This means that, if we took several independent samples from the population and calculated the mean for each of them, the distribution of these means would form a *bell curve*. In other words, the means would be symmetrically distributed around their overall mean, rather than being skewed in a particular direction. Figure 9.4 shows a normal distribution (also known as a bell curve or Gaussian distribution). It shows how frequently different values occur. As Fig. 9.4 indicates, values that are close to the mean occur much more frequently than values at either end of the distribution. Thus there is a higher likelihood of values occurring that are close to the mean than those that are at extreme ends of the distribution. It is this likelihood that is used in statistical testing to draw conclusions about whether a certain finding is likely to have occurred assuming random chance. If the likelihood is very small, we usually assume the result has not come about randomly and that some form of systematic influence is taking place.

Thus, statistical tests that assume normal distributions will only deliver meaningful results if the sample means are in fact normally distributed. It is therefore important to test assumptions prior to undertaking any statistical testing. This can be done by visually inspecting the data (e.g. histograms, Q-Q plots), by exploring descriptive parameters (e.g. *skewness* and *kurtosis* values) or by undertaking tests such as the Kolmogorov-Smirnov test or Shapiro-Wilk test, which test whether a given distribution differs significantly from normality.

Figure 9.5 shows a histogram and a Q-Q plot which can be used to visually check how well the data fit a normal distribution. A normal distribution has been added to the histogram. In this case we can see that the data roughly follow the normal distribution, but the distribution is not very smooth. In the Q-Q plot, how well the values fit the line indicates whether the distribution has the same shape as a normal distribution. Again, we see a relatively good but not perfect fit. The Kolmogorov-Smirnov test for these data is significant, indicating significant deviations from normality. The Shapiro Wilk test is non-significant. Overall, this shows that data are often complex and seemingly contradictive, and multiple factors need to be taken into account during analysis and interpretation.

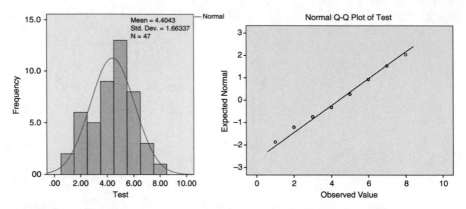

Fig. 9.5 Histogram and Q-Q plot. Both plots are useful for visually inspecting a dataset for deviations from normality

If assumptions are not met, alternative testing methods may need to be sought, such as non-parametric tests (see Sect. 9.3.7) or other robust estimation methods [42]. If deviations from assumptions are not accounted for, conclusions from statistical models can be biased.

9.3.6   Parametric Tests

Parametric tests are a family of tests that are based on assumptions about the underlying distribution of the sample means, as mentioned in Sect. 9.3.5. Most tests assume that the sampling distribution of the mean is normally distributed or follows some other well-known form (e.g. Bernoulli). The main advantage of parametric over non-parametric tests is that they tend to have higher statistical power, i.e. they require smaller sample sizes. We will now explore some of the most commonly used parametric tests and provide examples for how these have been used in smartphone evaluations.

9.3.6.1   t-Test

Student's t-test is one of the most widely known and used statistical tests. The test is used to compare two means. The two means can either belong to two separate groups (e.g. comparing the intervention group and the control group) or to the same sample (e.g. comparing before and after the intervention). In the former case, an *independent t-test* is used and in the latter case, a *dependent t-test* is needed.

If the two means come from the same population, we would expect them to be roughly the same. They might differ a little by chance, but we would not expect large differences by chance. The t-test is used to test whether the distribution of the difference between the two means is "significantly different" from the mean difference we would expect by random chance [8]. In other words, we test whether the difference between the two means is likely to have occurred under the assumption that the null hypothesis is true. The output of the test is a probability (the "p value") which denotes the probability of the difference between the two means having occurred assuming the null hypothesis. If this probability is sufficiently small (usually a conventional cut-off of *0.05* is used), the null hypothesis is rejected. In other words, if the *p value* is smaller than *0.05* (or another specified cut-off like *0.01*), the null hypothesis qualifies to be rejected. This is usually seen as an indication that the observed difference between the two means has not occurred by chance.

The t-test involves several assumptions including normality, homogeneity of variances, and independence of errors (for more details see e.g. [8]).

Example: Using the t-test to evaluate the effectiveness of a smartphone app for improving healthy lifestyles

Garcia-Oritz et al. [10] aimed to test the effectiveness of an app which was designed to promote healthy lifestyles in the general population in primary care. They conducted a randomised, multicentre clinical trial with a 12-month follow up with two study groups and 883 participants in total. Both groups received counselling by a research nurse on benefits of the Mediterranean diet and physical activity, but the intervention group also received training in the use of the app. Physical activity was measured using an accelerometre sensor and the 7-day Physical Activity Recall (PAR) questionnaire. Adherence to the Mediterranean diet was measured by an adherence screening questionnaire. The independent t-test was used for the comparison of means between the two groups and the dependent (or "paired") t-test was used to assess changes within the same group from baseline to follow-up.

In terms of diet adherence, both groups showed an increase, but this was not significant ($p = 0.46$). There was no significant difference between the two groups at 12-month follow up in physical activity as measured by the Physical Activity Recall (PAR) questionnaire. In PA evaluated by accelerometer, there was a decrease in both groups but this was not significant.

It is noteworthy that assumptions are not discussed in the article, so it is difficult to assess the validity of the findings.

9.3.6.2   Analysis of Variance (ANOVA)

Analysis of variance (ANOVA) is used when there are more than two groups to compare, for example when the evaluation design includes several comparison groups. It is important to note that ANOVA is an omnibus test, meaning that it allows the comparison of several means in a single test.

The output of the ANOVA is an F-value and an associated p-value. The test will return a significant result if any two means differ significantly, and a non-significant result if none of the means differ. However, the output will not show which two means differ, nor whether there are more than two means that differ. A post-hoc analysis (e.g. using Tukey's test) is needed to tease out where the significant differences lie.

The advantage of the ANOVA is that, as an omnibus test, it reduces the inflation of *type I error* (discussed further in Sect. 9.3.9), as opposed to conducting a t-test for each individual mean comparison.

A one-way ANOVA involves varying only one independent variable. For example, when comparing app users who show high, low or no engagement with the app in terms of user satisfaction, the independent variable is "level of engagement". A two-way ANOVA involves two independent variables, for example, comparing users' satisfaction in terms of *level of engagement* and *gender*. With the two-way ANOVA we can test the effects of each independent variable separately, and also the interaction effects of the two independent variables, e.g. to assess whether level of engagement has a stronger effect on user satisfaction in men than in women.

Example of using ANOVA to evaluate a healthy eating app

Helander et al. [15] evaluated an app that was designed to promote healthy eating through self-monitoring and peer feedback. Users of the app uploaded photos of their meals which they then self-rated on an 11-point healthiness scale (self-monitoring). Users were also able to rate other users' photos (peer feedback).

Data were used from 189,770 people who had downloaded and used the app at least once. They compared four groups: "Actives" (people who had taken ≥ 10 photos), "Semi-actives" (people with 2–9 photos), "Non-actives" (people with one photo), and "drop-outs" (people with no photos).

Using ANOVA, they found significant differences between Actives, Semi-actives and Non-actives in average healthiness rating from peers for the first picture ($F_{2,58167} = 225.9, p < .001$). This suggests that app engagement matters, and more needs to be done to engage less active users to bring about improvements in health outcomes.

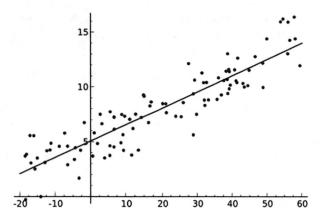

Fig. 9.6 Linear regression plot. (From https://en.wikipedia.org/wiki/File:Linear_regression.svg (Public domain))

9.3.6.3   Linear Regression

Linear regression can be used to study relationships between two or more variables [16]. In its most basic form, regression analysis examines the relationship between two variables (the *dependent variable* or *outcome* and the *independent* or *explanatory variable*) and plots a line that best fits the data points, as shown in Fig. 9.6.

The relationship between two variables (x and y) is modelled in a simple linear regression:

$$y = \beta_0 + \beta x_i + \epsilon_i$$

for n data pairs $(x_i, y_i), i = 1, \ldots, n$

y: the dependent variable (that you are trying to predict)
x: the explanatory variable (the predictor)
β_0: y-intercept
ϵ: residual error term (differences between actual and predicted values)

For more than two variables, multiple linear regression is used and takes the following form:

$$y_i = \beta_0 + \beta_1 x_{i1} + \ldots + \beta_p x_i p + \epsilon_1$$

p: number of explanatory variables

Regression shows how much one variable (y) changes as another variable (x) changes. Because it allows you to include several explanatory variables in the model, regression allows you to *control* for extraneous variables. This helps limit bias by controlling potential confounding variables such as age, socioeconomic status, and education level. Essentially, this means you can assess the relationship between two variables (e.g. length of app usage and improvements in self-reported health) after effects of other variables (e.g. age) have been accounted for. The main outputs of regression analysis are:

- (standardized) beta coefficients, which show how much the dependent variable changes with each unit change in the explanatory variable, e.g. "for each additional week of usage of a smartphone, there is a decrease in BMI of 0.5"
- R^2: the proportion of variance in the dependent variable that can be explained by the explanatory variables
- F-ratio with p-value, which indicate whether the model is a good fit for the data; a significant p-value indicates a good fit (it tests the null-hypothesis that all regression coefficients are equal to zero)

Example: Using linear regression to evaluate the effect of a smartphone app on medical trainees' knowledge

Fralick et al. [9] conducted a prospective, controlled, pre-post study to evaluate a smartphone app which contained local bacterial resistance patterns (antibiogram) and treatment guidelines. The intervention group consisted of medical trainees who received the app; this was compared with a control group of medical trainees who did not have access to the app. Trainees completed a knowledge test at baseline and four weeks later.

Regression analysis was used to test whether change in knowledge (dependent variable) was predicted by group allocation (explanatory variable). Potential confounders (sex, baseline knowledge, baseline confidence) were included in the model.

The analysis revealed that app use was associated with a 1.1 point higher change in knowledge score compared to the control group ($\beta = 1.08, t(1) = 2.08, p = 0.04$).

It is important to note that linear regression should only be used with dependent variables that are at least interval-scaled; it is not suitable for ordinal or nominal dependent variables.

Logistic regression is a specific form of regression analysis that can be used to predict a nominal *binary* dependent variable such as *overweight/not overweight* or *adhered to guidance/did not adhere to guidance*. If the dependent variable is nominal with more than two levels (e.g. normal weight, overweight, obese) then *multinomial regression* can be used. For an ordinal dependent variable, an *ordinal regression* can be used.

9.3.7 Non-parametric Tests

Non-parametric tests are tests that do not require the data to fit a certain distribution. Non-parametric tests require less assumptions to be met than parametric tests, although they are not assumption-less. The tests essentially work by first ranking the data from lowest to highest scores. The analysis is then carried out on the ranks rather than the raw data. This eliminates the effect of outliers [8]. For example, imagine you have the data points 1, 4, 9 and 27. The 27 is clearly an outlier. When we rank the data, their ranks would be 1, 2, 3, 4, thus removing the extremeness of the outlier. We now explore some of the most commonly used non-parametric tests.

9.3.7.1 Mann-Whitney U Test and Wilcoxon Signed-Rank Test

The Mann-Whitney U test [23] is the non-parametric counterpart of the t-test for independent samples. The counterpart of the t-test for dependent samples is the Wilcoxon signed-rank test [43]. Both tests work by ranking data and then analysing the ranks. In the Mann-Whitney test, for example, the data for both groups that are being compared are put together and then ranked. If there is no difference between the groups, we would expect a similar mix of high and low ranks in the groups. If there is a difference, however, we would expect to see a larger number of high ranks in one group than the other. Using this method, the effect of outliers and skew are mitigated [8].

The outputs of the Mann-Whitney and the Wilcoxon signed-rank test are a test statistic (U and W_s respectively) and a p-value.

Example: Using the Wilcoxon signed-rank test to assess the applicability of data obtained from a wearable activity tracker to medical research.

Lee et al. [21] aimed to assess whether data obtained from wearable activity trackers (Fitbit) would differ from data obtained from actigraph units. Actigraphy is an established method for monitoring human rest and activity cycles in medical research. They asked 16 healthy adults to wear both a Fitbit and an actigraph unit (Actiwatch) over a period of two weeks.

To assess whether data from the two devices differed significantly, the authors used a correlation and the Wilcoxon signed-rank test. It was necessary to use this test because both measures were obtained from the same individual, hence the data samples were related and not independent. The correlation (Spearman's correlation) between the data from the two sources was also reported (this is an indication of the strength of the relationship between the two variables).

(continued)

Overall, most variables measured with Fitbit and Actiwatch correlated significantly and showed no significant difference using Wilcoxon's signed-rank test, indicating that Fitbit could potentially be used in medical research instead of Actiwatch. For example, sleep start times for the two devices were significantly and highly correlated ($r = 0.869$, $p < 0.001$), and the Wilcoxon signed-rank test showed no significant difference between their values ($p > 0.05$) [21].

9.3.7.2 Kruskall-Wallis Test and Friedman Test

The Kruskall-Wallis test and the Friedman test are the non-parametric counterparts of the one-way ANOVA for independents samples and the one-way ANOVA for dependent samples, respectively. Like the previously discussed non-parametric tests, the Kruskall-Wallis and the Friedman test are based on ranks. Akin to the ANOVA, both these tests are omnibus tests, meaning they tell us whether the sample means stem from different populations, but not which particular means differ. The output of the Kruskall-Wallis test is the H test statistic and a p-value, and the output of the Friedman test is the test statistic Q and a p-value.

Example: Using the Kruskall-Wallis test to compare different categories of mental health apps in terms of user adoption

Huang et al. [17] conducted an observational study, analysing apps identified via the Android app store. They identified and collected metadata for 274 mental health apps. The authors used the Kruskall-Wallis test to assess whether different categories of apps (e.g. books & reference, lifestyle, medical, health & fitness) differed in terms of ratings, reviews, and installs. They found significant differences in all three variables indicating that apps in the different categories differed. Post-hoc tests revealed that apps in "books and references" had significantly lower ratings, installs and amount of reviews than apps in other categories.

9.3.8   *Analysing Categorical Data: Chi-Square Test, Fisher's Exact Test and McNemar's Test*

So far, we have discussed tests that require at least ordinal data for the outcome variable (i.e. the dependent variable). When dealing with a categorical outcome, a different set of tests is required. For categorical outcomes, we cannot use summary descriptives like the arithmetic mean because this would be meaningless. For example, if you are interested in comparing two groups of app users on whether they are from a rural or urban geographic area, you could allocate a code of 1 to urban and a code of 2 to rural; however these values are arbitrarily chosen and numerically do not mean anything.

Say for example a researcher wishes to compare people who used their app for 1 month or more with people who discontinued app usage within the first month. The researcher may want to determine whether the two groups differ in terms of whether they reside in an urban or rural area. In other words, the researcher would like to know whether users from rural areas are more or less likely than users from urban areas to discontinue app usage in the first month. This means we have two nominal-scaled variables.

A good starting point for categorical data is usually a matrix such as the one shown in Table 9.1. Statistical tests for categorical data operate on the basis of comparing *expected values* that you would expect in the different categories based on random chance with *observed values*. Expected values are calculated by multiplying the row totals by the column totals and dividing by the total sample size. In the example in Table 9.1, for example, the expected count in cell 1 (rural location, app users who use the app for more than a month) would be:

$$\frac{(281 + 520) \times (281 + 126)}{(281 + 520 + 126 + 448)} = 237.1$$

Once this has been done for all cells, expected and observed values can be compared. The chi-square test generates a statistic (χ^2) and a p-value which tests whether expected and observed values differ significantly.

One should note that the chi-square test is not accurate in smaller samples. A conventionally used cut-off is that the expected frequency in each cell should be at least 5. If any cell has an expected frequency below 5, a Fisher's exact test can be used instead.

Table 9.1 A 2 × 2 matrix depicting categorical data

	App users who use the app for >1 month	App users who discontinue use within 1 month
Rural location	281	520
Urban location	126	448

If the data are dependent or paired (e.g. if you are comparing data from before to after an intervention on a nominal outcome), then McNemar's test should be used.

Example: Using the chi-square test to evaluate a smoking cessation app

Ubhi et al. [39] aimed to evaluate an app which was designed to help smokers stay smoke-free for 28 days ("SmokeFree28" or "SF28"). They analysed data from 1170 app users. An important part of their evaluation was to compare their app users to a nationally representative sample of smokers in England who had tried to quit in the past year. This helped them determine whether their sample was representative of the wider population and thus whether their findings were externally valid.

They used the chi-square test to compare app users with the nationally representative sample on a number of categorical variables, e.g. gender and occupation as well as continuous variables that had been categorised (e.g. by dividing age up into age brackets). Overall they found that their app users had a higher likelihood than the national sample of being younger, having a non-manual occupation, and being female, thus raising concerns about external validity [39].

9.3.9   Multiple Testing and Inflation of Error

There are two basic errors that can occur in statistical hypothesis testing. *Type I error* occurs when an effect is found where in reality none exists (false positive), and *type II error* occurs when no effect is found when in reality there is one (false negative). More accurately put, Type I error occurs when the null hypothesis is true, and the researcher incorrectly rejects it. Type II error occurs when the null hypothesis is not true, and the researcher fails to correctly reject it. It is important to keep the probability of both errors as low as possible to reduce the risk of false conclusions.

When a series of hypothesis tests are conducted (also known as *multiple testing*), the risk of type I error can become inflated. What this essentially means is that, as more tests are conducted, the risk of finding a significant result by pure chance is increased. Therefore, any tests that are conducted should always be preceded by careful consideration of existing evidence and theory. Multiple tests should not be undertaken in an attempt to "fish" for a significant p-value. Instead, analyses should be carefully planned prior to running the study based on the research question and/or hypotheses.

Inflation of error can be dealt with in different ways. Traditionally, the Bonferroni method is used which involves adjusting the probability level at which a p-value is viewed as significant, by dividing the significance level by the number of tests. For example, when conducting 5 tests at a significance level of 0.05, the Bonferroni method would result in an adjusted significance level of $0.05/5 = 0.01$. However, because the Bonferroni method is very conservative, it risks increasing type II error, i.e. missing existing effects. This method has been criticised for being unnecessary or even deleterious to sound statistical inference [12, 30]. Other methods such as the false discovery rate (FDR) [2] are less conservative than the Bonferroni method and may be more suitable. Another approach altogether is not to undertake any adjustment and simply state clearly why all tests have been undertaken, to demonstrate that this is derived from theory-based consideration (rather than an attempt to "fish" for significant p-values) [12, 30].

9.3.10 Effect Sizes

Despite being termed "significant", p-values that meet the significance criterion alone do not give useful insights into the *meaningfulness* of the findings. In some cases, even minuscule differences between groups can lead to "significant" results, which would however most likely make no difference to the lived experience of actual people.

Consider the following example: Suppose a researcher used data from users of a health app to compare self-reported health (measured on a 7-point Likert scale) in two groups, e.g. people who used the app for at least one month vs. people who used it less than one month. If there are 2000 users (a small number for most apps) with 1000 in each group, then a power analysis (e.g. using G*Power, a tool to compute sample size calculations) reveals that, assuming a pooled standard deviation of 1.5, a mean difference as small as 0.17 would lead to a significant p-value.

Taking this back to the outcome measure used, this means that e.g. an average score of 2 in one group on the 7-point Likert scale compared to a score of 2.17 in the other group would lead to significant results. It is questionable whether such a small difference would make a difference to the actual lived experience of people. Therefore, we need to consider not only statistical significance but also how (clinically) *meaningful* the findings are.

This is why reporting *effect sizes* is of critical importance. Effect sizes are measures giving an indication of the magnitude of the measured effect. Essentially, p-values tell us the probability of the outcome occurring under random chance, while effect sizes give us an idea of how large/strong this effect is. Effect sizes can be unstandardised (e.g. simply reported the difference in means between two groups) or standardised. Standardised effect sizes are useful because they allow comparison across studies. For example, *Cohen's d* standardises the mean difference by dividing by the pooled standard deviation:

$$d = \frac{M_2 - M_1}{s_{pooled}}$$

Unstandardised effect sizes are often easier to interpret. For example, stating that there was a difference of 2 between two groups on a 7-point Likert scale is relatively intuitive to interpret.

There are different ways of calculating effect sizes depending on the analysis used and the study design. For further details see e.g. Field [8], Cohen [7] or Grissom and Kim [13].

9.3.11 Confidence Intervals

Effect sizes – and other descriptive statistics like means or correlations – should always be reported together with a *confidence interval*. A confidence interval is a range of values around a statistic (e.g. a mean) within which the "true" population value is believed to lie with a certain probability (usually 95%) [8]. As we can never measure the entire population and are limited to measuring a given sample, there is always some degree of error within the data, meaning that statistics derived from the sample are never 100% accurate and do not perfectly reflect the true population value.

Confidence intervals are useful because they (a) give an indication of the variability of the results and (b) they can give an indication of how different two values are likely to be in the population. If confidence intervals of two statistics (e.g. two means from two different groups) overlap, it is likely that the two values are the same in the population. Conversely, if the confidence intervals do not overlap, this indicates the two values are derived from different population. It is useful to include confidence intervals in graphs in form of error bars to help visually explore the data, as shown in Fig. 9.7.

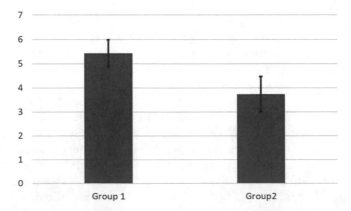

Fig. 9.7 A graph showing two means with error bars indicating 95% confidence intervals. The confidence intervals do not overlap, indicating the two means are different

9.4   Data Science

The field of *data science* has been growing steadily in response to the increasing amount of *big data* available. This is also true in the field of *Health Data Science*. Traditional methods do not always scale to big data analysis and this has led to the introduction of new methods, supported by increases in computational power and performance. This is especially important as much of these big data come in the form of text data, images and other unstructured formats. In her paper in the Journal of the American Medical Informatics Association, Meyer [25] highlights the need for more researchers and healthcare workers trained in data science techniques, including Machine Learning, to address this need

Developing a mobile health intervention is an endeavor that requires substantial input from people with very diverse skill backgrounds. Some background in health and life sciences (domain knowledge) is essential given that we are dealing with a health-related intervention. This may include health care professionals like doctors and nurses, psychologists, biologists, or population health experts to name a few.

In addition to this there is an engineering requirement. Without an app there is nothing to deliver the intervention to the intended target group. Certain personnel are needed to create the applications. This can include people like app developers, computer scientists, data managers and software engineers. With this blend of expertise you can build and deploy your intervention.

There is however also a third group of people that can add real value to such a project. This group is made up of those with expertise in data science and can include e.g. mathematicians, bio/heath informaticians, statisticians and data scientists. The last few groups are extremely useful for evaluating the intervention to determine if it was indeed successful. This can have a scientific/clinical focus in terms of whether the intervention actually helped people in some way (e.g. improved their quality of life) and how we can demonstrate/prove this. This may show clinical value or may be useful from a research perspective.

What this means in practical terms is that, when considering the design of an intervention, you also need to consider the skill set of your team. Team science is an effective way of carrying out work on such projects. Although each member may be an expert in their particular domain, they also need some exposure to the other domains so they can become conversant in the others and thus more effective. This chapter focuses on the data science and analytics domain. Even if your expertise is not in this area, an understanding of the methods of evaluation and analysis may still be of value. If you are in the engineering camp for example, you may consider what information you record and how you store it to make the job of the analyst or researcher easier. Conversely if you are a health specialist/clinician you may also want to think about which clinical/biological aspects are required to properly evaluate the success of the intervention and how the results of such analysis/evaluation can translate into new scientific knowledge or changes to practice.

In this section we provide some brief information that underpins many data science and Machine Learning methods before providing an overview of Machine Learning with some examples of commonly used algorithms. The type of analysis approach that you use will depend on the type of the data your intervention collects as well as its quantity and format and the analysis outcome you are trying to achieve.

9.4.1 Linear Algebra

Many data science and Machine Learning methods are based on linear algebra. This is because complex problems can often be simplified into a series of linear equations that can be rapidly solved through computation. An understanding of this topic although not essential is very helpful in order to truly understand what is going on and make more informed decisions (e.g. adjusting model hyperparameters). Certainly a professional data scientist should understand the relevant elements of linear algebra to be most effective in their role. A brief introduction is provided here.

9.4.2 Linear Equations

Linear (line) equations by definition will not have any square roots or powers in the equation. These equations can exist in multiple dimensions. In 2D they are represented with a line and in 3D as a plane. A straight line graph has the form:

$$y = mx + c$$

Where y is the dependent variable, x is the independent variable, and c is the *intercept*, the point where the line crosses the y-axis. Finally m is the *gradient* or the steepness of the line (0 would be a flat line on the x-axis). Figure 9.8 shows an example of changing the values of c and m. The gradient is determined by $\frac{\text{change in y}}{\text{change in x}}$.

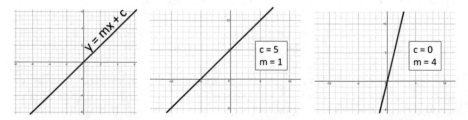

Fig. 9.8 Left: formulae for straight line, middle: the intercept is 5 (crosses y-axis at 5), right: the steepness is 4

Systems of linear equation are where >2 equations work together. One way of solving systems of linear equation is to use matrices.

9.4.3   Vectors and Matrices

One of the central components involves the use of *vectors* and *matrices*.

$$1, \begin{bmatrix} 1 \\ 2 \end{bmatrix}, \begin{bmatrix} 1 & 2 \\ 3 & 4 \end{bmatrix}, \begin{bmatrix} [1\ 2] & [3\ 4] \\ [5\ 6] & [7\ 8] \end{bmatrix}$$

From left to right: A scalar (single value), a vector, a matrix and a tensor

There is some difference in the representation behind terms such as array and vector depending on the discipline within which you work. In the context of physics vectors refer to a quantity with a magnitude and a direction and are usually represented graphically with arrows. In computer science a vector is a one dimensional set of values. Arrays store values of the same type and have a fixed size. A vector on the other hand can store heterogeneous values and has a dynamic size. An example of creating and outputting a vector in R can be seen in Listing 9.1 and 9.2. In Python the *numpy* library is used with the *array* function to create a vector (Listing 9.3 and 9.4).

```
1  a <- c(1,2,3,4)
2  print(a)
```

Listing 9.1   Creating a vector in R

```
1  [1] 1 2 3 4
```

Listing 9.2   R output of vector

```
1  from numpy import array
2
3  a = array([1,2,3,4])
4  print(a)
```

Listing 9.3   Creating a vector in Python

```
1  [1 2 3 4]
```

Listing 9.4   Python output of vector

Matrices are often used to store information (e.g. how training data is organised before applying a model). They can also be used to reduce complex problems in higher dimensions to linear problems that are easier to compute and solve (using a linear approximation). Let's say you wanted to create a matrix called M that had 2 rows and 3 columns with the numbers 1 to 6 $M = \left(\begin{smallmatrix} 1 & 2 & 3 \\ 4 & 5 & 6 \end{smallmatrix} \right)$. We could implement this in either Python (Listing 9.5–9.6) or R (Listing 9.7–9.8).

```
1  import numpy as np
2
3  M = np.matrix([[1,2,3], [4,5,6]])
4  print(M)
```

Listing 9.5 Creating a matrix in Python

```
1  [[1 2 3]
2   [4 5 6]]
```

Listing 9.6 Python output of matrix

```
1  M <- matrix(c(1,2,3,4,5,6), nrow=2, ncol=3, byrow=TRUE)
2  print(M)
```

Listing 9.7 Creating a matrix in R

```
1        [,1] [,2] [,3]
2  [1,]    1    2    3
3  [2,]    4    5    6
```

Listing 9.8 R output of matrix

If we had a matrix M:

$$M = \begin{bmatrix} 1 & 2 \\ 3 & 4 \\ 5 & 6 \end{bmatrix}$$

We could refer to specific values using subscript notation where i is the row index and j is column index ($M_{i,j}$):

$$\begin{bmatrix} M_{1,1} & M_{1,2} \\ M_{2,1} & M_{2,2} \\ M_{3,1} & M_{3,2} \end{bmatrix}$$

Note that indexing for arrays, lists, matrices etc. starts at 1 in R and at 0 in Python

If a matrix has the same shape as another, they can be summed. To do this we simply add the values in the corresponding positions. I.e.

$$\begin{bmatrix} 1 & 0 \\ 2 & 4 \end{bmatrix} + \begin{bmatrix} 3 & 6 \\ 3 & 4 \end{bmatrix} = \begin{bmatrix} 1+3 & 0+6 \\ 2+3 & 4+4 \end{bmatrix} = \begin{bmatrix} 4 & 6 \\ 5 & 8 \end{bmatrix}$$

Matrix multiplication works in a slightly different way. To multiply matrices we need to ensure that the number of columns in the first matrix are equal to the number of rows in the second. In this case we multiply and add corresponding values:

$$\begin{bmatrix} 1 & 0 \\ 2 & 4 \end{bmatrix} \times \begin{bmatrix} 3 & 6 \\ 3 & 4 \end{bmatrix} = \begin{bmatrix} (1 \times 3) + (0 \times 3) & (1 \times 6) + (0 \times 4) \\ (2 \times 3) + (4 \times 3) & (2 \times 6) + (4 \times 4) \end{bmatrix} = \begin{bmatrix} 3 & 6 \\ 18 & 28 \end{bmatrix}$$

We can implement this in R and Python. Note that we cannot just use the conventional multiplication operator. In both cases we have to explicitly use the *dot product* operator/function. If we don't do this in both cases the values will simply be multiplied by their corresponding values (i.e. 1×3, 0×6, 2×3 and 4×4) giving a result of $\left(\begin{smallmatrix} 3 & 0 \\ 6 & 16 \end{smallmatrix} \right)$, which is element-wise multiplication.

```
A <- matrix(c(1,0,2,4), nrow=2, ncol=2, byrow=TRUE)
B <- matrix(c(3,6,3,4), nrow=2, ncol=2, byrow=TRUE)
M <- A %*% B
print(M)
```

Listing 9.9 Multiplying 2 matrices in R using the dot product

```
       [,1] [,2]
[1,]      3    6
[2,]     18   28
```

Listing 9.10 R output of multiplication

```
import numpy as np

A = np.matrix([[1,0], [2,4]])
B = np.matrix([[3,6], [3,4]])
M = np.dot(A, B)
print(M)
```

Listing 9.11 Multiplying 2 matrices in Python using the dot product

```
[[ 3   6]
 [18  28]]
```

Listing 9.12 Python output of multiplication

These techniques are also frequently applied to geometry and computer graphics. One trick that web developers use is to replace some of the transformation functions with matrices to improve performance. If we had some Cascading Style Sheet (CSS) code (used to style HTML elements on web pages) such as that in Listing 9.13 which draws a red box on the screen (Fig. 9.9) that is 100px^2 and positioned at the top of the screen, we could use the *translate* function to move the block 100px to the right and 100px down by adding the code in Listing 9.14 (Fig. 9.10).

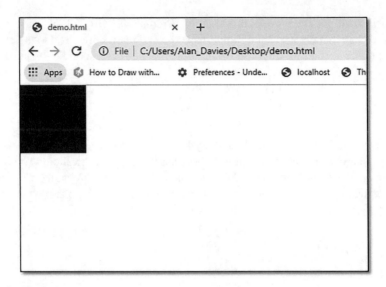

Fig. 9.9 The red block in the top left hand corner of the screen

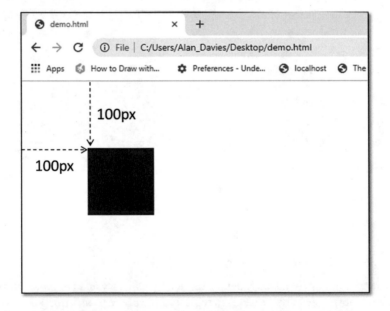

Fig. 9.10 The red block re-positioned 100px left and down using the *translate* function

There are many other geometric transformations, such as rotating, translating, skewing and scaling, all of which use matrix manipulations under the hood.

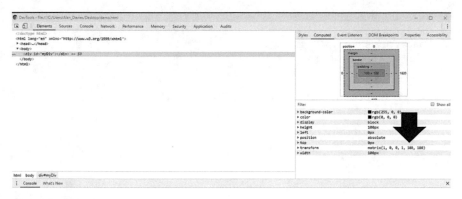

Fig. 9.11 The computed style showing the matrix values on the developer console in Google Chrome. Google Chrome is a trademark of Google LLC

```
#myDiv {
    position : absolute ;
    top :0;
    left :0;
    width :100px ;
    height :100px ;
    background−color :  red ;
}
```

Listing 9.13 A 'div' HTML element positioned top left of screen

```
#myDiv {
    position : absolute ;
    top :0;
    left :0;
    width :100px ;
    height :100px ;
    background−color :  red ;
    transform :  translate (100px ,  100px );
}
```

Listing 9.14 The element with the added transform

After doing this a developer can then use the 'developer tools' and determine the *computed style* (Fig. 9.11). We can see that the computed style also shows us the matrix values *matrix(1, 0, 0, 1, 100, 100)*. A developer could then copy this into the code replacing the original translate function (Listing 9.15). This would improve the performance of the transformation. This would be useful if there were multiple complex transformations occurring (e.g. a hybrid (progressive) web app that uses CSS animations, such as a game).

```
#myDiv {
    position : absolute ;
    top :0;
    left :0;
```

```
5      width:100px;
6      height:100px;
7      background-color: red;
8      transform: matrix(1, 0, 0, 1, 100, 100);
9  }
```

Listing 9.15 The translate function replaced with the matrix values directly

9.4.4   Special Matrices

There are also "special" types of matrices that can be useful for various purposes. One such type is the *inverse* of a matrix. The basic idea is that as there is no such concept as dividing by a matrix, the inverse of a matrix is used instead. If you wanted to solve a simple equation such as $5x = 18$ you would divide both sides of the equation by 5 i.e. $\frac{5x}{5} = x$ and $\frac{18}{5} = 3.6$ so $x = 3.6$. Because one cannot divide by a matrix you can achieve a similar goal with multiplication. In the previous example this would be the same as multiplying both sides of the equation by one fifth i.e. $\frac{1}{5}5x$ and $\frac{1}{5}18$. One divided by a number is referred to as the number's *reciprocal*. For matrices this is written with a minus 1 in superscript after the matrix i.e. $I = M \times M^{-1}$. To have an inverse, a matrix must be square ($n \times n$). To determine the inverse of a matrix:

$$\begin{bmatrix} 1 & 3 \\ 2 & 4 \end{bmatrix}^{-1}$$

We can divide 1 by the *determinant*, which is found through the difference of the multiplication of the diagonals. The answer is then multiplied by each value in the matrix after we swap the diagonal values round and make the remaining numbers negative.

$$\begin{bmatrix} 1 & 3 \\ 2 & 4 \end{bmatrix}^{-1} = \frac{1}{(1 \times 4) - (3 \times 2)} \begin{bmatrix} 4 & -3 \\ -2 & 1 \end{bmatrix}$$

We can then multiply the value by each element to get the inverse matrix:

$$= -0.5 \times \begin{bmatrix} 4 & -3 \\ -2 & 1 \end{bmatrix} = \begin{bmatrix} -2 & 1.5 \\ 1 & -0.5 \end{bmatrix}$$

To do this using R we can apply the solve function and pass in the matrix i.e. *solve(M)*. This will produce the identity matrix for a given matrix. For Python add a dot and the capital letter I to the matrix i.e. *M.I* to produce the equivalent. Of course in practice you would rarely need to determine the inverse of a matrix as code and libraries exist for solving linear equation systems rapidly and computationally effectively without having to use inversions, such as Python's *linalg.solve* function in the *numpy* and *scipy* packages. For example if you had a series of related equations, such as:

$$7x + 5y - 3z = 16$$

$$3x - 5y + 2z = -8$$

$$5x + 3y - 7z = 0$$

We could solve these using matrices. To do this you add the values to a matrix. As there is $7x$ in the first equation, the first element of the matrix contains a 7, then a 5 and then -3 and so on. A single value like x would be represented with a 1 and no value with a 0:

$$A = \begin{bmatrix} 7 & 5 & -3 \\ 3 & -5 & 2 \\ 5 & 3 & -7 \end{bmatrix} ; x = \begin{bmatrix} x \\ y \\ z \end{bmatrix} ; B = \begin{bmatrix} 16 \\ -8 \\ 0 \end{bmatrix}$$

So to determine the values x, y, z we could use the inverse so $Ax = B$ becomes $x = A^{-1}B$. Instead of this we can automate the process using computational techniques (Listing 9.16). We do this because it can be computationally intensive to compute using the inverse and inverting can also lead to numerical instability.

```
import numpy as np

A = np.matrix([[7,5,-3], [3,-5,2], [5,3,-7]])
B = np.array([16,-8,0])

print(np.linalg.solve(A, B))
```

Listing 9.16 Using *linalg* to solve a series of equations

This gives an output of 1, 3 and 2 so $x = 1$, $y = 3$, $z = 2$. Which we can verify by plugging in the results into the original equations:
Equation 1:

$$7(1) + 5(3) - 3(2) =$$

$$(7 + 15) - 6 =$$

$$22 - 6 = 16$$

Equation 2:

$$3(1) - 5(3) + 2(2) =$$

$$(3 - 15) + 4 =$$

$$-12 + 4 = -8$$

Equation 3:

$$5(1) + 3(3) - 7(2) =$$

$$(5 + 9) - 14 =$$

$$14 - 14 = 0$$

Another common operation to carry out on matrices is to *transpose* them. This refers to creating a new matrix where the columns are changed into rows. Matrices that are transposed are denoted with a superscript letter T, for example M^T. An example of a matrix transposition in R can be seen in Listing 9.17 with the output in Listing 9.18.

```
M <- matrix(c(1,0,2,4), nrow=2, ncol=2, byrow=TRUE)
print(M)
print(t(M))
```

Listing 9.17 R example of transposing a matrix

```
       [,1] [,2]
[1,]     1    0
[2,]     2    4

       [,1] [,2]
[1,]     1    2
[2,]     0    4
```

Listing 9.18 R output of matrix before and after transposing

9.4.5 Machine Learning

There is a currently a lot of hype around Machine Learning. Machine Learning works well with large amounts of data and has been used to good effect for things like recommender systems for tailoring suggestions, for example by suggesting movies to watch or goods advertising based on finding patterns from users' previous behaviours. The application of Machine Learning in the medical, pharmaceutical

Features   Labels

Age	Sys BP	Dia BP	HR	BMI	HbA1c	Diabetes
47	135	75	101	20.5	49	1
56	145	62	87	25.2	48	1
65	138	55	97	18.3	67	0
24	120	65	76	19.1	52	1
33	150	80	88	22.6	42	0
46	124	76	57	20.6	73	1

Examples/records

Fig. 9.12 Fictitious sample data from 6 people with a classification of diabetes (1) or no-diabetes (0)

and health domain however is less clear despite being mentioned prominently in strategic documents and reports, such as the Topol review that discusses Machine Learning in the light of predictive analysis [28]. Part of the reason for the relatively slow (but now quickening) uptake in the health and pharmaceutical industries is down to the lack of access to datasets. Many Machine Learning models require large datasets to perform well. Accessing such data and at volume is not easy given ethical and technical issues. Added to this is the fact that many Machine Learning models also suffer from a lack of explainability, especially when compared to some other well established statistical methods. Providers may be reluctant to make critical healthcare or clinical trial decisions based on a model that might have good performance but has low explainability. This is also problematic in terms of providing a rationale for such decisions. The sensitive and important nature of healthcare and potential for litigation if delivered badly is another reason that adoption has been slower than the hype might suggest. The majority of Machine Learning devices in healthcare seem to surround the diagnostic imaging and genetics fields [19]. Another category involves the use of Natural Language Processing (NLP) for the analysis of unstructured text data (e.g. clinical notes) [19]. There is however a drive to leverage such methods for use in the healthcare arena, and such methods have been successfully applied to analyse data collected from mHealth interventions and wearable devices.

We have discussed *regression* previously in this chapter. Many Machine Learning algorithms can be used for regression problems. Another useful task Machine Learning is good at is that of *classification*, i.e. determining what class (category) data belong to. This is often achieved by training a model on a subset of the available data (Fig. 9.12). In Machine Learning we tend to split a dataset into *features*; these are the columns that contribute to the label classification. We normally represent

$$
X = \begin{pmatrix}
47 & 135 & 75 & 101 & 20.5 & 49 \\
56 & 145 & 62 & 87 & 25.2 & 48 \\
65 & 138 & 55 & 97 & 18.3 & 67 \\
24 & 120 & 65 & 76 & 19.1 & 52 \\
33 & 150 & 80 & 88 & 22.6 & 42 \\
46 & 124 & 76 & 57 & 20.6 & 73
\end{pmatrix}
\qquad
y = \begin{pmatrix}
1 \\ 1 \\ 0 \\ 1 \\ 0 \\ 1
\end{pmatrix}
$$

Fig. 9.13 Splitting the features X from the labels y

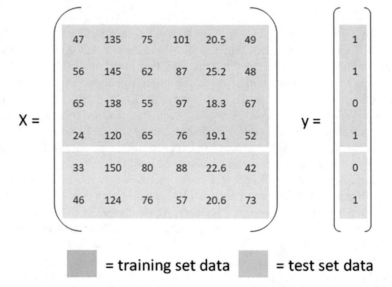

= training set data   = test set data

Fig. 9.14 Splitting data into training and test sets

these features with a capital letter X. The labels are also separated and referred to with a lower case letter y (Fig. 9.13).

Once this split is made, we can then split the data further into a *training set* and a *test set* (and sometimes also into a *validation set*) as seen in Fig. 9.14.

Typically more data are used for a training a model than for testing (approx 25% for testing, but this does vary). Once a model has been trained on a dataset, we can introduce new data to the model to see how well it performs with these new data. This way we get a feel for the *generalizability* of the model. This is an example of *supervised* Machine Learning. In supervised Machine Learning we have some data with known labels that we can provide for training to 'teach' the algorithm by example what feature properties the different classes expect. There are also *unsupervised* Machine Learning algorithms that can be used when we don't know what these labels are, for example clustering methods. Unsupervised learning is also a useful tool for data exploration and analysis. Finally there is also *reinforcement* learning. This method uses reward in a specific environment to improve the actions the algorithm takes. An example of this was used to beat a human champion at the very difficult game called 'Go' which has many more permutations than chess, making brute force methods impractical. The algorithm (AlphaGo) was able to train itself to beat human experts. This was the first time a computer program was able to beat a human at this game [34]. In December 2019, a Reinforcement learning model called "AlphaStar" successfully beat one of the world's top professional players of StarCraft 2, a real-time strategy game. Previous artifical intelligence algorithms had struggled to deal with the complexity of the game.

One of the main challenges with Machine Learning when trying to model real world data is the *bias variance trade-off*.

When a trained model has a high amount of bias, it is said to be *underfitted* to the data (it fails to model the relationships between features and the target), whereas if a model has a high amount of variance, it is said to be *overfitted* to the data (the model is learning noise in the data and is too precise). The tradeoff comes from being able to minimise both of these errors and learning a model that can generalize beyond its training data. This book does not have the scope to discuss the entire field of Machine Learning and as such we will just mention a few examples of some of the commonly used models to highlight the variety of approaches available followed by a short section on how the performance of these algorithms can be assessed. First we will briefly examine some considerations that apply to most Machine Learning models.

9.4.5.1   Dimensionality Reduction

Many large data sets can have a very high number of features. This can make the performance of algorithms slow and increases complexity. Many of the features may not even contribute (or at least significantly contribute) to an overall classification. This is often referred to as the *curse of dimensionality*. One can think of this in terms of graphs. In 2 dimensions (2D), we can plot 2 features, one on the x-axis and the other on the y-axis. If we increase this to 3 features, we can use a third dimension (3D) where we can use the z-axis to represent depth. Representing 4 or more features becomes significantly more complex and cannot be plotted easily. As more and more higher dimensions are used the complexity increases. To help with this problem there are different methods known as *dimensionality reduction* methods. A common example of this is *Principle Component Analysis* or PCA.

9.4.5.2   Regularisation

A way to prevent over-fitting of a model to a data set is to use *regularisation*. Two of the common approaches are referred to as L_1 and L_2 regularisation respectively. They work by penalizing complex models to prevent over-fitting. The first L_1 works by penalizing model weights in proportion to the summation of the values of the model weights. This can be used to remove features that are less relevant. The L_2 regularisation helps to reduce the effect of outliers on a model's weights. It works by penalizing the weights in proportion to the weight's sum of squares. This is known to improve generalization for linear models.

9.4.5.3   Cross Validation

This is essentially a way of evaluating models by training them on subsets of the data. This can help in the detection of model over-fitting. One method is known as k-fold cross-validation and involves splitting data into k sets. These splits are also known as *folds*. The model is trained on all but one of the folds. The remaining fold is then used for evaluating the model. This process is then repeated a number of times with random subsets of the data. The general process involves randomly shuffling the data, splitting it into k-folds, training on all but one of the groups and using the remaining group for testing. This is then repeated. The value of k is often set to the size of the dataset or the value of 10 (which has been determined through prior experimentation).

9.4.6   Decision Trees

Decision tree algorithms have been around for decades. Some of the most powerful Machine Learning models are based on Decision Trees, such as *Random Forest* and *Gradient Boosting Trees*. Decision tree algorithms are also one of the more explainable of the methods. In order to understand how these methods work it is first necessary to consider how individual decision trees work. A statistician called Leo Breiman from the University of California coined the term *CART*, which stands for **c**lassification **a**nd **r**egression **t**rees. These algorithms are capable of carrying out both regression and classification tasks. The first thing to note is that unlike a conventional tree that grows upwards, these trees tend to be represented from the top down or sideways.

Figure 9.15 displays an example of a decision tree that could be used to determine whether or not to lend money to someone based on their income and rental expenses. The first node (Income < 25K) is termed the *root* node representing the entire sample that is further subdivided. Sub-nodes that are further divided are called *decision* nodes. Nodes with proceeding nodes are also called *parent* nodes with subsequent nodes referred to as *child* nodes. If a node has no child nodes it is termed

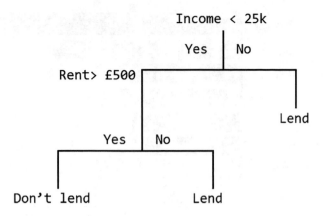

Fig. 9.15 Decision tree diagram

a *leaf* or *terminal* node. And finally a sub-section of a tree is called a *branch* or *sub-tree*. The splitting of data is performed via recursive greedy binary splitting. This means a repeated action is used to split data into 2 parts. The greedy element refers to the way the best decision is made at the current step, rather than considering future splits that might lead to an overall better tree. This is achieved by comparing every feature and value until the best split can be achieved. The way this is done is dependent on if you are using the algorithm for regression or classification. In the former case the mean square error (MSE) or sum of squared errors (SSE) are typically used to find the optimal split. In the case of classification the class error rate, cross entropy or most commonly the Gini index/impurity is used. If the index is 0 then all the cases belong to a specific target category.

$$Gini_i = \sum_{k=1}^{K} \hat{p}_{mk}(1 - \hat{p}_{mk})$$

Some advantages of these methods include not having to scale data prior to algorithm application. They work with small data sets and it is relatively easy to understand the output and related visualisations. The main disadvantage is that they are prone to over-fitting and so don't generalize well. This can be rectified somewhat by *pruning* more complex trees into smaller trees that generalize better. This also has the added advantage of increasing performance. They are also quite sensitive to small variations in training data. This can lead to very different trees being built. And they are also sensitive to training set rotation, which can be mitigated by performing a PCA.

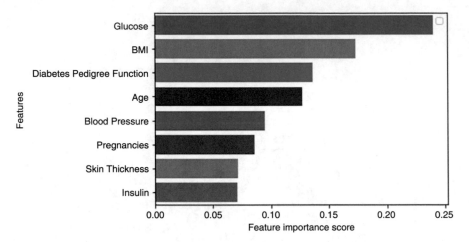

Fig. 9.16 Feature importance of features from the public domain Pimi Indians diabetes dataset
https://www.kaggle.com/uciml/pima-indians-diabetes-database

9.4.6.1 Improving Decision Trees

To overcome some of the limitations, multiple trees can be combined into a forest
of trees called a *random forest*. This brings together the combined power of lots
of weaker classifiers to create a much more powerful classifier. The decrease in
impurity can also be averaged and the features then ranked. This can then also be
used as a means of determining and removing unnecessary features. Figure 9.16
shows a plot of Feature importance derived from the 'Pimi Indians diabetes' dataset
that contains labelled data about diabetes status. We can see in the plot that the
features *Glucose* and *BMI* (Body Mass Index) are considered to be among the most
important features for predicting diabetes status.

9.4.7 Support Vector Machines (SVM)

Another popular method that can be used for both classification and regression is
called Support Vector Machines (SVM). When we want to partition data points in a
dataset into distinct categories (classes) for classification, we could imagine drawing
a dividing line (decision boundary) to separate the data. Take for example the data
in Fig. 9.17. Where would you draw the line? Here we have added two arbitrary
lines to the sub image on the left. Both separate the data, but if we were to add new
data (e.g. the red data point on the image on the right), the choice of dividing line
will influence which class the new data is considered to belong to. A Support Vector
Machine can be used to improve this situation. SVMs work by adding margins to the

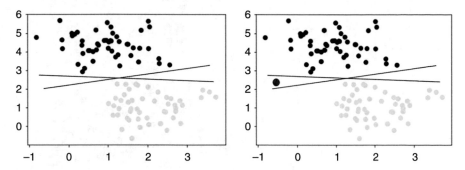

Fig. 9.17 (Left) arbitrary lines dividing the data, (right) adding a new data point (red dot) to the data

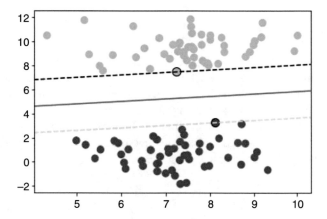

Fig. 9.18 Maximum margin boundary between two classes

lines that extend to the nearest data points in the classes. The line with the maximum margin is considered to be the optimal separation of the data.

Not all of the training data points are important or essential for determining the decision boundary between classes. The ones that are situated on the border between classes are known as *support vectors* (circled data points in the image below). This is where the name Support Vector Machine comes from.

When used for classification, SVMs work by partitioning data into separate groups (classes) using a hyperplane. This is often drawn in diagrams in 2D with a line separating the classes. The hyperplane is actually a flat surface that exists in higher dimensional space. The boundary between classes is placed halfway between them and is called the maximum margin boundary/hyperplane. This is seen in Fig. 9.18 with the separation of the 2 classes. The solid line between the 2 dashed lines is the maximal margin hyperplane between the two classes.

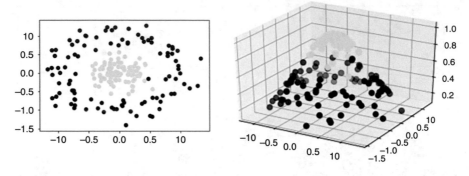

Fig. 9.19 Using extra dimensional space to separate data classes

9.4.7.1 The Kernel Trick

The kernel trick can be used to approach problems that are non-linear (cannot be separated with a straight line), as shown for example in the image on the left in Fig. 9.19. We can project our data into extra dimensional space in order to make the data linearly separable, as seen in the image on the right in Fig. 9.19.

There are different *kernels* (mathematical functions) available that work with different types of data. Two examples of available kernels are the *Polynomial kernel* that is often used with image processing:

$$K(x_i, x_{i'}) = (1 + \sum_{j=1}^{p} x_{ij} x_{i'j})^d$$

When we increase the polynomial degree (d), we increase the complexity of the decision boundary by adding additional higher order terms.

Another example of available kernels is the *Radial Basis Function* (RBF) kernel:

$$K(x_i, x_{i'}) = exp(-\gamma \sum_{j=1}^{p} (x_{ij} - x_{i'j})^2)$$

This is also known as the Gaussian RBF kernel. The width of the kernel can be adjusted by changing the γ (gamma) value which is defined as $\frac{1}{2\sigma^2}$. A large gamma value reduces the standard deviation (σ) leading to a narrow RBF kernel and vice versa. Increasing the gamma may cause the model to overfit the data; too small a gamma value and the model may underfit. Tuning parameters like the gamma are one of the ways you can improve the performance of your model. Other kernel options include linear, poly and sigmoid.

Reasons to use SVM:

- Linear classification
- Non-linear classification (with the 'kernel trick')
- Regression problems
- Outlier detection
- Works with small to medium sized datasets

9.4.7.2 Soft Margin Classification

Using a hard margin to classify has two inherent issues: it only works with linearly separable data and it is sensitive to outliers. We can loosen the restrictions of the margin classification and switch from hard to soft margin classification. To do this we can vary the hyperparameter called C. Increasing the value of C will make the margin more narrow and the number of margin violations will increase and vise versa. The C hyperparameter can also be reduced to try and regularise an over-fitting model.

Example: Using Machine Learning and wearable data to detect stress and anxiety in Autism

Masino et al. [24] carried out some work exploring the possibility of detecting stress (caused by a stress inducing task) and no-stress states in people with Autistic Spectrum Disorder (ASD). In a lab-based setting they used wearable sensors to collect heart rate and RR interval data (distance between R wave peaks on the ECG waveform) ($N = 38$, $ASD = 22$, non-$ASD = 16$). In their paper they use both Logistic Regression and Support Vector Machines (SVM). Findings show that the SVM model performed better with 91% accuracy suggesting that Machine Learning methods such as SVM can be used to analyse consumer-grade wearable device data in order to classify individuals' state of stress [24].

9.4.8 k-Nearest Neighbors (k-NN)

K-NN is a non-parametric Machine Learning algorithm capable of solving both classification and regression problems. The algorithm works by classifying new data

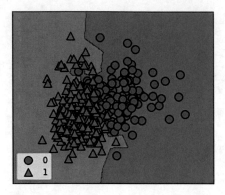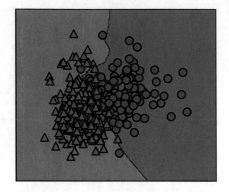

Fig. 9.20 Two features of a dataset plotted against each other with k = 1, and k = 12

based on their closest similarity to the training data points provided. The k in the name k-NN relates to the number of neighbors in the training set that are used to determine similarity.

Features are treated as coordinates in multidimensional feature space. For example, if you compared 2 features they would be represented in 2D (two-dimensional) feature space like a graph with one feature on the x-axis and the other on the y-axis (Fig. 9.20).

The simplest form is $k = 1$ seen in the left graph in Fig. 9.20. The boundary gets progressively smoother with the introduction of more neighbors $k = 12$. k-NN is an example of *instance-based learning* also known as *lazy learning*. This is so called because it relies on the raw training data to make predictions rather than explicitly generalizing. This means that the training phase is considerably faster than the prediction phase. k-NN can deal with multi-class problems (e.g. more than 2 classification categories). The distance between points is determined with various distance metrics such as the Euclidean distance (straight line distance between 2 points):

$$D(q, p) = \sqrt{\sum_{i=1}^{n}(q_i - p_i)^2}$$

9.4.8.1   What Value Should I Use for k?

The lower the value of k the more likely under-fitting is to occur and vise versa. A common starting point is to set k to the square root of the number of records in your training set. Figure 9.21 illustrates a visual example of k set to 3. The new test data point identified by the star looks at the 3 nearest points giving a $\frac{2}{3}$ probability of being classed as the 'triangle' class.

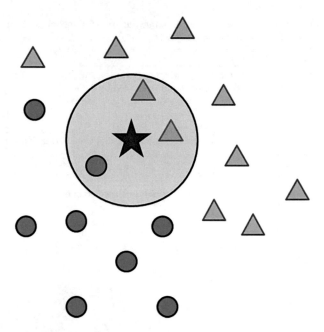

Fig. 9.21 Illustration of k = 3 Nearest Neighbors to classify a new data point

9.4.9   Evaluating a Model

Different Machine Learning models will have different ways of evaluating the model's performance. There are however some common outputs that are used for many of the models produced. Some of the common evaluation metrics are displayed in Table 9.2.

Another way of summarising the classification performance is to use a *confusion matrix* as seen in Fig. 9.22. Here we can see how many times the classifier made certain classifications. For example, 52 times the classifier predicted a value of 0 that was correctly classified. In 3 cases it predicted a 0 and it should have been a 1 and so on. We are looking for higher numbers in the cells that match the predicted and actual values than the other diagonals that show missclassifications.

A popular way of visualising performance is with a Receiver Operating Characteristic (ROC) curve (Fig. 9.23). We can use the ROC curve to plot the true positive and false positive rates against one another using different threshold values. Multiple models can be compared on the curve and the best one chosen. Good performance is indicated by a curve that hugs the left vertical and top horizontal position of the graph (e.g. has the most area under the curve). The plot shows the trade-off between both the sensitivity and specificity of a model. The closer the curve to the 45 degree dashed line, the worse the model's performance is. The area under the curve (AUC) is often used to quantify and compare different models.

Table 9.2 Some commonly used Machine Learning metrics for model performance. *TP* true positive, *TN* true negative, *FP* false positive, *FN* false negative

Metric	Description
Accuracy	One of the most frequently used metrics. Accuracy refers to the number of correctly made predictions divided by the total number of possible predictions and is usually displayed as a percentage $Accuracy = \frac{TP+TN}{TP+TN+FP+FN}$
Precision/positive predictive value	Percentage of positive classifications that were correct. How precise were we? $Precision = \frac{TP}{TP+FP}$
Recall/sensitivity	The proportion of actual positives classified correctly $Recall = \frac{TP}{TP+FN}$
F1-score	A harmonic mean of the precision and recall
Support	Number of times a class occurs in a ground truth (number of correct target values)

Fig. 9.22 A confusion matrix

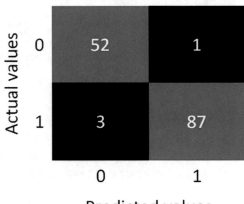

Actual values / Predicted values

	0	1
0	52	1
1	3	87

9.4.10   Model Selection

Choosing which type of model to use will depend on what type of data you have, how much data you have, and what you are trying to do with these data (classification, regression, clustering, or dimensionality reduction). Python's scikit-learn Machine Learning module has a useful 'cheat sheet' to help you determine which model to use based on the features of the data and the desired task. This can be seen in Fig. 9.24.

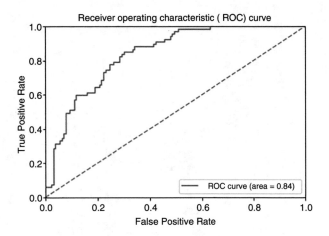

Fig. 9.23 Receiver operating characteristic (ROC) curve

9.4.11   Natural Language Processing (NLP)

There are many forms of text data used in healthcare. This includes clinic notes, referral letters, reports and medical notes themselves to name just a few. This type of data has the potential to be analysed by NLP methods. This can range from more basic analyses such as the frequency of certain words appearing in a document to more advanced methods like n-gram analysis and topic modelling. As with many automated methods, what you put in (the model's input) will impact on what you get out (the model's output). Text data can be represented as a *corpus* which contains raw text strings with additional metadata.

Another form is the *document term matrix*, a sparse matrix represented with rows for documents and columns representing terms. The *bag of words* pre-processing technique is often used on a corpus of documents to prepare the data for text mining methods. The first step is to split the document into a set of *tokens*. This can be achieved for example by splitting words based on the spaces between them or other punctuation. The next step is to build up a *vocabulary* of words before finally *encoding* them into a sparse matrix [27].

Figure 9.25 shows a word cloud visualisation where the frequency of a word occurring in the text is denoted by its relative size. These types of output can be used in place of histograms to communicate the main words used. In this instance the word cloud was generated from an interview with experts on electrocardiograms (ECGs). The image on the right (from the same study) shows how the words can be clustered to group them.

An example of an application that is based on pre-processed corpus data is *sentiment analysis*. This approach looks at the emotion behind certain words (the emotional tone). This sort of analysis is often applied to social media data (e.g. Twitter messages on a certain topic). There are several popular choices of lexicon for such purposes (Table 9.3). An example using the *Bing* lexicon on some comments

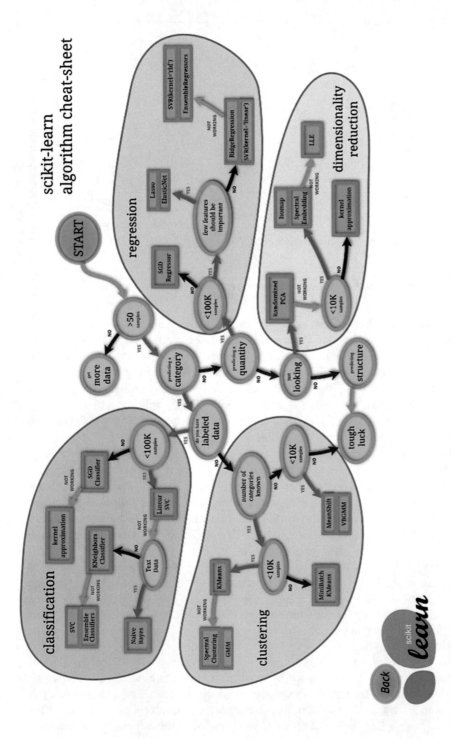

Fig. 9.24 The scikit-learn algorithm cheat sheet from https://scikit-learn.org/stable/tutorial/machine_learning_map/index.html. Follow the link to view an interactive version of this diagram

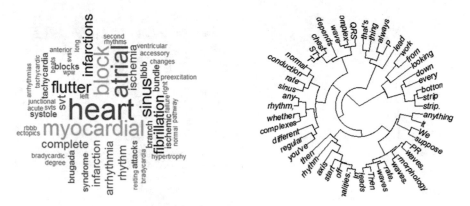

Fig. 9.25 (Left) word cloud, size equates to frequency. (Right) hierarchical word clustering

Table 9.3 Set of commonly used lexicons containing words with associated sentiment

Sentiment lexicons	Description
Bing	Binary word classification positive or negative sentiment
AFINN	Uses a score from −5 to +5 (negative scores are negative sentiments, positive scores are positive sentiments)
NRC	Binary word classification (yes/no) for categories: Anger, anticipation, disgust, fear, joy, sadness, surprise, and trust

posted on a bioinformatics MOOC (Massive Open Online Course) can be seen in Fig. 9.26. The words on the left of the figure are words that appeared in the comments identified as having a negative sentiment. The words on the right show positive sentiment words. The size of the bar shows each word's contribution to the overall sentiment.

N-gram analysis can also be used to model text data. The *n* in n-gram denotes adjacent words or characters that have a length of *n*. For example each word in a sentence can be an n-gram or each letter in a word. An *n* of 1 is called a uni-gram, 2 is a bi-gram, 3 a tri-gram and so on. They are used to statistically represent the structure of text. This is helpful when the sequence of letters or words is important. Figure 9.27 shows an example sub-section of a visualisation of tri-grams showing how words are related to other words from the MOOC comments. Here we can see connections between certain words in the comments.

We may also want to identify topics (themes) in the text in an automatic way. A popular method for this is to use the *term frequency inverse document frequency* or *tf-idf* for short. This method re-scales features, giving them more importance depending on the frequency of their occurrence in a certain document but not across all the documents [27]. This takes the form (where tf = term frequency (i in j), df = document frequency (documents containing i) and N is the total number of documents):

$$\text{tfidf}_{i,j} = \text{tf}_{i,j} \times \log\left(\frac{N}{\text{df}_i}\right) + 1$$

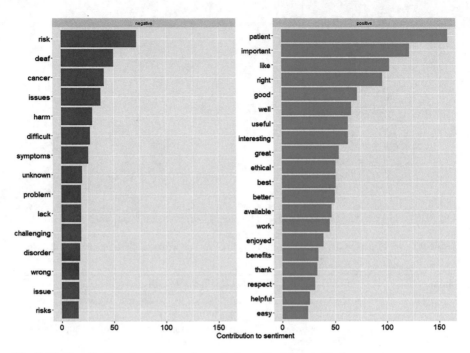

Fig. 9.26 Contribution of word to sentiment (red negative/blue positive)

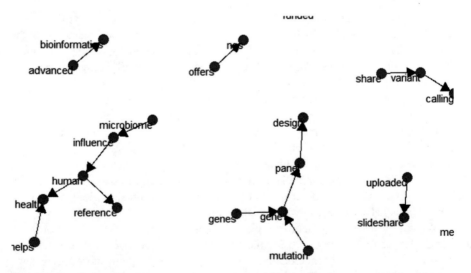

Fig. 9.27 Sub-section of plot showing tri-gram analysis on MOOC comment posts made by participants of the course

9.5   Which Tools to Use?

Having used many different tools to analyse data we would advocate the use of
software such as R and Python for data science and statistics. This is partly because
they are both extraordinarily well supported with libraries for advanced techniques,
but also because they are freely available to download and use. They can also handle
the processing of large amounts of data. Both R [31] and Python have interactive
notebooks available that allow code, text, math notation and other resources to be
presented and shared in a single document (Fig. 9.28) and are becoming increasingly
useful for data science reporting.

According to a survey of over 23k professionals working with data that was
run by Kaggle (The 2018 Machine Learning and Data Science Survey), the top
programming language used on a regular basis was Python (83%), followed by SQL
(44%) and R (36%) [14]. There is an ongoing debate over which language between
R and Python is the best. In the opinion of the authors, who regularly use both of
these languages interchangeably, both are valid and can largely do the same things.
We would tend to veer towards using R with the *tidyverse* (a set of data science
packages sharing a design standard) for statistical analysis and Python for Machine

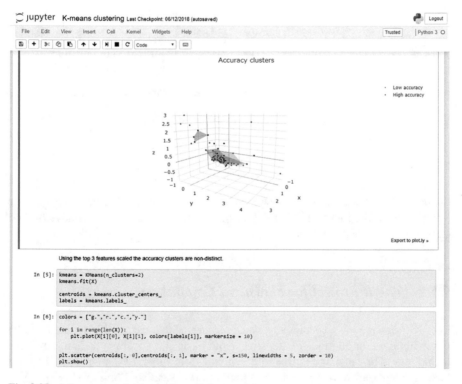

Fig. 9.28   A Jupyter notebook running a Python script

Learning and when building analysis into a larger system (such as a web server). To some degree the tool chosen will relate to the task at hand, the budget available, familiarity of the tool and the background and experience of the people using the tool. Below is a breakdown of some programming languages and statistical tools that can be used for data analysis.

9.5.1 Python

Python is a free fully featured general purpose programming language that supports both functional and object orientated programming paradigms available from https://www.python.org/. Python is a very popular language for Machine Learning and data science. We recommend the Anaconda distribution (https://www.anaconda. com/distribution/) as this comes with a variety of pre-installed libraries and additional tools for data science including *Jupyter notebooks*. An example of Python code to carry out a t-test can be seen below. We present the same analysis in the following examples for comparison.

```
1 import os
2 import pandas as pd
3 from scipy import stats
4
5 data_file = pd.read_csv(os.getcwd() + "\scoredata.csv")
6 print(stats.ttest_ind(data_file['group1'], data_file['group2'],
      equal_var=False))
```

Listing 9.19 Python code example running a t-test on scores from 2 groups

```
1 Ttest_indResult(statistic=-0.65297154869724483, pvalue
      =0.51665335081032071)
```

Listing 9.20 Python code output

We start by reading in the data as a CSV (comma separated values) file and print the results of the t-test function *stats.ttest_ind()* providing the 2 groups that we want to compare to the function. We see that the output (Listing 9.20) displays the test statistic and associated p-value.

9.5.2 The R Project for Statistical Computing

The R language was specifically designed for statistical analysis and includes many libraries for all kinds of statistics, from basic statistical methods to advanced techniques. The language is free to download from https://www.r-project.org/ and has an integrated development environment (IDE) called *RStudio* (Fig. 9.29). A sample of R code can be seen in Listing 9.21.

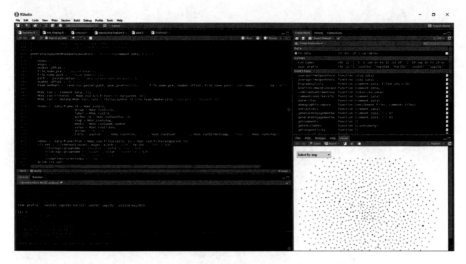

Fig. 9.29 RStudio running some analysis on data for a research study on user engagement on a bioinformatics MOOC (RStudio and Shiny are trademarks of RStudio, PBC)

```
1  library(tidyverse)
2
3  score_data <- read_csv(paste0(getwd(), "/langs/scoredata.csv"),
       col_names = TRUE, na = c("NA"))
4  print(t.test(score_data$group1, score_data$group2))
```

Listing 9.21 R code example running a t-test on scores from 2 groups

```
1   Welch Two Sample t-test
2
3  data:   data_file$group1 and data_file$group2
4  t = -0.65297, df = 51.963, p-value = 0.5167
5  alternative hypothesis: true difference in means is not equal to
       0
6  95 percent confidence interval:
7   -16.994875    8.650048
8  sample estimates:
9  mean of x mean of y
10   34.10345    38.27586
```

Listing 9.22 R code output

Again we begin by loading the CSV data, calling the *t.test()* function and passing in the 2 groups. The output (Listing 9.20) is much richer than that of Python providing more associated statistical detail by default. We can see however that the test statistic (*t*) and the p-value are the same as the Python output.

9.5.3 Julia

Julia is a relatively new language (https://julialang.org/) that was designed for performance and allows for parallel and distributed computing. Although currently not as well utilised as Python or R in the field, Julia is gaining in popularity and may be very useful for performance essential analysis tasks.

```
using CSV, HypothesisTests , DataFrames

score_data = CSV.File(string(pwd(), "//scoredata.csv")) |>
    DataFrame
print(UnequalVarianceTTest(vec(score_data[1]), vec(score_data[2])
    ))
```

Listing 9.23 Julia code example running a t-test on scores from 2 groups

```
Two sample t-test (unequal variance)

Population details:
    parameter of interest:    Mean difference
    value under h_0:          0
    point estimate:           -4.172413793103445
    95% confidence interval: (-16.9949, 8.65)

Test summary:
    outcome with 95% confidence: fail to reject h_0
    two-sided p-value:           0.5167

Details:
    number of observations:   [29,29]
    t-statistic:              -0.6529715486972448
    degrees of freedom:       51.963011928433744
    empirical standard error: 6.38988605464955
```

Listing 9.24 Julia code output

As in Python and R, Julia works in a similar way. Here we again load the data from the CSV file and call the *UnequalVarianceTTest()* function (Listing 9.23). The output like that of R has a lot of useful information provided by default (Listing 9.24).

9.5.4 SPSS

Created by IBM, the Statistical Package for Social Sciences (SPSS) is good for most standard inferential and descriptive statistical tests. SPSS provides a graphical interface where tests can be selected and run from menus. SPSS provides rich detail in its statistical output reports (Fig. 9.30).

SPSS is not a programming language and as such only performs statistical tests. It is a commercial piece of software available from https://www.ibm.com/uk-en/

Group Statistics

	Group	N	Mean	Std. Deviation	Std. Error Mean
Test	1.00	24	4.3750	1.37722	.28112
	2.00	24	4.2917	2.03190	.41476

Independent Samples Test

		Levene's Test for Equality of Variances		t-test for Equality of Means					95% Confidence Interval of the Difference	
		F	Sig.	t	df	Sig. (2-tailed)	Mean Difference	Std. Error Difference	Lower	Upper
Test	Equal variances assumed	2.640	.111	.166	46	.869	.08333	.50106	-.92524	1.09191
	Equal variances not assumed			.166	40.450	.869	.08333	.50106	-.92899	1.09565

Fig. 9.30 SPSS output after running an independent t-test

analytics/spss-statistics-software. To run the same analysis we first load the file using the graphical user interface (GUI) and then use menus to select the required test from the available options. The results are then displayed in tabular summary (Fig. 9.30).

9.5.5 JASP

JASP (https://jasp-stats.org/) supports both frequentist and Bayesian analysis, is free to install and use and works in a similar way to SPSS in that analyses are carried out primarily via the graphical user interface (Fig. 9.31).

Again the test is chosen from a list of available tests via menu buttons with the output displayed in a tabular summary that can be copied directly. The tables support the APA (American Psychological Association) reporting style which is widely used in the behavioral and social sciences fields.

9.6 Qualitative Data Analysis

We will now provide an introduction to qualitative analysis in the context of evaluating health apps.

Qualitative data analysis can be undertaken using various tools. It can involve hands-on methods using materials such as sticky notes, pen and paper to organise the material and visually create categories and links. Often, however, data are first brought into electronic format (e.g. by transcribing interview recordings verbatim or typing up observation notes) and then analysed using software like QSR NVivo. It is important to note that software such as NVivo can help you to organise the data, but it cannot undertake analysis and creation of themes and categories for you. This process requires active, interpretive and often creative input of the researcher. Most qualitative analysis methods involve *coding* the data. This essentially means

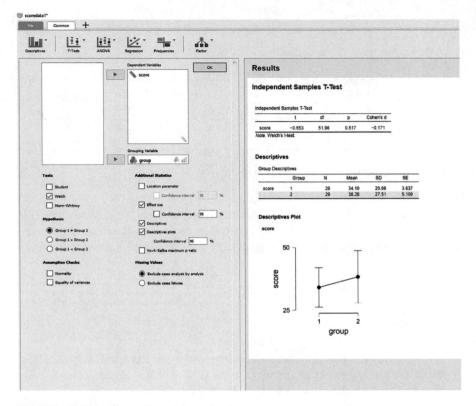

Fig. 9.31 JASP running a t-test and associated output

that labels or *codes* are attached to data snippets (e.g. lines of text), and these are then grouped into broader categories to create more conceptual themes.

9.6.1   Epistemology and Ontology

Qualitative research can be conducted using different epistemological lenses. *Epistemology* refers to our understanding of how we develop knowledge and theory. An *inductive* approach aims to build knowledge from the bottom up, using empirical observations to develop theory. A *deductive* approach, on the other hand, begins with a theory and uses this to develop a hypothesis which can then be tested using empirical data (top-down) [32]. One can furthermore differentiate between *abductive* and *retroductive* reasoning [3]. Abductive reasoning involves finding the simplest and mostly likely explanation for a phenomenon. Unlike deductive reasoning, this explanation is not positively verified but simply inferred. In terms of qualitative research, the abductive research strategy involves first describing concepts using participants' language and meanings, and these lay accounts are then "abducted" into technical accounts using the researcher's categories. In retroductive reasoning, evidence and theory are linked in an iterative, continually evolving and dynamic process; this essentially involves trying out different models until the best "fit" for the data is found.

Epistemology is also concerned with the question of whether research findings are independent of the researcher – i.e. the researcher is neutral and findings are objective – or whether phenomena are influenced by the process of being researched, resulting in findings that are not value-free.

The epistemological underpinning of your research will depend on your research questions, aims, and your overall approach to research. Qualitative research is often viewed as exclusively inductive but this is not the case. Arguably, researchers would struggle to free themselves and their interpretations of all prior knowledge, meaning that previous experiences will always influence the interpretation of the data in some form. Moreover, qualitative studies can specifically aim to explore participants' accounts in the context of existing models and theories. For example, Mueller et al. [26] qualitatively analysed how lung cancer patients' accounts of their experiences leading up to diagnosis matched intervals described in the Pathway to Diagnosis Model [40], thus at least partly using a deductive approach.

Ontology is concerned with the nature of reality and how we can access it. There are essentially two opposing perspectives, with different variants within each perspective. *Realism* purports that there is an external reality which exists independently of our beliefs and understanding. Variants include *naive realism* which assumes this external reality can be observed and reported accurately, and *subtle realism* which assumes that an external reality exists but it can only be known through socially constructed meanings [32]. In contrast, *idealism* holds that there is no such external reality and that the social world is made up of socially constructed meanings. Variants of idealism differ in whether they assume there is a form of social reality through shared constructed meanings (*subtle/collective/contextual idealism*) or whether there is no shared social reality, only individual constructions (*relativism or radical idealism*).

When using qualitative research in the context of app evaluations, it is important to consider epistemological and ontological questions because this will affect your approach, analysis, interpretation, and how you present and disseminate the findings. For example, you may wish to consider how the investigator might influence the findings. If you think findings may be "value-mediated" by the researcher (rather than findings being neutral, objective and value-free), you may wish to take certain actions such as encouraging the researcher to keep reflective notes on the research process, or incorporating the views of several researchers to invite a variety of different interpretations.

For a detailed and practice-oriented overview of qualitative research and the different underlying philosophical stances, see for example *Qualitative Research Practice: A Guide For Social Science Students and Researchers* by Ritchie et al. [32].

We will now briefly introduce three commonly used approaches in the context of health app evaluation.

9.6.2   Thematic Analysis

Thematic analysis (TA) involves coding data by identifying *themes* and *sub-themes* in the data. In practice this involves reading and re-reading the interview text multiple times (or repeatedly listening to recordings) to identify, code and re-code the data. Codes tend to be initially descriptive and then progress into more conceptual themes. This can be a lengthy process and requires some skill and expertise from the research team.

For example, consider the following two quotes from two different participants:

> *"The visualisation doesn't really show all the information, in fact it's often hard to read because of the font size."* [P1]
>
> *"Yeah I don't like using the visualisation tool. To be honest – I don't really understand what it's showing me."* [P3]

Both of these quotes mention *visualisation*, and this could be a potential theme. If we examine this a little deeper we might also note that they are both talking about problems or barriers with interpretation and therefore the theme could be something like *interpretation barriers* or *interpretation problems*.

Another example can be seen in Fig. 9.32 which shows a primary theme ("barriers to making an interpretation") and associated sub-themes. This work explored healthcare practitioners' views on interpreting electrocardiograms (ECG/EKGs). Here the participants are represented in the rows and the columns refer to the sub-themes. Quotes from the participants are pasted into the related cells.

Software such as NVIVO can be used to help carry out qualitative analysis. Such software allows one to drag quotes into themes (nodes) which produces some structural organisation as well as numerical counts for the number of people mentioning the theme. Various other useful visualisations such as wordclouds and tree diagrams are also included.

Thematic analysis is a widely used method in qualitative research and is perhaps one of the more accessible methods to researchers who are not experts in qualitative methods [4].

9.6.3   Framework Analysis

Framework Analysis is a specific form of thematic analysis. As such, it aims to identify recurring and important themes in the data. Framework Analysis is distinct in its rigorous, methodical approach to qualitative data analysis. It was developed by Spencer et al. [36] for the purpose of applied policy research, however it lends

Interview coding matrices (1.0 Barriers to making an interpretation)

	1.0 Barriers to making an interpretation					
	1.1 Presentation of the ECG	1.2 Artefact	1.3 Forgetting skills over time	1.4 Fear, panic or pressure (stress) associated with making an interpretation	1.5 Finding it difficult to make an interpretation	1.6 Errors and mistakes
P2F			Being taught the system did help, but I find unless I'm regularly reading ECGs and have instruction I forget how to use the system and interpret them.	I suppose when looking at them in first and second year I'd panic and not know where to look.	Really hard, but I've always found ECGs difficult!	I'm not sure I've really had enough experience to make any significant errors. I suppose lead inversion? And not knowing which waveform is which.
P5M				The simple things, like AF/VT are noticed quite easily. But congenital problems, like long QT, right heart failure etc, require more time and are harder to interpret. having clinical history.	If I don't know the patient history it can be problematic, as some patients have other problems that different tests can detect – ECG can give lots of information but they can also mistake stuff. For example if an athlete comes in with 40 bpm, we would assume bradycardia. But this would be wrong, for	
P13M						I suppose limb lead errors, like inversions.
P16F				Stressful, the majority of it's easy it's just knowing what the answers are	people of Afro-Caribbean descent have ECGs that naturally have ST ele... it loo...	Believe it or not I've never made any errors until today!

Fig. 9.32 Main theme '1.0 Barriers to making an interpretation' and associated sub-themes

itself well to any field of inquiry as long as the research addresses specific questions and/or a-priori issues it wishes to address. It is less well suited for very explorative research with no pre-defined research questions or aims.

FA involves the following five stages:

1. **Data familiarisation**: The researchers will first need to familiarise themselves with the data to obtain an overview and generate initial ideas. This typically involves reading transcripts, listening to audio-recordings or reading observational notes. Throughout this process the researchers should keep notes on any recurring or important themes.
2. **Development of a theoretical framework:** Based on a combination of the themes identified in Step 1 and the interview protocol, the researcher will then proceed to develop a hierarchical index of topics and sub-topics which are to be further explored.

	Medication graph	Registration pages	Sliders
Participant 1	Prefers graph 1	Commented that there might be some potential embarrassment around reporting alcohol use and exercising (needs to be handled sensitively)	Struggled with sliders; tended to tap rather than slide; switched off daily reminder (small toggle switch) when actually meant to switch it on; despite these difficulties described the sliders as "not bad"
Participant 2	Able to interpret graph 1, but doesn't like the second graph because too busy, too much on it	Required clarification on "daily reminder"; might need more explanation	Struggled to use sliders, especially setting it/leaving it at zero; despite this also described sliders as "fine"
Participant 3	Commented that we need to make sure the graph is big enough; avoid using colours esp. green/red because some people might not be able to see this clearly; suggested using open and closed circles for medication taken/not taken	None	Also struggled to leave the sliders at zero; generally not used to sliders

I1:	We've been playing around a bit with, trying to put some sort of information in the graph about your medication as well. So, this is a first idea of what we came up with and we were wondering what you thought of that.
R:	Yes, I quite agree with that. Like you say, down here and up to there, is where you've took your medication and then when you've stopped taking it, they just go sky-high.
I1:	So, you would be able to see that from this graph?
R:	Yes, definitely.
I1:	What do you think of this version?
R:	No. There's too much of it.

Fig. 9.33 Example framework matrix. The matrix shows participants in the rows, while sub-topics are placed in the columns. Text that is highlighted in yellow is linked to the original interview transcript, shown on the right

3. **Indexing data:** This index is then applied to the data (e.g. the interview transcripts) by labelling sections of text according to the topic or sub-topic occurring within it.

4. **Summarising data into thematic frameworks:** The labelled data are now organised into framework matrices. Participants are placed in rows and sub-topics make up the columns. The labelled data (e.g. snippets of text) are summarised into the cells of the matrix, keeping as close to the participants' original wording as possible. Matrices can be created with NVivo, using the *Summary Link* function to link the summarised text to the original text excerpt. Figure 9.33 shows a framework matrix created for a usability evaluation of a smartphone app for symptom management. As the figure shows, participants have been placed in the rows, and the columns show topics discussed by the participants, such as *Medication graphs* (we displayed different graphs to show how reported symptoms varied with medication intake), the *registration pages* (the pages participants needed to complete in order to set up the app on their phone) and *sliders* (participants struggled with this feature and it was therefore explored in detail).

5. **Synthesising data:** The matrix can now be used to generate themes by comparing data across participants and across columns. Themes are usually initially descriptive and are then categorised into more conceptual themes.

Example: Using Framework Analysis to explore patients' experiences of using a smartphone application to increase physical activity

Casey et al. [6] embedded a qualitative evaluation of an app designed to enhance physical activity in primary care within a wider RCT to evaluate the app's effectiveness. They interviewed 12 participants. The sample was selected *purposively* (a common sampling method in qualitative research) to ensure it included both intervention and control participants as well as a range of people with different ages, sex, baseline activity levels, and smartphone literacy. Framework analysis was used to analyse the data. The interview protocol included questions on participants' expectations, their experiences of using the smartphone app, what they thought and felt and how they reacted in different situations (e.g. when the step count was lower than their goal), and barriers and facilitators to physical activity. Four members of the research team (a nurse, two GPs, and one clinical engineer) reviewed the data and contributed to the analysis in order to enhance rigour and reflexivity.

Using Framework Analysis, the authors explored participants' accounts and identified "building blocks" of apps which appeared to have the potential to bring about behaviour change in terms of physical activity, such as "awareness and knowledge", "feedback" and "goal setting".

9.6.4 Grounded Theory

Grounded Theory is one of the most widely known and used qualitative analysis approaches. It was originally developed by Glaser and Strauss in 1967 [11]. The aim of Grounded Theory is to develop theories about social phenomena based on qualitative data from participants who have experienced these social phenomena [36].

At the time, the prevalent form of research was deductive logical which means that theories were developed first and then used to generate hypotheses which could be tested using quantitative methods. Glaser and Strauss discovered that there was no established method to develop theory based on data itself, and therefore developed Grounded Theory with the aim of bridging this theory-research gap.

The key characteristic of this approach is an inductive strategy: the researcher aims to develop a theory that is *grounded* within the data. Themes are viewed as *emerging* from the data rather than being constructed by the researcher. This notion of the researcher as a passive observer of the data was later challenged, and differing philosophical perspectives have since been put forward by grounded theorists.

Grounded Theory often entails coding "line-by-line", meaning that each line of data (e.g. each line in a transcribed interview) must be assigned an individual code that captures its meaning. The coding process involves moving from initially descriptive codes to increasingly analytical categories. Grounded Theory also often involves *memo-writing*, which entails keeping detailed written notes on the codes and categories and any decision-making processes.

It is important to note that Grounded Theory is unlikely to be a suitable approach for app evaluation. It was developed for the purpose of developing theory rather than answering specific research questions. Grounded Theory is more frequently used for app development and app improvement.

Leung et al. [22] discuss how Grounded Theory can be used to facilitate app development and evaluation for underrepresented mental health care consumers. The authors suggest that Grounded Theory can be used to analyse data collected post-launch (e.g. event data within the app, surveys, interviews with app users) to explore and build concepts and theories about the causes of different social problems the users are experiencing. This information in turn can help develop new features within the app to address the experienced problems. Instead of focusing on specific aims and outcomes, the Grounded Theory approach allows the researcher to explore underlying root causes of social problems, thus helping to generate a theoretical basis for improving the app. This is particularly important when targeting "seldom heard" or "hard-to-reach" user groups, for whom existing psychosocial theories of health behaviour may not be representative.

> **Example: Using Grounded Theory to evaluate PTSD Coach, a smartphone app for post-traumatic stress symptoms**
>
> Kuhn et al. [20] developed PTSD Coach, a smartphone app designed to help users with post-traumatic stress disorder (PTSD) understand and self-manage their symptoms. The app was already widely available (130,000 downloads across 78 countries) before the evaluation commenced. As such, a more controlled study approach (such as an RCT) was not possible. Instead the authors sought to examine user satisfaction, perceived helpfulness, and usage patterns in a smaller sample of 45 veterans receiving treatment for PTSD. The veterans used the app for several days and then participated in focus groups where they discussed their experiences of using the app. Trained researchers observed the focus groups and took detailed notes. The observation notes were then analysed using a Grounded Theory approach.
>
> Based on the analysis, the authors conclude that participants found value in the use of the app. The focus groups also helped highlight how the app could be improved.
>
> It is debatable whether the authors used a true Grounded Theory approach as they mention specific pre-conceived hypotheses (while a Grounded Theory researcher should remain unbiased and neutral) and the outcomes of the analysis are descriptive rather than theoretical and conceptual. This example highlights the difficulty in implementing Grounded Theory in mHealth research.

9.6.5 Content Analysis

Content analysis is used to analyse documents and communication artifacts of varying formats such as text, pictures, audio and video. The main advantage of this approach is that it is less invasive because it relies on using existing documents to explore a given issue or phenomenon. The findings are therefore not likely to be altered through the process of being investigated, as would be the case in observational or interview studies, where participants may alter behaviour or responses when under investigation. There are, however, other sources of bias, for example if the researcher does not use a systematic approach to identify relevant documents.

Content analysis can be quantitative or qualitative. In its quantitative form, content analysis involves coding the data and then performing analysis on the codes (e.g. assessing frequencies and identifying patterns). In its qualitative form, the codes are used to analyse meanings of content within the document.

Epistemologically, content analysis generally employs a deductive approach, as codes tend to be driven by research aims and hypotheses, though more data-driven approaches are also possible.

Because content analysis is used to analyse data across different documents, it is not typically used in the evaluation of individual apps. It is more commonly used to perform evaluations across apps. It can be used, for example, to analyse textual data in app descriptions provided in app stores or to analyse content within apps. This information can be used to describe apps, and this can also be compared to other documents such as clinical guidelines, evidence-based protocols or behaviour change techniques [18].

Example 1: Using content analysis to evaluate adherence to evidence-based guidelines among diabetes self-management apps

The following is an example of using content analysis to convert qualitative data into quantitative data using codes.

Breland and Yeh [5] aimed to assess the extent to which existing diabetes self-management apps address self-management behaviors recommended by the American Association of Diabetes Educators. Apps were identified by searching for "diabetes" in the Apple App Store and then assessed for eligibility based on their description pages. This yielded 227 apps. For each of the 7 behaviours recommended by the American Association of Diabetes Educators, apps then received a binary rating of either 1 (if they promoted the behaviour) or 0 (if they did not promote the behaviour). For example, for the recommended behaviour "healthy eating", apps received a score of 1 if they provided information about diabetes-appropriate nutrition or if they provided

(continued)

means for tracking food intake. The authors were then able to use these codes to describe content across apps, assess the extent to which guidelines were adhered to, and compare different app groups in terms of adherence using statistical tests.

Example 2: Using content analysis to assess acceptability of a mobile application for type 2 diabetes

The following is an example of qualitative content analysis. Torbjørnsen [38] conducted interviews with adults who had used a digital diabetes diary app for one year. The interview study was embedded within a larger RCT to evaluate the effectiveness of the app. First, text segments from interview transcripts that were relevant to the research aim (i.e. understanding the app's acceptability to users) were selected and labelled using codes. These codes were then categorised into themes and sub-themes. These themes were then interpreted in the frame of the Acceptability Model. This could be viewed as a combination of inductive and deductive approaches, although the selection of "relevant" text excerpts from the start means this approach is largely deductive. Importantly, the extraction and analysis of only the excerpts of text that were relevant to the research question – and thus the removal of the majority of the context – distinguishes this approach from a thematic analysis, which has a stronger emphasis on context.

9.7   Summary of Key Points

We have introduced a few common data analysis methods and tools from qualitative and quantitative paradigms to provide an overview of methods that you might use on your data depending on the aim (e.g. evaluation of effectiveness or of feasibility), the nature of the data itself and your skills, abilities and interest in certain approaches. All of the methods discussed have their pros and cons and their selection and use is ideally decided upon before data are collected rather than afterwards so that the data collection phase can appropriately fit the method applied for analysis. Please see the further reading section to delve deeper into any of the methods covered here (and the ones that weren't).

• Any form of data analysis first requires data preparation and cleaning in order to manage missing/incomplete data, inconsistencies, and noise

- Before statistical tests are conducted, clear aims and objectives, an answerable research question and wherever possible a testable hypothesis should be formulated, and inherent assumptions of tests should be tested before any analyses are conducted
- Statistical tests can be used to test whether relationships between variables or differences between groups are "statistically significant", but causal relationships can only be inferred if an appropriate experimental study design with random allocation is used
- The quality of a model's output depends heavily on its input ("garbage in, garbage out"). Therefore the most important aspect of any analysis is the quality of the data
- There are many tools and software libraries, both commercial and open source that provide users with a plethora of easy to apply analysis methods
- Qualitative analyses are useful for identifying recurring and important themes in people's reports of their subjective experiences; this is especially useful when exploring unintended and unexpected outcomes

9.8 Quiz

1. What is the measurement scale of "number of app users who deleted the app within 1 day of downloading"?

   (a) Nominal
   (b) Ordinal
   (c) Interval
   (d) Ratio

2. To assess how much individual data points differ from the average, you would use:

   (a) Standard deviation
   (b) Arithmetic mean
   (c) Confidence intervals
   (d) Effect sizes

3. A researcher wished to assess the effect of an educational app on medical trainees' medical domain knowledge. Medical knowledge was assessed before and after participants used the app for two weeks. Which tests would be suitable for this study design?

   (a) Independent t-test or McNemar test
   (b) Dependent t-test or Wilcoxon signed-rank test
   (c) ANOVA or independent t-test
   (d) Dependent t-test or Mann-Whitney test

4. A researcher wished to assess the relationship between app usage (measured as number of times a user opened the app per day) and the presence of a notification feature within the app. Two groups were compared (with/without the notification feature). The researcher wanted to assess this relationship independently of other variables that might affect the outcome, such as the age of the users, their familiarity with technology, and the operating system they used. Which of the below analysis methods would be best suited?

   (a) Independent t-test to test for differences between users using the app with-/without the notifications combined with t-tests to test for differences between the groups in age etc.
   (b) ANOVA to test for differences across the groups and controlling for variables like age
   (c) Linear regression, predicting app usage using presence of notifications as a predictor, and including variables like age in the model to control for them

5. Which analysis method is better suited for qualitative research with specific research questions?

   (a) Grounded Theory
   (b) Framework Analysis

6. Machine learning methods that use distance metrics often require that feature scaling is applied to the data first to compensate for data of different magnitudes.

   (a) True
   (b) False

7. Would we want a Machine Learning model to fit our data precisely?

   (a) Yes
   (b) No

8. Dimensionality reduction is important because...

   (a) It removes noise and improves the performance of a model
   (b) It has to be run for every Machine Learning algorithm
   (c) It increases multicollinearity effects

Answers to the quiz can be found in "Solutions to Quizzes".

9.9 Exercises

1. Using a tool of your choice, with regard to the data in the table below (Table 9.4):

   (a) Calculate the *mean* and *standard deviation*

Table 9.4 Data for X and Y

X	Y
12	45
32	35
64	13
32	53
37	23
23	10
7	45

    (b) Run an independent t-test on the data (X and Y)

    (c) Is there a statistically significant difference between X and Y?

2. Using the *np.linalg.solve* function from Python's numpy module, solve the following as a system of linear equations using matrices

$$2x + y - 2z = 35$$

$$x - y - z = 0$$

$$x + y + 3z = 12$$

3. Read the following open-access paper:

Torbjørnsen, A., Ribu, L., Rønnevig, M., Grøttland, A., & Helseth, S. (2019). *Users' acceptability of a mobile application for persons with type 2 diabetes: a qualitative study.* BMC Health Services Research, 19(1), 641. http://doi.org/10.1186/s12913-019-4486-2

Based on the paper, answer the following questions:

    (a) What qualitative analysis method did the authors use?

    (b) Did the authors use an inductive or deductive approach?

    (c) What data collection method was used?

    (d) How were participants recruited?

    (e) How was the end point for data collection determined?

Recommended Reading

1. Braun V, Clarke V. Using thematic analysis in psychology. Qual Res Psychol. 2008;3(2):77–101.
2. Jiang F, Zhi H, Dong Y, Li H, Ma S, Wang Y, Dong Q, Shen H, Wang Y. Artificial intelligence in healthcare: past, present and future. Stroke Vasc Neurol Neurology. 2017;e000101.
3. Field A, Miles J, Field Z. Discovering statistics using R. Los Angeles: Sage; 2012.
4. James G, Witten D, Hastie T, Tibshirani R. An introduction to statistical learning with applications in R. London: Springer; 2015.
5. Géron A. Hands-on machine learning with scikit-learn & tensorflow. Beijing: O'Reilly; 2017.

6. Ritchie J, Spencer L. Qualitative data analysis for applied policy research. In: Huberman AM, Miles MB, editors. The qualitative researcher's companion. London: Sage; 2002. p. 305–30.
7. Field A. Discovering statistics using SPSS. 3rd ed. Sage Publications Ltd., London; 2014.
8. Greenland S, Senn SJ, Rothman KJ, Carlin JB, Poole C, Goodman SN, Altman DG. Statistical tests, P values, confidence intervals, and power: a guide to misinterpretations. Eur J Epidemiol. 31(4):337–50; 2016.
9. Wilcox RR. Introduction to robust estimation and hypothesis testing. Amsterdam/Boston: Academic; 2012.

References

1. Allen M. Hypothesis formulation. In: The SAGE encyclopedia of communication research methods. Thousand Oaks: SAGE Publications, Inc; 2017. https://doi.org/10.4135/9781483381411.n238
2. Benjamini Y, Hochberg Y. Controlling the false discovery rate: a practical and powerful approach to multiple testing. J R Stat Soc Ser B. 57:289; 1995. https://doi.org/10.2307/2346101
3. Blaikie N. Approaches to social enquiry: advancing knowledge. 2nd ed. Cambridge: Polity; 2007.
4. Braun V, Clarke V. Using thematic analysis in psychology using thematic analysis in psychology. Qual Res Psychol. 3:37–41; 2008. https://doi.org/10.1191/1478088706qp063oa
5. Breland JY, Yeh VM, Yu J. Adherence to evidence-based guidelines among diabetes self-management apps. Transl Behav Med. 3(3):277–86; 2013. https://doi.org/10.1007/s13142-013-0205-4
6. Casey M, Hayes PS, Glynn F, OLaighin G, Heaney D, Murphy AW, Glynn LG. Patients' experiences of using a smartphone application to increase physical activity: the SMART MOVE qualitative study in primary care. Br J Gen Pract J R Coll Gen Pract. 64(625):e500–8; 2014. https://doi.org/10.3399/bjgp14X680989
7. Cohen J. Statistical power analysis for the behavioral sciences. 2nd ed. Hillsdale: Lawrence Earlbaum Associates; 1988.
8. Field A. Discovering statistics using SPSS. 3rd ed. London: Sage Publications Ltd; 2014.
9. Fralick M, Haj R, Hirpara D, Wong K, Muller M, Matukas L, Bartlett J, Leung E, Taggart L. Can a smartphone app improve medical trainees' knowledge of antibiotics? Int J Med Educ. 8:416–20; 2017. https://doi.org/10.5116/ijme.5a11.8422
10. Garcia-Ortiz L, Recio-Rodriguez JI, Agudo-Conde C, Patino-Alonso MC, Maderuelo-Fernandez J-A, Repiso Gento I, Puigdomenech Puig E, Gonzalez-Viejo N, Arietaleanizbeaskoa MS, Schmolling-Guinovart Y, Gomez-Marcos MA, Rodriguez-Sanchez E, EVIDENT Investigators Group, and Mobilizing Minds Research Group. Long-term effectiveness of a smartphone app for improving healthy lifestyles in general population in primary care: randomized controlled trial (Evident II Study). JMIR mHealth uHealth. 6(4):e107; 2018. https://doi.org/10.2196/mhealth.9218
11. Glaser BG, Strauss AL. The discovery of grounded theory: strategies for qualitative research. London: Weidenfeld and Nicolson; 1967.
12. Greenland S, Senn SJ, Rothman KJ, Carlin JB, Poole C, Goodman SN, Altman DG. Statistical tests, P values, confidence intervals, and power: a guide to misinterpretations. Eur J Epidemiol. 31(4):337–50; 2016. https://doi.org/10.1007/s10654-016-0149-3
13. Grissom RJ, Kim JJ. Effect sizes for research: a broad practical approach. Mahwah: Lawrence Erlbaum Associates; 2005. https://books.google.co.uk/books?id=4C49CGkNxLAC
14. Hayes B. Programming languages most used and recommended by data scientists; 2019. https://businessoverbroadway.com/2019/01/13/programming-languages-most-used-and-recommended-by-data-scientists/

15. Helander E, Kaipainen K, Korhonen I, Wansink B. Factors related to sustained use of a free mobile app for dietary self-monitoring with photography and peer feedback: retrospective cohort study. J Med Internet Res. 16(4):e109; 2014. https://doi.org/10.2196/jmir.3084

16. Hoffman JIE. Linear regression. In: Basic biostatistics for medical and biomedical practitioners. London: Academic; 2019. p. 445–89. https://doi.org/10.1016/B978-0-12-817084-7.00027-9

17. Huang H-Y, Bashir M. Users' adoption of mental health apps: examining the impact of information cues. JMIR mHealth uHealth. 5(6):e83; 2017. https://doi.org/10.2196/mhealth.6827

18. Jake-Schoffman DE, Silfee VJ, Waring ME, Boudreaux ED, Sadasivam RS, Mullen SP, Carey JL, Hayes RB, Ding EY, Bennett GG, Pagoto SL. Methods for evaluating the content, usability, and efficacy of commercial mobile health apps. JMIR mHealth uHealth. 5(12):e190; 2017. https://doi.org/10.2196/mhealth.8758

19. Jiang F, et al. Artificial intelligence in healthcare: past, present and future. Stroke Vasc Neurol. 2(4):230–43; 2017. https://doi.org/10.1136/svn-2017-000101

20. Kuhn E, Greene C, Hoffman J, Nguyen T, Wald L, Schmidt J, Ruzek J. Preliminary evaluation of PTSD coach, a smartphone app for post-traumatic stress symptoms. Military Medicine. 179(1):12–18; 2014. https://doi.org/10.7205/MILMED-D-13-00271

21. Lee H-A, Lee H-J, Moon J-H, Lee T, Kim M-G, In H, Cho C-H, Kim L. Comparison of wearable activity tracker with actigraphy for sleep evaluation and circadian rest-activity rhythm measurement in healthy young adults. Psychiatry Investig. 14(2):179–85; 2017. https://doi.org/10.4306/pi.2017.14.2.179

22. Leung R, Hastings JF, Keefe RH, Brownstein-Evans C, Chan KT, Mullick R. Building mobile apps for underrepresented mental health care consumers: a grounded theory approach. Soc Work Ment Health. 14(6):625–36; 2016. https://doi.org/10.1080/15332985.2015.1130010

23. Mann HB, Whitney DR. On a test of whether one of two random variables is stochastically larger than the other. Ann Math Stat. 18(1):50–60; 1947. https://doi.org/10.1214/aoms/1177730491

24. Masino AJ, Forsyth D, Nuske H, Herrington J, Pennington J, Kushleyeva Y, Bonafide CP. M-Health and autism: recognizing stress and anxiety with machine learning and wearables data. In: Proceedings – IEEE symposium on computer-based medical systems; 2019. p. 714–9. https://doi.org/10.1109/CBMS.2019.00144

25. Meyer MA. Healthcare data scientist qualifications, skills, and job focus: a content analysis of job postings. J Am Med Inform Assoc. 26(5):383–91; 2019. https://doi.org/10.1093/jamia/ocy181

26. Mueller J, Davies A, Jay C, Harper S, Blackhall F, Yvonne Summers, Harle A, Todd C. Developing and testing a web-based intervention to encourage early help-seeking in people with symptoms associated with lung cancer. Br J Health Psychol. 24(1):31–65; 2018. https://doi.org/10.1111/bjhp.12325

27. Muller A, Guido S. Introduction to machine learning with python: a guide for data scientists. Beijing: O'Reilly; 2017.

28. National Health Service. The topol review: preparing the healthcare workforce to deliver the digital future. Technical report; 2019. https://topol.hee.nhs.uk/wp-content/uploads/HEE-Topol-Review-2019.pdf

29. Nissen F, Quint JK, Morales DR, Douglas IJ. How to validate a diagnosis recorded in electronic health records. Breathe (Sheffield, England). 15(1):64–8; 2019. https://doi.org/10.1183/20734735.0344-2018

30. Perneger TV. What's wrong with Bonferroni adjustments. BMJ (Clinical research ed.) 316(7139):1236–8; 1998. https://doi.org/10.1136/bmj.316.7139.1236

31. R Core Team. R: a language and environment for statistical computing; 2017. https://www.r-project.org/

32. Ritchie J, Lewis J, McNaughton-Nicholls C, Ormston R. Qualitative research practice: a guide for social science students and researchers. 2nd ed. London: Sage Publications Ltd; 2013.

33. Shiffman S. How many cigarettes did you smoke? Assessing cigarette consumption by global report, time-line follow-back, and ecological momentary assessment. Health Psychol Off J Div Health Psychol Am Psychol Assoc. 28(5):519–26; 2009. https://doi.org/10.1037/a0015197

34. Silver D, Huang A, Maddison CJ, Guez A, Sifre L, Van Den Driessche G, Schrittwieser J, Antonoglou I, Panneershelvam V, Lanctot M, Dieleman S, Grewe D, Nham J, Kalchbrenner N, Sutskever I, Lillicrap T, Leach M, Kavukcuoglu K, Graepel T, Hassabis D. Mastering the game of go with deep neural networks and tree search. Nature. 529(7587):484–9; 2016. https://doi.org/10.1038/nature16961

35. Snik F, Rietjens JHH, Apituley A, Volten H, Mijling B, Di Noia A, Heikamp S, Heinsbroek RC, Hasekamp OP, Smit JM, Vonk J, Stam DM, van Harten G, de Boer J, Keller CU. Mapping atmospheric aerosols with a citizen science network of smartphone spectropolarimeters. Geophys Res Lett. 41(20):7351–8; 2014. https://doi.org/10.1002/2014GL061462@10.1002

36. Spencer L, Ritchie J, O'Connor W, Morrell G, Ormston R. Analysis in practice, chapter 11. In: Qualitative research practice: a guide for social science students and researchers, 2nd ed. London: Sage Publications Ltd; 2013. p. 295–343.

37. Tedesco S, Sica M, Ancillao A, Timmons S, Barton J, O'Flynn B. Accuracy of consumer-level and research-grade activity trackers in ambulatory settings in older adults. PLOS ONE. 14(5):e0216891; 2019. https://doi.org/10.1371/journal.pone.0216891

38. Torbjørnsen A, Ribu L, Rønnevig M, Grøttland A, Helseth S. Users' acceptability of a mobile application for persons with type 2 diabetes: a qualitative study. BMC Health Serv Res. 19(1):641; 2019.

39. Ubhi HK, Michie S, Kotz D, Wong WC, West R. A mobile app to aid smoking cessation: preliminary evaluation of SmokeFree28. J Med Internet Res. 17(1):e17; 2015. https://doi.org/10.2196/jmir.3479

40. Walter F, Webster A, Scott S, Emery J. The Andersen model of total patient delay: a systematic review of its application in cancer diagnosis. J Health Serv Res Policy. 17(2):110–8; 2012. https://doi.org/10.1258/jhsrp.2011.010113

41. White RW, Horvitz E. Experiences with web search on medical concerns and self diagnosis. In: AMIA … annual symposium proceedings/AMIA Symposium. AMIA Symposium; 2009. p. 696–700. http://www.pubmedcentral.nih.gov/articlerender.fcgi?artid=2815378&tool=pmcentrez&rendertype=abstract

42. Wilcox RR. Introduction to robust estimation and hypothesis testing. Amsterdam: Academic; 2012.

43. Wilcoxon F. Individual comparisons by ranking methods. Biom Bull. 1(6):80; 1945. https://doi.org/10.2307/3001968

44. Zhang S, Zhang C, Yang Q. Data preparation for data mining. Appl Artif Intell. 17(5–6):375–81; 2003. https://doi.org/10.1080/713827180

Solutions to Quizzes

Chapter 1

Q1. An app which allows users to send text messages to their healthcare professionals would be considered. . .
   (d) all of the above

Q2. Which of the following items is **not** an example of ecological momentary assessment (EMA)?
   (b) An app asks users to rate their breathlessness levels after they have undertaken a physical exercise at a clinic as part of a study.

Chapter 2

Q1. Which one of the following is **not** a common reason why projects fail?
   (c) Using an iterative design methodology

Q2. A minimal viable product (MVP) is. . .
   (b) A minimal end-to-end slice of functionality that adds some value

Q3. The Agile manifesto promotes self organising teams with a flatter structure where individuals are valued and trusted.
   (a) True

Q4. Which of the following are typical roles in a Scrum team?
   (c) Scrum master, Product Owner, Development team

© Springer Nature Switzerland AG 2020
A. Davies, J. Mueller, *Developing Medical Apps and mHealth Interventions*, Health Informatics, https://doi.org/10.1007/978-3-030-47499-7

Q5. A product backlog...
  (a) contains a list of all the project's current requirements

Q6. Pair programming and code review are only used in Agile software design methods/frameworks.
  (b) False

Q7. A user story should contain the following components...
  (b) Type of user, feature or goal and value/reason

Q8. Data flow diagrams can be used to show the logical flow of a conditional expression (if/then/else).
  (b) False

Q9. Which of the following is **not** a correct Git statement:
  (c) git pull then push with commit

Chapter 3

Q1. Which statement best describes the Behaviour Change Wheel?
  (a) A framework which postulates that policy factors, intervention functions and different sources of behaviour interact to change behaviour

Q2. Which of the following is crucial to the person-based approach for digital intervention development? Several may apply.
  (a) Qualitative research to elicit users' views
  (b) Review of available evidence
  (d) Review of relevant behaviour change theories
  (e) User testing of the intervention

Q3. Which of the following statements is most accurate?
  (d) Health apps may be classed as medical devices depending on their functions, features, and intended use, and therefore national regulatory frameworks for medical devices may apply

Chapter 4

Q1. When applying test driven development (TDD), we first...
  (b) Start by writing a test

Q2. Which of the following is **not** a commonly included sensor included in most mobile smartphones
  (b) Radiation detector

Q3. The MVC pattern is commonly used with web development projects
  (a) True

Q4. The main development languages for iOS development include
  (b) Objective-C and Swift

Q5. Basic web apps are able to interface easily with the hardware components of a mobile device
  (b) False

Q6. The most commonly downloaded apps are...
  (c) Games

Chapter 5

Q1. When designing an app to collect and use geo-spatial data, it is preferred that:
  (b) We collect only the level of information that is absolutely necessary

Q2. Apart from the first block, the hash in a block chain block...
  (a) points to the hash of the previous block

Q3. The first block in a blockchain is called the
  (b) genesis block

Q4. The most secure protocol for sending data to a server is with the
  (a) HTTPS

Q5. Under the GDPR pseudonymised data is still considered to be personal data.
  (a) True

Q6. MongoDB is an example of...
  (b) an unstructured database

Q7. SQL queries should ideally be made by joining strings together (concatenation).
  (b) False

Q8. Public keys should never be shared.
  (b) False

Chapter 6

Q1. Which of the following is **not** a preattentive attribute?
(c) Fixation duration

Q2. The most suitable visualisation type to compare two categories of information is...
(a) A bar chart

Q3. Which of the following are good reasons to use visualisations
(a) To explore the structure and relationships in our data
(b) To communicate results to different users

Q4. People reason better when given information in the form of
(b) Frequencies

Q5. Which of the following should **not** be routinely applied to visualisations
(c) Multiple statistical and textual annotation to provide context

Chapter 7

Q1. Which of the following is **not** a commonly used requirements gathering method?
(c) Data flow diagrams

Q2. Sample sizes for usability studies use a power analysis to determine the correct sample size?
(b) False

Q3. Which of the following image tags is considering accessibility?

```
<img src="dog.png" alt="Image of a dog" />
```

(b) Line 2

Q4. Physiological methods to detect human emotional states include:
(a) Eye-tracking
(b) Electroencephalography
(c) Electrocardiogram
(d) Electromyogram

Q5. Capturing event data from how users interact with an app provides useful insights into behaviour and usage patterns
(a) True

Chapter 8

Q1. Which of the following designs could you use to evaluate the clinical effectiveness of an mHealth intervention? (several may apply)
    (a) A randomised controlled trial
    (b) A cluster-randomised controlled trials
    (c) A randomised controlled trial

Q2. What type of study is a natural experiment?
    (b) An observational study

Q3. A researcher wished to compare the effect on activity levels of an app with daily reminders versus weekly email reminders. Participants were randomised to one of two groups. One group first used the app for 1 month, then received the email reminders for 1 month. The other group first received the emails and then the app. Physical activity was tracked in both groups using a wrist-worn activity tracker. This study design is a...
    (c) Cross-over trial

Q4. What type of health economic evaluation would be most suitable to evaluate the cost-effectiveness of a health app funded by a country's national health service? (several may apply)
    (a) Cost-utility analysis
    (b) Cost-effectiveness analysis

Chapter 9

Q1. What is the measurement scale of "number of app users who deleted the app within 1 day of downloading"?
    (d) Ratio

Q2. To assess how much individual data points differ from the average, you would use:
    (a) Standard deviation

Q3. A researcher wished to assess the effect of an educational app on medical trainees' medical domain knowledge. Medical knowledge was assessed before and after participants used the app for two weeks. Which tests would be suitable for this study design?
    (b) Dependent t-test or Wilcoxon signed-rank test

Q4. A researcher wished to assess the relationship between app usage (measured as number of times a user opened the app per day) and the presence of a notification feature within the app. Two groups were compared (with/without the notification feature). The researcher wanted to assess this relationship independently of other variables that might affect the outcome, such as the age of the users, their familiarity with technology, and the operating system they used. Which of the below analysis methods would be best suited?

(c) Linear regression, predicting app usage using presence of notifications as a predictor, and including variables like age in the model to control for them

Q5. Which analysis method is better suited for qualitative research with specific research questions?

(b) Framework Analysis

Q6. Machine learning methods that use distance metrics often require that feature scaling is applied to the data first to compensate for data of different magnitudes.

(a) True

Q7. Would we want a Machine Learning model to fit our data precisely?

(b) No

Q8. Dimensionality reduction is important because...

(a) It removes noise and improves the performance of a model

Index

© Springer Nature Switzerland AG 2020
A. Davies, J. Mueller, *Developing Medical Apps and mHealth Interventions*, Health
Informatics, https://doi.org/10.1007/978-3-030-47499-7